Anatomy and Physiology for Veterinary Technicians and Nurses

A Clinical Approach

Second Edition

Lori Asprea
Long Island University, Rockville Centre, NY, USA

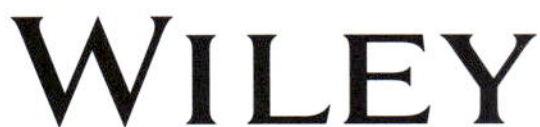

Library of Congress Cataloging-in-Publication Data Applied for:
Paperback ISBN: 9781394229208

Cover Design: Wiley
Cover Images: Courtesy of Lori Asprea

Set in 9.5/12.5pt STIXTwoText by Straive, Pondicherry, India

Printed in Singapore
M127220220725

Contents

Preface   *x*
Acknowledgments   *xi*
About the Companion Website   *xii*

Section 1   Anatomy   *1*

1   Directional and Anatomical Terms   *3*
Introduction   *3*
Directional Terms   *4*
Additional Terminology   *4*
Review Questions   *11*

2   Anatomy of the Common Integument   *13*
Introduction   *13*
Skin   *13*
Pads   *15*
Haircoat   *16*
Claws   *18*
Hooves and Horns   *18*
Review Questions   *20*

3   Anatomy of the Senses   *21*
Introduction   *21*
General Senses   *21*
Special Senses   *22*
  Anatomy of Taste   *22*
  Anatomy of Smell   *22*
  Anatomy of Hearing   *23*
  Anatomy of Equilibrium   *24*
  Anatomy of Vision   *25*
Review Questions   *28*

4   Skeletal Anatomy   *29*
Introduction   *29*
Vocabulary   *29*
Bone Categories   *29*
The Skeleton   *31*
The Appendicular Skeleton   *31*
  The Thoracic Limb   *31*
  The Pelvic Limb   *33*
  The Pelvis   *34*

The Axial Skeleton   *36*
  The Skull   *36*
    The Ribs and Sternum   *38*
    The Vertebrae   *40*
      The Named Vertebrae   *41*
Equines   *42*
  Bovines   *43*
  Bird Bones   *43*
  The Bone That Isn't   *43*
Review Questions   *44*

5   Joint Anatomy   *47*
Introduction   *47*
Movement   *47*
Joint Types   *48*
  Fibrous Joints   *48*
  Cartilaginous Joints   *48*
  Synovial Joints   *49*
The Skull   *50*
The Ribs and Vertebral Column   *51*
The Pelvis and The Hip   *51*
The Shoulder and Thoracic Limb   *51*
The Pelvic Limb   *52*
Review Questions   *53*

6   Muscle Anatomy   *55*
Introduction   *55*
Cellular Anatomy   *55*
Skeletal Muscle   *57*
  The Head and Neck   *58*
  The Thorax   *58*
  The Dorsum   *60*
  The Abdomen   *60*
  The Pelvis   *60*
  The Limbs   *61*
    The Thoracic Limb   *61*
    The Pelvic Limb   *62*
  Smooth Muscle   *63*
Review Questions   *64*

7   Anatomy of the Nervous System   *67*
Introduction   *67*
The Neuron   *67*
The Synapse   *68*
The Meninges   *68*
The Brain   *69*
  The Cerebrum   *69*
  The Cerebellum   *70*
  The Brainstem   *70*
  Diencephalon   *70*
  The Blood–Brain Barrier   *70*

Cranial Nerves   *71*
The Spinal Cord   *72*
Peripheral Nervous System   *73*
Review Questions   *74*

8   Anatomy of the Endocrine System   *77*
Introduction   *77*
The Hypothalamus   *77*
The Pituitary   *77*
Pineal Gland   *78*
The Peripheral Endocrine System   *78*
   The Thyroid   *78*
   The Parathyroid   *78*
   The Adrenals   *79*
   The Pancreas   *79*
   The Gonads   *79*
   The Kidney   *80*
   The Gastrointestinal Tract   *80*
   The Thymus   *80*
Review Questions   *81*

9   Anatomy of the Urinary Tract   *83*
Introduction   *83*
The Kidneys   *83*
   The Nephron   *84*
The Ureters   *86*
The Urinary Bladder   *86*
The Urethra   *87*
Avian   *87*
Review Questions   *88*

10   Cardiovascular Anatomy   *89*
Introduction   *89*
The Heart   *89*
   The Exterior of the Heart   *90*
   The Interior of the Heart   *91*
Peripheral Circulation   *92*
   Arteries   *92*
   Veins   *93*
   Lymphatics   *93*
The Named Arteries   *94*
The Named Veins   *96*
Review Questions   *98*

11   Respiratory Anatomy   *101*
Introduction   *101*
Entry into the Respiratory System   *101*
The Larynx   *102*
The Trachea and Lungs   *103*
The Pleura   *104*
The Anatomy of Breathing   *104*
Species Differentiation   *104*

Clinical Considerations   *105*
Review Questions   *106*

12   Gastrointestinal Anatomy   *107*
Introduction   *107*
Canines and Felines   *107*
   The Oral Cavity   *107*
   Dentition   *108*
   The Pharynx and Esophagus   *110*
   The Stomach   *111*
   The Liver   *112*
   The Intestines   *112*
Species Variation   *114*
Review Questions   *116*

13   Reproductive Anatomy   *119*
Introduction   *119*
The Female   *119*
The Male   *122*
Review Questions   *125*

Section 2   Physiology   *127*

14   The Cell and Hematology   *129*
Introduction   *129*
Mammalian Cell Anatomy   *129*
The Production of Energy   *130*
Mammalian Cell Boundaries   *131*
Hematology   *132*
   Red Blood Cells   *132*
   Platelets   *132*
   White Blood Cells   *132*
Review Questions   *134*

15   Functions of the Common Integument   *137*
Introduction   *137*
Skin   *137*
   Protection   *137*
   Thermoregulation   *138*
   Hydration   *139*
   Other Functions   *139*
   Clinical Considerations   *139*
Glands   *140*
Hair   *141*
The Pads   *142*
Claws, Nails, and Hooves   *142*
Antlers, Horns, and Beaks   *142*
Review Questions   *143*

16 Sensory Physiology *145*
Introduction *145*
Receptors and Signals *145*
The Visual System *146*
   Structures of the Eye *146*
   Function of the Eye *147*
Proprioception and Equilibrium *148*
The Auditory System *149*
The Olfactory System *149*
The Gustatory System *150*
The Tactile System *150*
Specialized Receptors *150*
Review Questions *151*

17 Osteology *153*
Introduction *153*
The Growth of Bones *153*
Bone Marrow *154*
Cartilage *155*
Avians *155*
Review Questions *156*

18 Physiology of Joints *159*
Introduction *159*
The Immoveable Joints *159*
The Moveable Joints *160*
   Connective Tissues *160*
   The Synovial Joint *161*
Review Questions *162*

19 Muscle Physiology *165*
Introduction *165*
Striated Muscle *165*
   The Generation of a Muscle Contraction *166*
   Skeletal Muscle versus Cardiac Muscle *167*
   Adenosine Triphosphate *167*
   The Basis of Speed *168*
Non-Striated Muscle *168*
Innervation *169*
Review Questions *170*

20 Neurophysiology *171*
Introduction *171*
The Neuron *171*
The Action Potential *173*
Signal Transmission *174*
Central and Peripheral Functions *175*
The Brain *175*
The Autonomic Nervous System *176*
Review Questions *178*

21 Endocrine Physiology *181*
Introduction *181*
Endocrine Glands *181*
Regulation of Hormones *181*
Hormone Types *182*
Hypothalamus and Pituitary Gland *183*
  The Anterior Pituitary *183*
  The Posterior Pituitary *184*
The Thyroid Gland *184*
Parathyroid Gland *186*
The Adrenal Gland *187*
The Pancreas and Insulin *188*
Other Endocrine Activities *189*
Prostaglandins and Pheromones *189*
Review Questions *190*

22 Renal Physiology *193*
Introduction *193*
The Nephron *193*
  Renal Excretion and Reabsorption of Water *195*
Acid–Base Balance *196*
Blood Pressure and the Renal System *196*
Uremia *197*
Anemia and the Kidney *197*
Species Differences *198*
Review Questions *198*

23 Cardiovascular Physiology *201*
Introduction *201*
Cardiac Muscle *201*
The Heartbeat *202*
  De- and Repolarization *202*
  Cardiac Conduction System *202*
  Rhythm *203*
Cardiac Output *204*
Flow Through the Heart and Back *205*
  Vasculature *206*
Blood Pressure *206*
Autonomic Nervous System Involvement *207*
The Lymphatic System *208*
Review Questions *209*

24 Respiratory Physiology *211*
Introduction *211*
The Basics *211*
Ventilation and Temperature *212*
Residual Capacity *213*
Thoracic Pressure *213*
The Nervous System and Respiration *213*
The Rhythmicity of Breathing *214*
Gas Exchange *214*
Hemoglobin *215*

Carbon Dioxide   *216*
Chemoreceptors   *216*
Mechanisms to Increase Oxygenation   *217*
Species Differences   *217*
Review Questions   *218*

25   Digestive Physiology   *221*
Introduction   *221*
The Entryway   *221*
   Teeth   *222*
   Moving Toward the Stomach   *222*
The Stomach   *223*
Entering the Small Intestine   *224*
The Colon   *226*
The Liver   *226*
Species Differentiation   *227*
Review Questions   *228*

26   Reproductive Physiology   *231*
Introduction   *231*
The Female   *231*
Hormonal Control   *232*
   Other Factors Affecting the Estrous Cycle   *233*
The Male   *233*
Fertilization and Pregnancy   *234*
Parturition   *235*
Review Questions   *236*

Appendix 1   Dissection Notes   *239*
Appendix 2   The Cranial Nerves   *241*
Appendix 3   Selected Muscle Origins and Insertions   *243*
Appendix 4   Common Abbreviations   *245*
Glossary   *251*
References   *255*
Index   *257*

Preface

The author and the illustrators have all been students at one point in their lives. Some of us have also been teachers and practitioners of veterinary science. We have long talked about putting together a book that reflects how we think about the subjects of anatomy and physiology. For one thing, we sought to have the anatomy and the physiology portions of the book as two separate sections. In some veterinary technology programs, anatomy and physiology are taught as separate courses or in separate portions. Even when they are combined, it can be more helpful to build on the foundation of a complete understanding of anatomy in order to understand the complexity of physiology.

We all agree that adding clinical scenarios makes the information more interesting and, thus, easier to remember. Anatomy and physiology are not part of our curriculum for the sake of theory. A good understanding of anatomy and physiology is the backbone of more advanced areas of study, such as pathology, nutrition, disease, and more. The aim of the study of these topics is to be able to apply this knowledge to daily practice in a clinic, hospital, or research facility.

In this second edition, we have tried to increase the materials included in each chapter, as well as include additional chapters that might be helpful. We have also presented all new case presentations, questions, and some critical thinking questions to stoke curiosity. We have also added more images, illustrations, figures, and appendices. We fervently hope that this work will be of use. We hope equally as much that you, the reader, will let us know what information you would like added or subtracted as we move forward.

We hope that you find this book worthwhile, not only for current study but also for frequent reference. There are also online components that will be of help for people who learn best with visual images rather than written narrative.

Acknowledgments

It is absolutely impossible to write and illustrate a book like this without the support and guidance of dozens of people. It is possible to go on for pages of excruciating detail thanking everyone who has helped us with this project. However, in deference to the reader, we shall endeavor to be brief.

The guidance of our teachers has sustained us and carried us to this moment. We thank the faculty and staff at all the colleges we have attended. We thank our family and friends for their tremendous forbearance. I particularly thank our students for their enthusiasm, their patience, and their encouragement, not to mention their perfect timing when it comes to asking that one last question . . .

Our good friends at Wiley are, of course, the ones who made this all happen. To Ritu and Atul, and the entire team of incredible people there, our deepest gratitude.

Lori Asprea would like to honor a few special people: the Veterinary Technology faculty at Long Island University; Dr. Seetha Tamma, a dear friend and advisor; the Schwarzman Animal Medical Center; Robin Gelman for her gorgeous illustrations; Olivia Davir for her beautiful artwork and help; my husband Brian, who seems to have an endless supply of patience and encouragement; and finally, Dr. Robin Sturtz, without whom not a single bit of this would have ever come to fruition. Robin Gelman would like to dedicate this book to her husband, Sam Gelman, her inspiration.

Lastly, we all would like to thank the animals in our lives that contribute so much love. Each animal that we have had the honor to know and care for fuels the passion for our field. They are the reason we have constant companionship, even when we work on projects like this, and they don't understand why we've been staring at the glowing screen for so long.

L.A.C.

About the Companion Website

This book is accompanied by a companion website:

www.wiley.com/go/asprea/anatomy_vettech2e

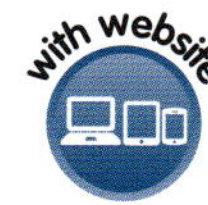

The website includes:
- Study questions
- Answer Keys
- Labelling quizzes
- A dissection video
- Chapter wise figures from the book
- Teaching PowerPoints

Section 1

Anatomy

1

Directional and Anatomical Terms

> **Clinical Case: Georgia, a 5-Year-Old Female Spayed Domestic Short Hair**
>
> *A veterinary technician is assisting a doctor with an appointment. While handling the patient, the technician notices a lump on the patient's hind leg, as shown in Figure 1.1. While reading this chapter, think about the appropriate terminology that should be noted in the patient record for an accurate description of the mass.*
>
> 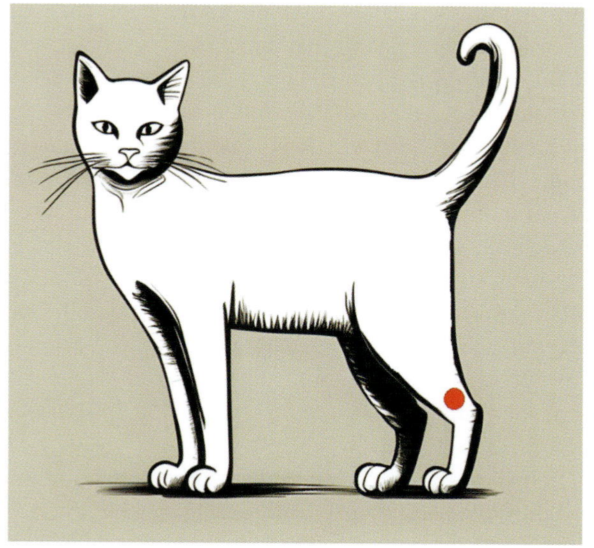
>
> **Figure 1.1** *Our clinical case with the area of concern noted in red on the hind limb.*

Introduction

The study of anatomy is, put simply, the study of the structure of organisms. It involves looking at architecture, at the different positions, shapes, and sizes of various living tissues. As one might imagine, the anatomy of different species has some things in common and some things that are quite diverse. The structure of the heart is very similar in dogs and cats; it is quite different in equines and reptiles. The kidneys of the dolphin look very different from those of the dog, although they function in the same way. By understanding the differences in anatomy among animals, we can have a greater appreciation for how their body systems function. This understanding is the basis of recognizing states of health and disease.

There are a number of different ways to organize how one looks at anatomy. Gross anatomy refers to features that can be seen with the naked eye. Developmental anatomy is the study of how anatomy changes as the fetus becomes a puppy or a kitten. Topographic anatomy refers to the relation to the parts of the whole (e.g., how the different parts of the kidneys and the connecting conduits make up the urinary system). Regional anatomy refers to the structures of a given area of the body; if one looks at the head, for example, as one unit, it will involve the study of all the muscles, blood vessels, bones, and other tissues that are present. Imaging anatomy refers to the anatomical features as they are seen on a good radiograph.

Anatomy and Physiology for Veterinary Technicians and Nurses: A Clinical Approach, Second Edition. Lori Asprea.
© 2026 John Wiley & Sons, Inc. Published 2026 by John Wiley & Sons, Inc.
Companion website: www.wiley.com/go/asprea/anatomy_vettech2e

Applied anatomy refers to the anatomy that is most important surgically or for medical treatment. In planning orthopedic surgery, for instance, it is necessary to know not only the structure of the bones but also the local muscles and blood vessels. Most of us use a systems approach when learning anatomy. For example, we study all the bones in the skeletal system, all the muscles in the muscular system, or all the organs in the urinary system.

One of the most important issues in studying anatomy is the understanding of directional terms. If one is asked to find a particular spot on an animal, describing it as "on the leg" is not precise enough. Describing a location using appropriate directional terms makes this much clearer. While the acquisition of vocabulary can be tedious, it is integral to effectively communicate with our clients, veterinarians, and other members of the patient-care team as well as keep accurate medical records. In other words, good anatomic vocabulary contributes to excellent patient care.

Directional Terms

Directional terms in veterinary medicine are very different from those used in human medicine. The human head is "up" from the hips, while it is "forward" in the dog. This is another reason why it is important to use the proper terms. It is also important to understand that many of these terms are used while referring to, or in relation to, anatomical landmarks to make the description clear. This is the same as when one is giving directions for travel. We don't say, "The store is far away on Main Street." We say, "The store is on Main Street, in between avenue A and avenue B, across from the diner." This tells us exactly where the store is using landmarks around it; in the same way, we use anatomical directional terms to be specific about which body part we are discussing.

Anatomical terminology has many unique terms, prefixes, and suffixes which are derived from Latin and Ancient Greek. As such, these terms for direction can correlate to the terms for the location on the body. Going toward the head is **cranial** or moving cranially, referring to the cranium or skull. Going in the opposite direction, toward the tail, is **caudal** or moving caudally, from the Latin word "caud" meaning tail. Going toward the top of the animal that faces the ceiling is moving in a **dorsal** direction, referring to moving toward the dorsum or "back/spine." From the top downward is moving in a **ventral** direction referring to the ventrum or ground-facing side of the animal from the Latin term for "belly." Moving toward the center or midline of the animal or a specific limb is considered **medial**, while moving from the midline toward the side of the animal is **lateral**.

On the appendages, such as the limbs and tail, or even pinna (ear flaps), we use some special terms. Closer to the body on the appendage is **proximal**, while moving away from the body on the appendage is moving in a **distal** direction (Figure 1.2). For example, the elbow is proximal (nearer to the body) than the **carpus** (wrist). Alternately, you could say the carpus is distal (further from the body) to the elbow. When using these terms to describe a lesion, mass, or injury, we could say, "There is an approximately 6 cm wound immediately distal to the **lateral** elbow on the right forelimb" (Figure 1.3). This tells us the size of the wound, that it is just below (or farther away from) the elbow on the lateral (outer facing) side of the animal on the right leg. Being described in such a way leaves no room for error when communicating with anyone on the patient care team or in written records.

There are other specialized terms used for direction on the limbs and head. Previously, we discussed that the term cranial was moving toward the head, but once we reach the head, a different term is used: **rostral**. Rostral is used in the place of cranial only on the head and means toward the nose, derived from Middle English and Old French to mean the "bony beak." The term rostral remains paired with caudal as its opposite on the head. As an example, one could say "The nose is rostral to the eyes" or "The ears are caudal to the nose" (Figure 1.3).

Additional Terminology

Features of the limbs also get special names. The front legs are referred to as the **thoracic limbs**, while the rear legs as the **pelvic limbs**. The shoulder and elbow in dogs are, in medical terms, the **scapulohumeral** and **humeroradioulnar** joints, respectively, although they are commonly referred to as shoulder and elbow in discussions with clients and others on the patient care team. The next joint distal to the elbow is the carpus, which is the equivalent of the human wrist. On the pelvic limb, the joint between the femur and tibia is the **femorotibial joint**, commonly known as the **stifle**, which is equivalent to the human knee. The next joint going distally is the **tarsus**. The common name for the tarsus is the **hock**, a term generally reserved for large animals, all of which is equivalent to the human ankle.

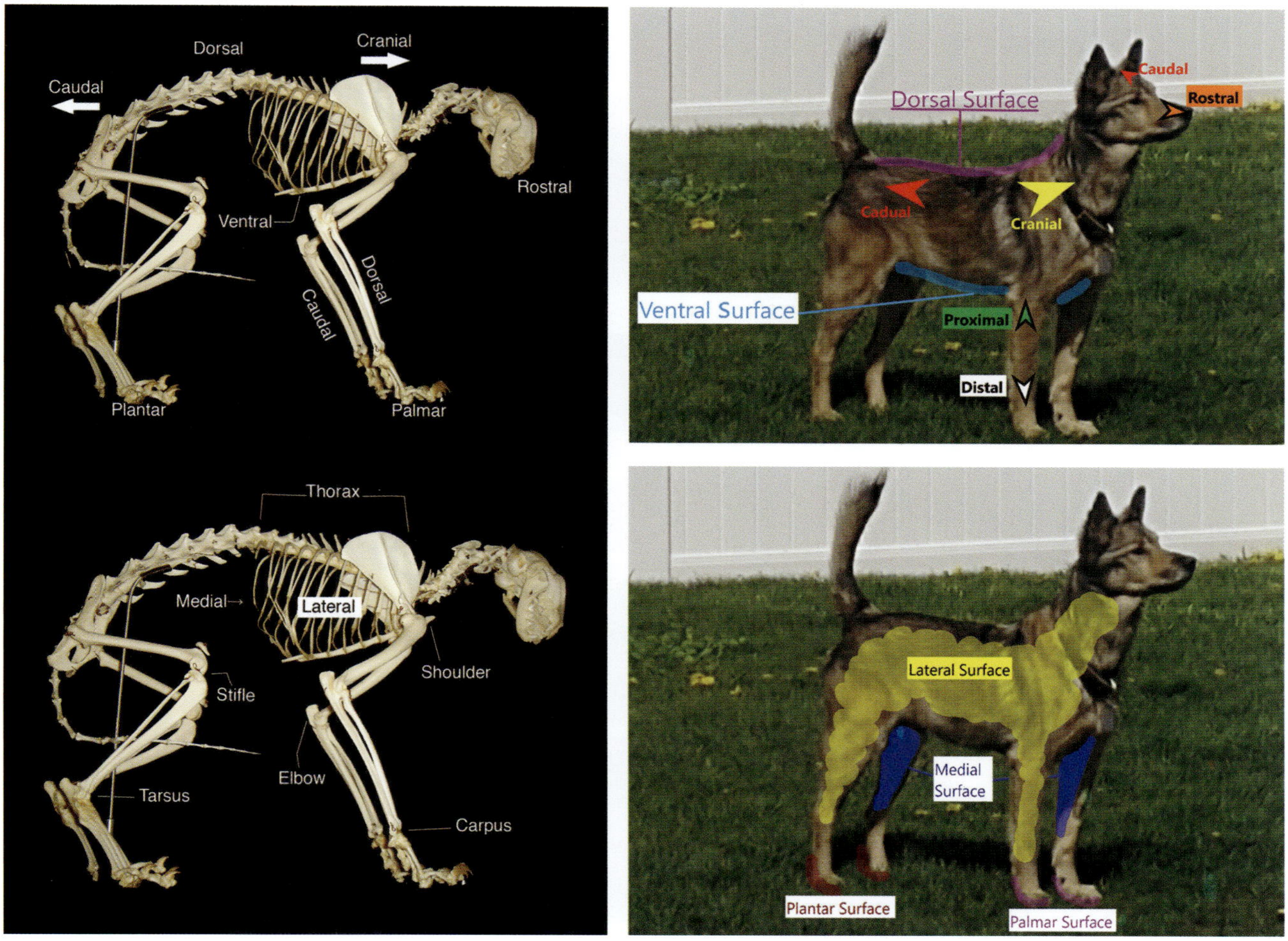

Figure 1.2 Directional terms as they pertain to the feline/canine skeleton. Also noted are some of the major joints.

Figure 1.3 A laceration is noted on this patient, described as "an approximately 6 cm wound immediately distal to the lateral elbow on the right forelimb." Note the importance of directional and location terms.

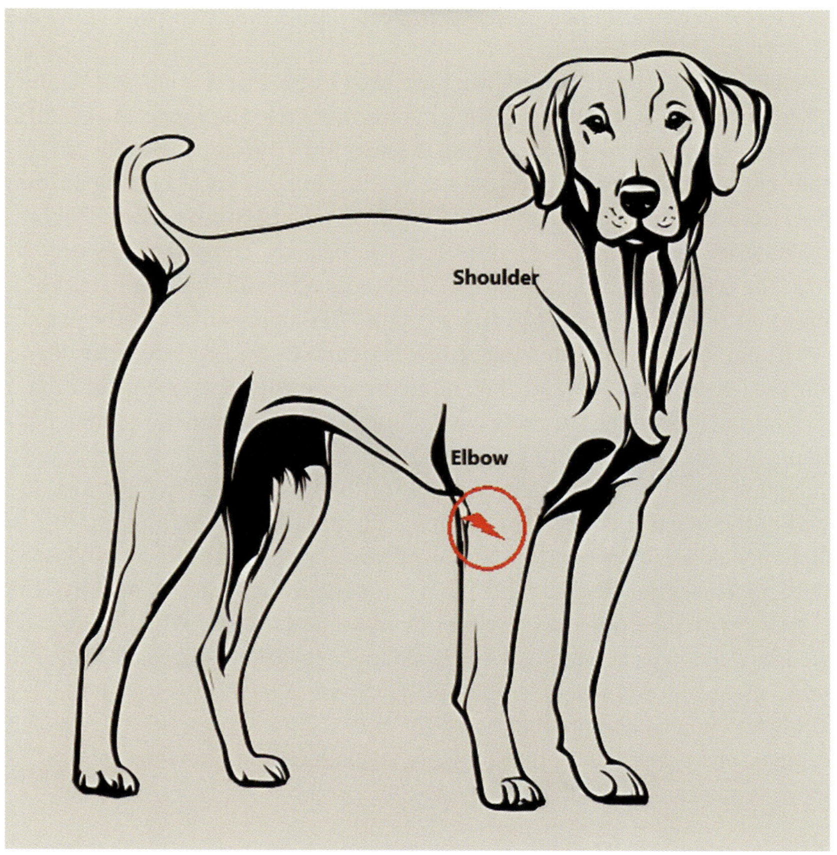

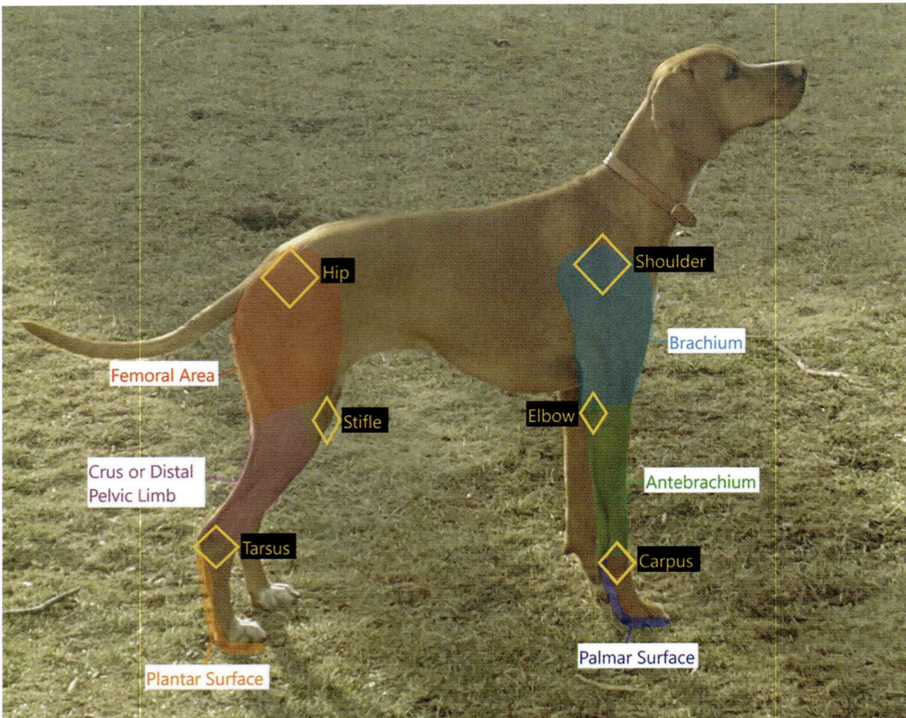

Figure 1.4 The different sections of the thoracic and pelvic limbs with the plantar and palmar surfaces noted.

The part of the thoracic limb from the shoulder to the elbow is referred to as the **brachium**; the area from the elbow to the carpus is referred to as the **antebrachium**. The area from the head of the femur (the proximal-most bone of the pelvic limb) to the stifle is called the **femoral area**. The area from the stifle to the tarsus is technically called the **crus**, although this term is not commonly used in a clinical setting; the distal pelvic limb is less precise but often used in general practice (Figure 1.4).

When considering the trunk, we have used terms like caudal, dorsal, and ventral. These terms also apply to the limbs. The front of the leg from the shoulder going distally to the paw is the dorsal section, with the back of that same area as the caudal section. On the thoracic limb, the area from the carpus distally, on the caudal surface, and around to and including the ventral surface of the paw that meets the ground is known as the **palmar surface**. On the pelvic limb, the analogous area from the tarsus to the bottom of the paw is the **plantar surface** (Figure 1.4).

There are specific names for other parts of the body. The part of the body that includes the chest and abdomen is referred to as the **trunk**. As discussed earlier, the proper name for the ventral part of the abdomen is the ventrum, while the proper name for the top of the trunk is the dorsum. The lateral surface of the part of the trunk caudal to the chest is the **flank**.

The part of the trunk from the neck to the caudal ribs is referred to as the **thorax**. The **abdomen** refers both to the outer surface (the skin) of the ventrum and to the space within it, extending from the caudal ribs to the pelvis. The space within the thorax is called the **thoracic cavity**, and the space within the abdomen is called the **abdominal cavity**. Note, however, that some of the features of each of these cavities are lined by a membrane. The **pleural membrane**, within the thorax, surrounds the lungs and lines the walls of the thoracic cavity. The area bordered by this membrane is considered to be within the **pleural cavity**. Similarly, the membrane surrounding some of the organs and lining the interior walls of the abdomen is called the **peritoneal membrane**, or **peritoneum**, and that space is called the **peritoneal cavity**. These cavities and tissues will be discussed again throughout the anatomy and physiology chapters of this text where relevant.

Along with directional and basic anatomical terminology, which allows us to accurately describe the location we desire, we also need to understand the medical language used to discuss these features. Veterinary medical terminology, like any other medical terminology, is a language in and of itself. It is based on a series of prefixes, suffixes, and root words that allow for endless combinations in an effort to accurately describe physiological processes, anatomical parts, diseases, syndromes, and a myriad of other things in medicine. Please refer to Tables 1.1–1.3 for the most common list of these terms along with examples of their use.

Table 1.1 Prefixes.

Term	Referring to	Example
a/an-	without, not	Anemia – without blood – refers to a low red blood cell count
ab	away from	Abductor – muscle(s) that moves the limb away from the body
ad	toward	Adductor – muscle(s) that move the limb toward the body
ante-	before, in front of	Antebrachium – before the brachium (lower portion of the limb)
anti-	against	Antibacterial – an agent (drug, cleanser etc.) against bacteria
auto-	self	Autoantibodies – antibodies against one's own tissues
brady-	slow	Bradycardia – slow heartbeat
bi-	two	Bilateral – both/two sides
bucco-	cheek	Buccal pouch – space in between cheek and gums – used for medicine administration
circum-	around or surrounding	Circumduct – moving a limb around in a circular way
crypto-	hidden	Cryptorchidism – one or both testicles are undescended and remain in the abdominal cavity
cyan-	blue	Cyanosis – mucous membranes or skin appearing blue due to lack of oxygen
cyt-	cell	Cytology – study of cells
dis-	apart, away	Dissect – cut apart
dys-	abnormal, bad	Dysplasia – abnormal growth
ex/exo-	out of, outside, external	Exoskeleton – an outer covering in invertebrates analogous to mammalian skeleton
endo-	inside	Endoscopy – to look or examine inside with a specialized tool
epi-	upon, on	Epiglottis – the covering on the trachea
erythr/o-	red	Erythrocyte – red blood cell
eu-	good	Eupneic – breathing well/normally. Euthanasia – good death
extra-	beyond, outside of	Extraocular – just outside the eye
hemi-	one half	Hemiplegia – paralysis of one side of the body
hetero-	different	Heterozygous – two different forms of one gene
home/o-	same	Homeostasis – a steady, balanced state maintained by living things
hyper-	excess, too much	Hyperthermia – too high of body temperature; febrile
hypo-	below, under, too little	Hypothermia – too low of body temperature
infra-	beneath	Infraorbital – beneath the bony orbit of the eye
inter-	between	Interdigital – in between the digits of the paw or hoof
intra-	inside, within	Intraocular – within the eye
iso-	equal, like	Isosthenuria – urine with the same concentration of protein-free plasma
leuk/o-	white	Leukocyte – white blood cell
lith-	stone	Lithotripsy – a procedure using sound waves to break up stones in the body
macro-	large, long	Macrophage – a type of large white blood cell
melan/o-	black	Melanocyte – a pigment-producing cell
meso-	middle	Mesoderm – the middle layer in a developing embryo
meta-	beyond	Metacarpus – the bones beyond the carpus
micro-	small, minute	Microhepatica – small liver
myo-	muscle	Myocardium – the muscle layer of the heart
necro-	death	Necrosis – tissue death
neo-	new	Neonate – newborn
pan-	everything, all	Panzootic – involving all animals

(Continued)

Table 1.1 (Continued)

Term	Referring to	Example
para-	next to, alongside	Parathyroid – an organ alongside the thyroid gland
peri-	around, enclosing	Pericardium – the tissue around the heart
poly-	many, multiple	Polydactyl – multiple (excessive) digits
post-	after	Postrenal – after the kidneys, referring to illness
pre-	before	Prerenal – before the kidneys, referring to illness
pseudo-	false	Pseudopregnancy – false pregnancy
re-	again, backward	Reflux – return of fluid backward from it should be – acid reflux from the stomach into the esophagus
retro-	backward, behind	Retropharyngeal space – area behind the pharynx
semi-	partially, half	Semilunar – half-moon shaped, referring to the cardiac valves
sub-	below, under	Sublingual – under the tongue. Subcutaneous – under the skin
supra-	above, over	Suprarenal– above the kidney
sy/syl/sym-	together, joined	Symphysis – a joint where two bones come together; pubic symphysis or mandibular symphysis
trans-	across, over	Transection – to cut across something
tachy-	rapid, swift	Tachycardia – fast heart rate
ultra-	extremely, beyond	Ultrasound – sounds beyond the limit we can hear; sound technology used for imaging

Table 1.2 Suffixes.

Term	Referring to	Example
-ac	pertaining to	Cardiac – pertaining to the heart
-algia	pain	Neuralgia – nerve pain
-ate	having, possessing	Caudate – having a tail
-blast/o/ic	bud, germ	Osteoblast – a cell that builds the matrix for bone
-centesis	puncture	Thoracocentesis – puncturing the thoracic cavity with a needle to remove air or fluid
-cyte	cell	Leukocyte – white blood cell
-cytosis	referring to cells, many	Leukocytosis – too many white blood cells
-ectomy	excision, removal	Orchiectomy – surgical removal of the testicles
-emesis	vomiting	Hematemesis – vomiting blood
-emia	blood, in the blood	Hyperphosphatemia – excess phosphorus in the blood
-genesis	origin, beginning of	Pathogenesis – the origin and development of the problem
-gram	drawn, written	Electrocardiogram – a graph of the heart's electrical function on the surface of the skin
-graph	to write	Electrocardiograph – the machine that creates the graph for the electrocardiogram
-ia	condition of	Hyperglycemia – the condition of having too much sugar in the blood
-iasis/osis/sis	condition of	Trichiasis – condition of having hair grow in the wrong direction (eyelash)
-ism	condition of	Hyperthyroidism – condition of having an overactive thyroid gland
-itis	inflammation of	Sinusitis – inflammation of the sinuses
-lith	stone	Cystolith – bladder stone
-logy	study of	Osteology – the study of bones
-lysis	break down, destruction	Hemolysis – destruction of red blood cells
-megaly	enlargement	Splenomegaly – an enlarged spleen

Table 1.2 (Continued)

Term	Referring to	Example
-meter	measuring device	Sphygmomanometer – a manual blood pressure measuring device
-oid	resembling, like	Fibroid – having a fibrous-like appearance
-oma	tumor, cancer	Lipoma – fatty tumor; carcinoma – a malignant tumor of epithelial cells
-ostomy	opening	Tracheostomy – an opening in the trachea, usually to help breathing
-otomy	incision	Laparotomy – an incision made into the abdominal wall/cavity
-pathy	disease	Enteropathy – disease of the small intestine
-penia	lack of, deficiency	Lymphopenia – deficiency of lymphocytes
-pexy	fixation	Gastropexy – surgically fixating the stomach to the body wall
-phagia/phagy	eating	Dysphagia – difficulty eating; polyphagia – eating too much
-plasia	growth, formation	Neoplasia – new growth, generally referring to a tumor
-plasty	surgical reconstruction	Episioplasty/Vulvoplasty – surgery to reconstruct the vulva
-plegia	paralysis	Hemiplegia – paralysis of one side of the body
-pnea	breath, respiration	Dyspnea – abnormal breathing
-rrhea	flow or discharge	Diarrhea – flowing watery feces
-rrhexis	rupture	Enterorrhexis – rupture of the intestine
-scopy	to examine with a tool	Gastroscopy – to look or examine inside the stomach with a specialized tool
-stasis	level, unchanging	Homeostasis – a steady, balanced state, maintained by living things
-stomy	creating an opening	Colostomy – a surgical hole in the colon for waste removal
-tomy	incising	Tracheotomy – cutting into the trachea
-tome	cutting instrument	Osteotome – a bone-cutting instrument
-trophy	growth	Hypertrophy – increased size or growth of tissue
-uria	presence in urine	Hematuria – presence of blood in the urine

Table 1.3 Root words.

Term	Referring to	Example
abdomin/o	abdomen	Abdominocentesis – puncturing (with a needle) into the abdominal cavity to remove fluid
aden/o	gland	Adenoma – a benign tumor of a gland
adip/o	fat	Adipose tissue – fatty tissue
arter/o	artery	Arteriole – a small artey
brachi	arm	Brachium – the upper portion of the forelimb. Antebrachium – the lower portion of the forelimb
brachy	short	Brachycephalic – shorter than the average skull length (example: English Bulldog, Pug)
bronch/o	bronchus	Bronchoscopy – using a special tool to see inside the bronchi/ main branches in the lungs
carcin/o	cancer	Carcinoma – cancer of the epithelial tissue, possible in many organ systems
cardi/o	heart	Cardiomegaly – an enlarged heart
carp/o	wrist	Metacarpus – the bones between the wrist and phalanges
cephal/o	head	Mesocephalic – an average- or medium-sized skull length (example: Labrador Retriever)
cerebell/o	cerebellum	Cerebellar hypoplasia – a disease in which the cerebellum fails to grow properly *in utero*
cerebr/o	brain, cerebrum	Cerebrospinal fluid – fluid that surrounds the entire brain and spinal cord
col/o	colon/large intestine	Colectomy – surgical removal of a part or all of the colon

(Continued)

Table 1.3 (Continued)

Term	Referring to	Example
cyt/o	cell	Cytotoxin – an agent toxic to living cells
cyst	pouch, bladder	Cystitis – an inflammation of the urinary bladder ("cyst" can refer to the gallbladder as well)
dactyl	digit	Polydactyl – a condition of too many digits per paw
derm/a/o	skin	Dermatology a branch of medicine focusing on the skin and integument
dextr/o	right side	Oculus Dexter (abbrev: OD) – right eye
dolich/o	long, narrow	Dolichocephalic – a longer than average skull length (example: Greyhound, Borzoi)
duct/o	to lead, to carry	Abduction – to lead the limb away from the body
encephala/o	brain	Encephalopathy – any disease or disorder of the brain
enter/o	intestine/small intestine	Gastroenteritis – an inflammation of the stomach and small intestine
esthes/o	nerve sensations	Feline hyperesthesia – a condition in which the patient is extremely sensitive to touch
gastr/o	stomach	Gastrotomy – a surgical incision into the stomach
gingiv/o	gum	Gingivitis – inflammation of the gums
gloss/o	tongue	Glossopharyngeal nerve – a cranial nerve that helps controls tongue movement and more
glyc/gluc/o	(blood) sugar	Hypoglycemia – too low level of sugar in the blood
gnath/o	jaw	Prognathism (mandibular) – a term for an underbite
hemat/o	blood	Hematopoiesis – formation of blood cells
hepat/o	liver	Microhepatica – an abnormally small liver
iatro	medicine, healing	Iatrogenic – illness caused by medical treatment or interventions
ile/o	ileum	Ileocecolic junction – where the ileum, cecum, and colon meet in the digestive tract
jejun/o	jejunum	Jejunostomy tube – a feeding tube placed directly into the jejunum of the small instesine
lingu/o	tongue	Sublingual – under the tongue
mammo/mast	mammary glands	Mastitis – inflammation and infection of the mammary gland(s)
metri/o/a	uterus	Pyometra – pus-filled uterus
nephro	kidney, nephrons	Nephrology – the study of the kidney and its functions
neuro	nerve, nervous system	Neurology – the branch of medicine that deals with the nervous system
ocul/o	relating to the eye, vision	Intraocular pressure – the amount of pressure inside the eye
onych/o	nail, claw	Onychectomy – a removal of the claws; a declaw
ophthalm/o	relating to the eye	Ophthalmoscope – a tool used to look into the eye to view the retina and other structures
orchi/o	testicle	Orchiectomy – removal of the testicle(s); a neuter
oro	mouth	Oropharynx – an area comprised of the mouth and throat
osseo, oste/o	bony	Osteosarcoma – a cancer of the bones
oto	ear	Otitis externa – an inflammation and infection of the outer ear
path	abnormal, disease	Pathology – a branch of medicine focused on the study and diagnosis of diseases
pharyng/o	pharynx	Nasopharyngoscopy – a procedure to look into the back of the nasal passages and throat
phleb/o	vein	Phlebotomy – removal of blood from veins, usually for laboratory testing
pneum/o	air, breathing, lungs	Pneumothorax – air in the thoracic cavity outside of the lungs
pod/o	foot	Pododermatitis – an inflammation and infection of the skin around the toes and foot
poiesis	creation, formation	Erythropoiesis – formation of red blood cells in the body
poikilo	irregular, varied	Poikilocytosis – an increase in abnormally shaped red blood cells
pulmo/n	lungs	Pulmonary thromboembolism – a blood clot that gets stuck in the blood vessels of the lungs
pyelo	renal pelvis	Pyelonephritis – an infection and inflammation of the renal pelvis and kidney

Table 1.3   (Continued)

Term	Referring to	Example
pyo	pus	Pyoderma – a skin infection that forms pus-filled blisters or pustules
ren/o	kidney	Adrenal gland – a gland next to the kidney
rhin/o	nose	Rhinoscopy – using a special tool to see into the nasal passages
sinister/o	left side	Auris Sinister (abbrev: AS) – left ear
stoma	mouth, opening	Urethrostomy – an opening made in the urethra to allow urine to pass out of the body
tars/o	ankle or eyelid	Tarsus – the "ankle." Tarsorrhaphy – partially or completely sewing the eyelids together
therm/o	heat	Hyperthermia – an elevated body temperature
thorac/o	thorax or chest	Thoracotomy – opening the thoracic cavity
trache/o	trachea	Rhinotracheitis – an infectious disease that causes inflammation of the nose and trachea
trich	hair	Trichobezoar – a mass of hair formed in the stomach, a hairball
ure/uro	urine or urea	Uroabdomen – urine freely floating in the abdomen as a result of urinary tract injury
ven	vein	Venule – a small vein

Clinical Case Resolution: Georgia

In the example at the beginning of this chapter, a problem was noted with Georgia's "hind leg." This language is not appropriately descriptive for a medical record. Using the terminology learned in this chapter, we should describe this finding as follows: The patient has an approximately 3 cm mass (to describe size) on the left pelvic limb (to describe the side of the patient and limb) proximal to the lateral tarsus (to describe the exact location on the limb).

Review Questions

1   Define the terms medial, rostral, and dorsal.

2   Which is more cranial, the thoracic limb or the pelvic limb?

3   The caudal paw area on the thoracic limb is referred to as the _______ surface.

4   True or false: The stifle is caudal to the tail.

5   Define the term "topographic anatomy."

6   Go back to the case about Georgia and look at the provided Figure 1.1. Describe the mass that was found in relation to the stifle using appropriate directional and anatomical terms.

7   Refer to Figure 1.3 where a laceration was described. Describe the injury in relation to the hip using appropriate directional and anatomical terms.

8   Which of the following terms refers to the liver?
    A Gastric
    B Hepatic
    C Pleural
    D Renal

9 Which of the following terms refers to inflammation?

A Sarcoma

B Hyperthyroid

C Bradycardia

D Pancreatitis

10 Which of the following terms refers to muscle?

A Leukocyte

B Myocardium

C Polydactyl

D Ultrasound

Extra terminology practice: Use Tables 1.1–1.3 to deduce the meaning of the incorrect answer choices for questions 8, 9, and 10. Example: Gastric – referring to the stomach from the root word "gastr/o."

2

Anatomy of the Common Integument

> **Clinical Case: Poppy, An Approximately 2-Year-Old Female Intact Mixed Breed Dog**
>
> *This patient is presented to the clinic for an initial examination. The owners report that they found Poppy 2 days ago on the street. Upon examination, it is noted that there are multiple spots of alopecia (missing hair) along the chest and forelimbs, along with erythema (reddened skin) and pruritus (itching). Poppy is also of a thin body condition.*

The term integument refers to a broad range of tissues. Knowing the composition and structure of these elements contributes to a broader understanding of the function of this system. This will lead to the ability to recognize what happens in disease states such as the one described above.

Introduction

The integument is a collective term for aspects of bodily structure that are formed of connective tissue and epithelia. Connective tissue is a collection of proteins, fibrous material, and ground elements that form many parts of the mammalian body. An epithelial cell has a specific microscopic structure. Features such as skin, skin glands, fur/whiskers, hooves, horns, and claws are epithelial structures that are parts of the integument. This chapter will focus on the anatomical parts of the integument where the physiological functions will be discussed in Chapter 15. The primary focus is on companion mammals, while certain species-specific characteristics are discussed throughout.

Skin

Mammalian skin is a complex organ that serves many functions and contains many important parts. The superficial-most, or outermost layer, is the **epidermis**. Deep to the epidermis is the **dermis**. There is a layer of fat and connective tissue deep to the dermis called the **subcutaneous** layer or the **hypodermis**. The subcutaneous layer is not skin but is a part of the integument. See Figure 2.1 for a depiction of these layers.

The epidermis has several important specialized cells as well as multiple layers. The specialized cells we can find in the epidermis are **keratinocytes, melanocytes, Merkel cells,** and **Langerhans cells**.

Keratinocytes are found throughout the epidermis but begin in the deepest layer. They produce **keratin**, a tough, fibrous, and waterproof protein that provides skin and other parts of the integument with their strength.

Another specialized cell in the epidermis is **melanocytes**. Melanocytes have their cell body at the deepest portion of the epidermis with finger-like projections reaching into the upper layers. See Figure 2.2 for the melanocyte structure. Melanocytes are responsible for producing **melanin**, which is a type of pigment that gives color to skin and hair, as well as feathers and scales.

Merkel cells are found in the junction where the deepest layer of the epidermis meets the dermis. Merkel cells are specialized sensory cells that perceive light touch. They are connected to nerve endings that can receive touch sensations and send that information to the brain for processing.

Anatomy and Physiology for Veterinary Technicians and Nurses: A Clinical Approach, Second Edition. Lori Asprea.
© 2026 John Wiley & Sons, Inc. Published 2026 by John Wiley & Sons, Inc.
Companion website: www.wiley.com/go/asprea/anatomy_vettech2e

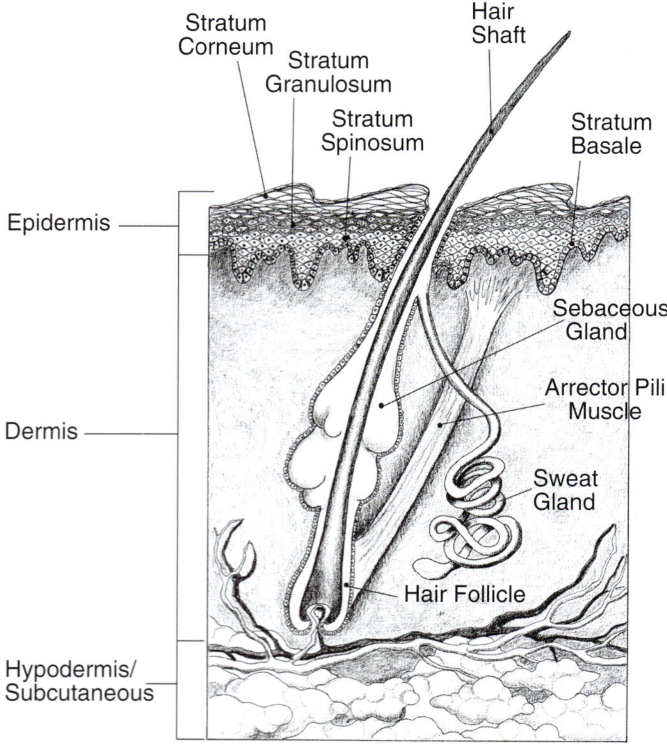

Figure 2.1 Layers of the skin. The epidermis ends at the stratum basale, and the dermis ends at the subcutaneous layer.

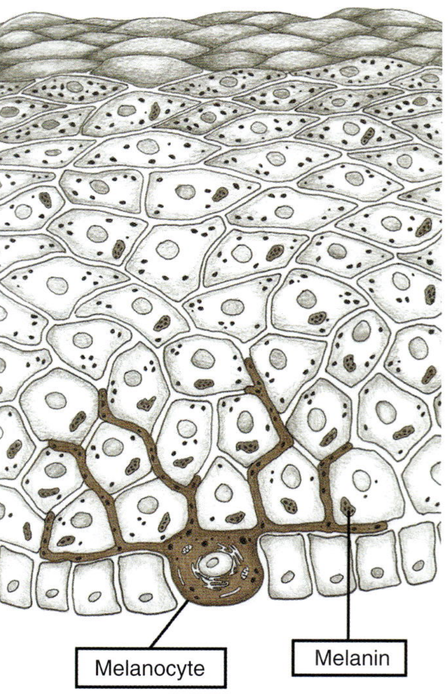

Figure 2.2 The melanocyte with the cell body in the deepest layer of the epidermis while projections reach up through the layers, depositing melanin. The amount and type of melanin creates a variety of colors.

The last specialized cell that can be found in the epidermis to be discussed is the **Langerhans cell**. The Langerhans cell can be found in the skin and many other areas of the body. The primary job of this specialized cell is to act as a bodyguard in the skin. It is able to recognize foreign invaders like viruses and bacteria and alert the immune system to take action, thereby protecting the body.

These specialized cells can be found in the layers of the epidermis. Although the epidermis is the outermost portion of skin, it too can be broken down into five individual layers. The deepest layer of cells that make up the epidermis is the **stratum basale** or **basal layer**. This layer is where new keratinocytes develop and undergo rapid division. These germinal cells will travel up through the layers of the epidermis undergoing keratinization. The next layer above the stratum basale is the **stratum spinosum** or the "spiny" layer. Here the keratinocytes that have moved up take on a spiny appearance microscopically, hence their alternate name. The next layer is the **stratum granulosum** where cells begin to lose their nuclei and **glycolipids** are introduced to help waterproof the skin. Above the stratum granulosum is the **stratum lucidum** or "clear" layer. This thin layer is comprised of a few rows of flattened cells and is only visible in thick-skinned areas like the foot pads. The final and outermost layer of the epidermis is the **stratum corneum**. This layer is comprised of dead cells that have completely keratinized or cornified. When you are looking at a patient or yourself, the layer of skin you see with the naked eye is the stratum corneum. Refer to Figure 2.1 to view these layers.

The epidermis has almost nothing in the way of blood vessels or nerve fibers. This is why a cat's head can be gently scratched without drawing blood. Anything that penetrates down to the level of the dermis, however, will cause pain and bleeding, as that is where the blood vessels and nerves are located. Along with blood supply and nerves, the dermis contains many other important structures such as lymphatics, hair follicles, sweat glands, sebaceous glands, and muscles.

The dermis is attached to the epidermis by way of the **basement membrane**. The basement membrane acts as a connection point to cement the epidermis and dermis together. The dermis itself is much more fibrous than the epidermis and is mostly composed of collagen, protein, and elastic fibers. Although not as cellular, the dermis has its own distinct layers: the **papillary layer** and the **reticular layer**.

The papillary layer of the dermis is just beneath the epidermis. It is comprised of loose connective tissue and helps form the **dermal papillae**. Dermal papillae are ridges or projections up toward the epidermis that have many functions, including nourishing hair follicles and supporting the epidermis. The papillary layer has blood vessels that provide nourishment and gas exchange, assist with thermoregulation, and remove waste products. This layer of the dermis also contains pain receptors to sense painful stimuli and specialized sensory structures called **Meissner's corpuscles**, which can perceive light touch. The reticular layer of the dermis is comprised of dense irregular connective tissues and makes up the majority of the thickness of the dermis. This layer is predominantly responsible for the dermis' strength and elasticity.

As previously discussed, the dermis contains many important structures. Two of these structures are specialized glands: **sweat glands** and **sebaceous glands**. Sweat glands produce a watery-like substance, while sebaceous glands produce a waxy substance. There are two types of sweat glands: **apocrine** and **eccrine**. In general, apocrine sweat glands are found in association with hair follicles, while eccrine glands are spread in other areas. Canines and felines have sweat glands primarily around the metacarpal and digital pads of the paw. A specialized form of sweat gland is the mammary gland.

Sebaceous glands produce **sebum**, which is a waxy, thick substance. Sebaceous glands also secrete **pheromones**, which are species-specific odors that have a great deal to do with socialization and reproductive behaviors. There are a number of sebaceous glands throughout the body in all mammalian species. The interdigital glands are important in ruminants. These are present in the area of the hoof where the digits begin to spread out from each other. The anal glands, present on either side of the anus, assume an important communication role in dogs and cats and will become quite familiar in clinical practice. Suborbital glands, present in the area of the medial canthus (place where the eyelids meet) of each eye, are used to mark territory by many antelopes.

Deep to the dermis is the hypodermis or subcutaneous layer (usually abbreviated as "sub-Q" or "SQ"). This layer is mostly composed of adipose tissue (i.e., fat) but also contains blood vessels and some nerves. When a cat or a dog picks up a neonate by the back of the neck, or the "scruff," it is not painful. This is because that area has a very thick layer of subcutaneous fat. The subcutaneous layer also allows for the skin to move somewhat freely over the animal without putting tension on the skin. In a healthy animal, this layer has a large water content; in a dehydrated animal, areas of thick subcutaneous tissue, such as the scruff, will maintain a tented appearance if pinched and released, rather than springing back to a normal position. This is one way we assess hydration status during a physical examination.

Pads

A thickened mass of epidermal layers is referred to as a **pad**. Dogs and cats have a pad on the palmar and plantar surface of each digit and a larger pad proximal to it called a metacarpal or metatarsal pad, depending on the limb. Carpal always refers to the thoracic limb, as it is derived from the term carpus, meaning wrist, while tarsal refers to the pelvic limb from tarsus or "ankle." There is also a small pad in cats just proximal to the carpus. This pad is usually associated with one of the skin glands and is often marked by a single tactile hair. Refer to Figure 2.3 for a diagram of the pads.

Figure 2.3 Pads of the feline and canine paw.

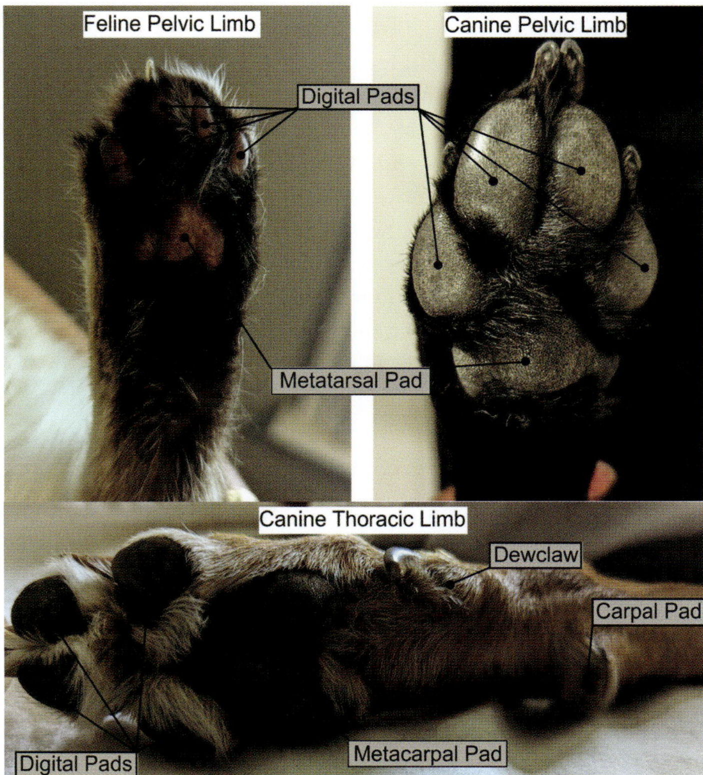

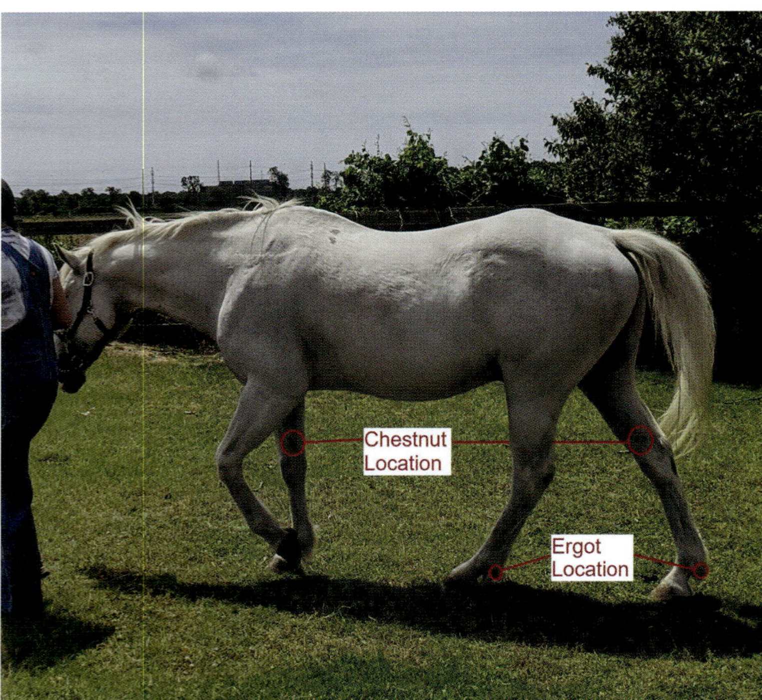

Figure 2.4 Chestnuts and ergots found on the distal equine limbs.

Horses have something similar to pads on their limbs, referred to as the **chestnut** and **ergot**. The chestnut is found on the medial surface, in the area of the carpus and tarsus. Interestingly, chestnuts are thicker in working horses than in light breeds, where they may be absent altogether. The ergot is found near the palmar and plantar surfaces of the limbs. A concentration of sebaceous glands in this area may be involved in scent marking (Figure 2.4).

Haircoat

The haircoat is an important feature of the integument. One of the attributes that defines an animal as a mammal is that it has hair. Hair is missing in specific spots on the body like the lips, paw pads, nipples, inner folds of the genitals, the nasal region, and hooves or horns, depending on the species. The haircoat is generally organized where the hair all slopes in a pattern away from the nose, apart from things like whorls (spiral hair patterns or "cowlicks") and some breed-specific differences like the Rhodesian Ridgeback, which has a strip of hair growing in the opposite direction along its dorsum as a breed standard. The word hair or fur is generally used interchangeably but can occasionally be used individually to denote coat type where hair can refer to a silkier coat with a long growth cycle and less shedding, whereas fur can refer to a coat with a shorter growth cycle and more shedding. Regardless of the length or texture of the coat, the anatomical construction of the follicle and resulting strand of hair is the same and for our purposes will be called hair. A discussion of the growth cycles can be found in Chapter 15.

In dogs and cats, the haircoat generally has several layers. The word **topcoat** is used to denote the outermost layer, and it is comprised of **guard hairs** or **primary hairs**. Guard hairs are longer and stiffer hairs that help to protect the skin and repel water. The word **undercoat** is used to denote the coat of hair underneath the topcoat. The undercoat is comprised of **secondary hairs** or **wool hairs**, which are shorter and softer than primary hairs. The trapping of air between the topcoat and the undercoat is an important method of thermoregulation, which is discussed in Chapter 15. When a dog or cat is combed, it is mostly the undercoat that comes off onto the comb.

Each individual hair arises from a **hair follicle** found in the skin. Hair follicles are like little pockets in the skin that help to anchor the hair in place while it grows and provide a connection from some glands to the surface of the skin. The visible portion of hair sticking out from the follicle is called the **shaft**, while the buried portion surrounded by the follicle in the skin is called the **root**. At the very base of the root is the hair **bulb** and **papilla**. The papilla contains a group of rapidly dividing cells that will keratinize to form the hair strand. The follicle is also paired with a muscle called the **arrector pili**, which allows the hair to stand up, which is an important communication tool in animals. Dogs and cats will raise the hair on their backs and tails to display fear or excitement. When this muscle contracts to squeeze the follicle and help the hair stand up, it also helps to move sebum from the follicle to the surface of the skin.

A single hair is made of three main layers: the **cuticle**, the **cortex**, and the **medulla**. It should be noted that the terms cortex and medulla can be found in multiple anatomical locations, as cortex generally refers to an outer tissue and medulla generally refers to the innermost or middle tissue. Here the cuticle of the hair is the outermost layer, then deep to that is the cortex, and finally in the center of the strand is the medulla. The cuticle is made of hard keratin and is one-cell layer thick. The keratinized cells are organized like shingles or scales, so the outside of the hair is slippery and will not tangle with other hairs. The cortex is the middle layer and is the thickest, comprised of hard keratin and containing the color component of the hair. The medulla is the innermost layer formed of soft keratin in loose layers. (Figure 2.5)

Although we can talk about a single strand of hair, it is important to note that most hair grows in small groups from **compound follicles**. These follicles are bunched together so that each hair strand has its own follicle, but they share a single opening on the skin. This results in not one single hair coming out of each single orifice (opening or pore) but anywhere up to 15 hairs coming out of each opening. These hairs are a mix of primary and secondary hairs, all coming together to form the haircoat.

There are specialized hairs called **tactile hairs** or **sinus hairs** that are thicker than guard hairs and are generally found in specific locations. Whiskers (**vibrissae**) are a type of tactile hair and can be found clustered on the face of most mammals. They can also be found on the limbs of some species as well. These specialized tactile hairs help sense motion and provide other sensory input, as the follicle is richly supplied with nerve endings. The actual hair itself does not have a nerve or blood supply, but when the tactile hair comes into contact with something, it will move slightly in the follicle, which triggers the nerve ending and thus turns the motion into a signal for the brain to interpret. As such, whiskers should not be removed or trimmed.

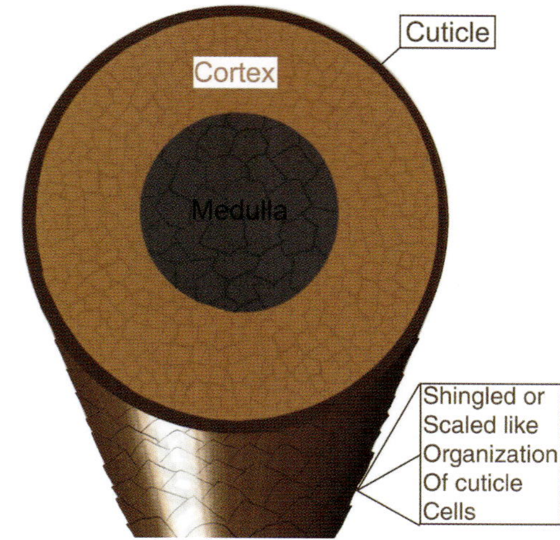

Figure 2.5 A single strand of hair showing the three layers: the cuticle, the cortex, and the medulla. Note the scale-like pattern on the cuticle to prevent matting.

Figure 2.6 Types of feathers. "Clipping" a bird's wings refers to trimming the primary feathers so that the bird cannot fly too high or too far if housed in a restricted area. Contour feathers are the outermost ones, giving the body its outline. Down feathers are closest to the body and provide good insulation.

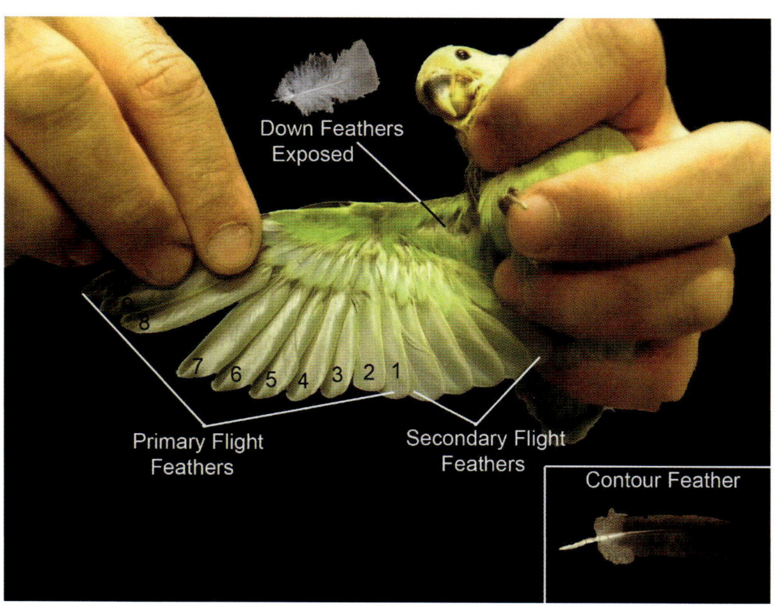

There are some breeds of cats and dogs that are "hairless." The adjective is a misnomer in that they usually have whiskers and often at least some body hair. These animals suffer from a high incidence of skin cancer and problems with thermoregulation, as the traditional haircoat is not in place. Careful counseling of clients with these animals is important, particularly regarding the use of sunscreen and the appropriate care of the skin.

Feathers are actually a specialized type of epidermis and can be thought of as the haircoat of the avian (see Figure 2.6). The contour feathers are the outer layer, giving the bird its silhouette. The down feathers are deep to the contour feathers and tend to be smaller and more tufted. Clipping a bird's wings actually means trimming the longest contour feathers, which are the primary flight feathers. If these are trimmed back to the level of the shorter (secondary) flight feathers, it will prevent the bird from flying long distances.

The general category of feathers includes **contour** and **down** feathers. Contour feathers are those on the exterior of the bird. Specialized contour feathers called primaries and secondaries are most involved in the aerodynamics of flight, helping to control direction and height while airborne. When referring to "clipping the wings" of a bird, the procedure is not that of removing the wings but of trimming the primary contour feathers such that the bird cannot fly very high or very far. This is a protective procedure for some captive birds. The down feathers are mostly related to insulation.

Claws

The claw is another type of integumentary tissue, and it is also composed of keratin. In some animals, including cats and dogs, there is often a digit with a claw on the medial surface of the limb called a **dewclaw**. The dewclaw does not make contact with the ground under normal circumstances but may help gain traction when animals turn when moving at faster speeds. Dogs usually have a dewclaw on all four limbs. Cats, on the other hand, rarely have a dewclaw on the pelvic limbs. As a result, cats with more than 18 digits are considered to be **polydactyl**: having more than the normal number of digits. Polydactyl animals need to be observed carefully in relation to the growth of the claws. All claws, particularly those that do not make contact with the ground, may grow so long that they impinge on the pad and can cause pain or even infection if not monitored for length.

Given that they are composed of keratin, there is no pain associated with trimming the claws themselves. However, there is a vein and nerves associated with the **distal phalanx**, which is the distal-most bone in each digit. This soft and sensitive area is commonly referred to as the "**quick**." This may be visible in some animals' claws if the claw is white or lightly colored. Cutting through the quick can cause significant pain and bleeding and should be avoided if possible. Avian and reptile claws are similar as well and can be trimmed with care.

Onychectomy, commonly called "declawing," which is performed on cats under some conditions, involves removing the distal phalangeal bone (Phalanx 3 or P3) as well as the claw itself. Failing to remove sufficient material can lead to regrowth of the claw; removing P3 as well ensures that this does not happen.

Hooves and Horns

Hooves and horns are also part of the integument. Similar to many structures we have discussed, the outer surface is composed of "dead" or keratinized tissue. Since there is no blood or nerve supply to this tissue, hooves, horns, and beaks can be trimmed without drawing blood if done properly.

Animals with hooves, or **ungulates**, have specialized thick layers of keratin on each foot. The hoof is comprised of three main parts: **the wall, the sole**, and **the frog**. The wall, comprised of thick hard keratin, is the external portion of the exposed part of the hoof when the animal is in a standing position. The sole is the palmar or plantar surface of the hoof. It is also made of keratin, and it is slightly curved inward to prevent direct contact with the ground. The frog is a triangular structure in the back center of the hood that serves as a digital cushion and helps promote blood circulation in the limbs. As discussed in the previous chapter, directional terms and landmarks help us to describe and note accurately. The hoof is no different in needing descriptors of its own. The front of the hoof is the **toe**, the back is the **heel**, and the sides are called

Figure 2.7 The anatomical terms for parts of the horse hoof.

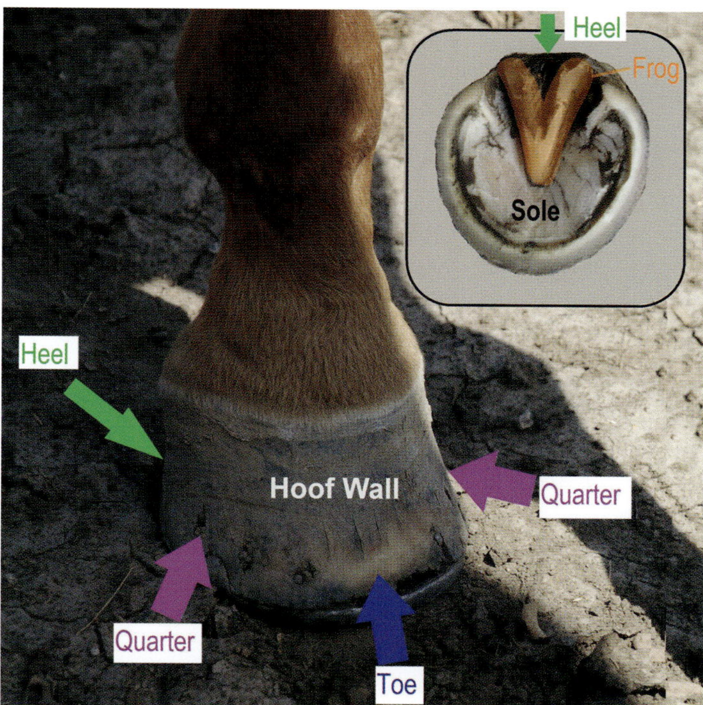

the **quarters** (Figure 2.7). The hoof has several layers, or **laminae**, which have an important function in ambulation. Inflammation between those layers can lead to a very painful condition called laminitis, one of the most frustrating causes of equine lameness; it is, unfortunately, a common problem in equines and often leads to intractable pain. The severity of the problem occasionally necessitates euthanasia.

Horn is also made from hard keratin and is a part of the integument. In some species (e.g., ruminants), the horn actually fits over the skull such that there is a space running through the center of the horn and down into the frontal sinus of the skull. This is important from a husbandry standpoint. If the animal is to be **dehorned** (has the horn permanently removed), and proper procedure is not followed, any contamination at the base of the horn can lead to sinus infection. Lapses in aseptic technique can be associated with encephalitis or inflammation of the brain. Both sinusitis and encephalitis are difficult to treat at best.

The difference between horn and antler is that antlers are shed, and horns are usually not. In cervids, the family including deer, elk, moose, and more, the antler is covered by a layer of softer epidermis called **velvet**, which eventually dies and falls away. The antler is hardened after it completes growing, and the velvet is shed. The antlers themselves are generally shed annually, coming off completely from the base to grow again next season.

Clinical Case Resolution: Poppy

In the beginning of this chapter, a newly adopted dog, Poppy was presented with alopecia, erythema, and pruritus. These can all be signs of multiple skin diseases, and a thorough physical examination along with diagnostic testing is required to make a diagnosis.

During the gross examination of the skin, it is noted that there is excessive flea dirt and live fleas present on the patient. Fleas are an external parasite and can often be found on animals living outdoors without preventative care. Fleas and their bites can cause intense pruritus. Fleas are also the intermediate host for the tapeworm, so it is safe to assume any animal that needs to be treated for fleas should also be treated for tapeworm.

In continuing the examination, it is decided to perform a skin scrape on Poppy. A skin scrape is performed by using a sterile scalpel blade to scrape a sample of skin off to be viewed under the microscope. This is usually done in an effort to diagnose mites that cause Demodectic mange or Sarcoptic mange. Demodex mites live in the hair follicles and generally affect very young or immunocompromised patients. Demodectic mites are normally found on the skin in small numbers but can take over and cause disease when an animal has an immature or poor immune system. These mites can cause hair loss, but generally no itching. Demodex is non-zoonotic (not contagious to people). Sarcoptic mites live in the epidermis and cause intense pruritus and alopecia. Sarcoptic mites are contagious and zoonotic. The skin scraping on Poppy reveals demodectic mange.

Poppy will be treated for fleas, tapeworm, and demodectic mange. She will also be put on a weight-gain diet and be rechecked in 1 week.

Clinical Case Critical Thinking

Use all of Poppy's case details to think about the following questions.

1) *It was noted that Poppy had pruritus, but was not diagnosed with sarcoptic mange, which usually causes this. Why do you think Poppy had pruritus?*
2) *It was mentioned that demodectic mange generally affects very young animals or immunocompromised animals. Was there anything about Poppy that might lead to her having a compromised immune system?*

Review Questions

1 An animal has a laceration that is bleeding, but the cut does not extend down to the muscle. What layers of skin are involved?

2 List three examples of sebaceous glands.

3 Do cats sweat?

4 Of the following areas, where would the stratum lucidum of the epidermis be the thickest?
A Eyelid
B Lip
C Digital pad

5 What is laminitis?

6 What is the difference between guard hairs and tactile hairs?

7 What is the difference between horns and antlers?

8 Which of the following is not painful?
A Laminitis
B Cutting the quick
C Demodectic mange

9 What is meant by clipping a bird's wings?

10 What do the following terms mean?
Pruritus
Alopecia
Erythema

3

Anatomy of the Senses

<table>
<tr><td>Clinical Case: Roo, An 8-Year-Old Female Spayed Hound Mix</td></tr>
<tr><td>Roo presents to the clinic for head shaking and scratching at her ear. The owners report she was recently swimming in a lake and at first, they thought she just had water in her ear. When she did not stop trying to scratch her ear and kept shaking her head, they brought her into the clinic for an evaluation.</td></tr>
</table>

Animals and humans alike use a variety of their senses constantly. There are general senses, and then more advanced senses. It is important to understand the anatomy of the sense organs in order to comprehend how they work, and how they function together.

Introduction

The basic senses are comprised of touch, pain, temperature, and proprioception. These senses focus on obtaining information about the environment but do not have dedicated sense organs, but rather a broad system used to gather and interpret information. The specialized senses are taste, smell, hearing, **equilibrium** or balance, and vision, each of which has its own complex organ system. Many of the senses use something called **modified neurons** to function. These specialized nerve cells have been altered in a way that allows them to convert external stimuli or chemical information into something that the nervous system and brain can process and interpret. Senses can be either **physical**, where the sense relies on physical stimuli from the environment, or **chemical**, where the sense relies on molecules in the environment, food, or substance to collect information.

General Senses

Touch is a tactile sense that involves gathering information from touch and pressure stimulation on the body. When something or someone comes into contact with the body, sensory neurons are responsible for taking the information in and communicating it to the central nervous system. This is a broad system that works throughout the whole body. Similarly, temperature and pain are perceived by these sensory neurons spread throughout the body to translate information to the central nervous system for processing. The central nervous system can then help the body to act if necessary. For example, if an animal is hot, they make seek shade or cooler areas. **Proprioception** is a general sense that allows the animal to perceive its movements and location within the environment. This system utilizes sensory neurons and the central nervous system along with stretch receptors in the skeletal muscles and joints. Feedback from these locations sends signals to let the animal understand its physical positioning and make purposeful movements.

Anatomy and Physiology for Veterinary Technicians and Nurses: A Clinical Approach, Second Edition. Lori Asprea.
© 2026 John Wiley & Sons, Inc. Published 2026 by John Wiley & Sons, Inc.
Companion website: www.wiley.com/go/asprea/anatomy_vettech2e

Special Senses

Anatomy of Taste

Taste, or the **gustatory sense**, is responsible for detecting the flavor of any substance put into the mouth. Generally, this is food, but animals ingest other substances as well, including the medications we often prescribe. Taste is a chemical sense and relies on particles from food or other ingested substances to function. The primary organs for taste are the tongue and parts of the mouth. Although these anatomical features serve other purposes, the portion that functions for this specialized sense is **taste buds**. Taste buds are found within the **papillae**, or bumps, on the tongue surface. Each papillae contains multiple taste buds, and each taste bud contains many specialized cells or modified neurons (Figure 3.1).

Anatomy of Smell

Smell, or the **olfactory sense**, is another chemical sense that allows the animal to gain information about the environment, food, other animals, etc. Smell is an extremely important sense for most animals, and they rely on this sense more heavily than the others. For example, dogs have on average over 100 million sensory receptor sites in their nose compared to only about 6 million in humans. The area of the brain called the **olfactory bulb** that processes smell is significantly larger and more developed in animals than in the human brain. In mammals, this powerful sense relies on the nose and specialized cells in the nasal cavity and sinuses, as well as a specialized organ called the **vomeronasal organ** or **Jacobson's organ**.

The anatomy of the nose, sinuses, and vomeronasal organ is critical in the sense of smell. The **nares**, or nostrils, have a central opening as well as an opening on the side of the nostril on the **alar fold** (Figure 3.2). Caudal to the nares are the nasal cavities on the left and right side which are divided by the **nasal septum**. In each nasal cavity are **nasal turbinates** or **conchae** which are a complex scrollwork of thin bone (Figure 3.3) covered by a mucous membrane made of epithelial tissue. Further caudal are similar structures called **ethmoturbinates** named such as they are turbinates close to the ethmoid bone in the skull at the back of the nasal cavity. This scrollwork pattern serves to increase the surface area of the nose while keeping it condensed to a small area. The concept of increased surface area will be discussed many times, as the anatomical design of many physical features relies on this. When thinking about this concept, think of the intestines. If you were to take the intestines out of a human and straighten them out, they would be about 20 feet of tubes, but by making them curl up on themselves and giving them lots of little folds, they can be fit into a much smaller area while still performing 20 feet worth of function. The same theory applies here to the turbinates with all of the swirls and folds. When air enters the nares, it travels through both nasal passages to the back of the nose and to the sinuses.

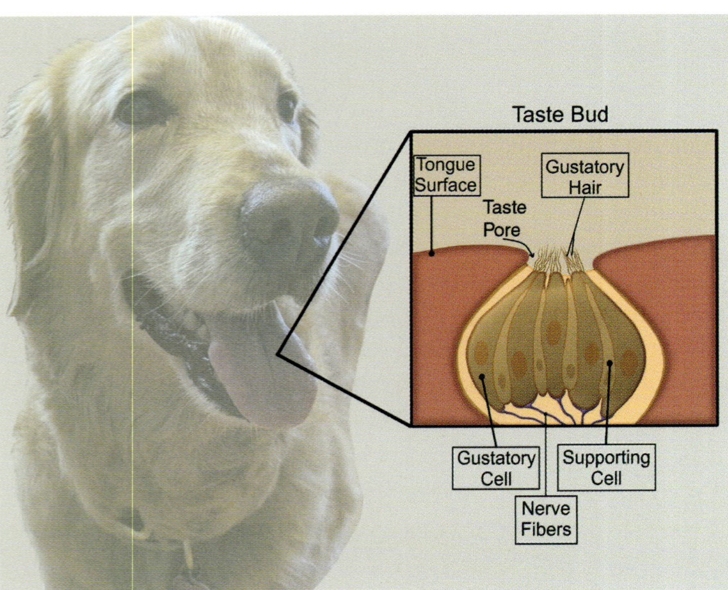

Figure 3.1 A single taste bud with gustatory cells to help perceive taste. The information collected by the gustatory cells is sent to the brain for processing. The tongue has over 1000 taste buds.

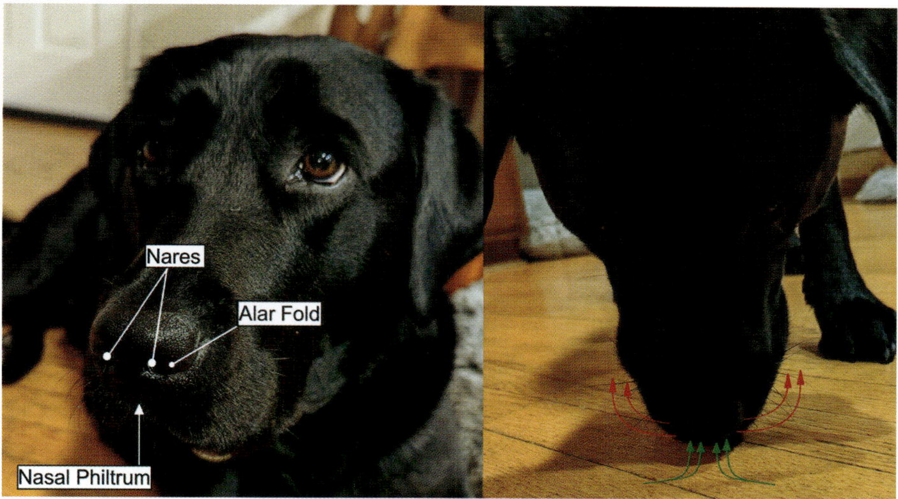

Figure 3.2 Nares and the external alar fold. Note that because of this anatomy, airflow when sniffing is not directed out the same way it came in, but rather in a cycle of in through the rostral portion of the nares and out through the lateral aspect under the alar fold.

Figure 3.3 A bisected cat skull showing the bony fold called nasal turbinates or nasal conchae. In the living animal, this bony scrollwork is covered with a highly vascularized mucous membrane.

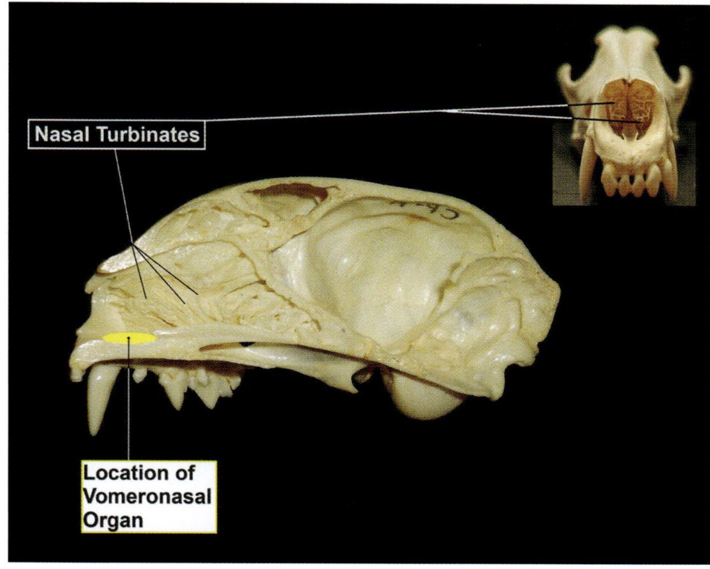

The act of sniffing is not the same act as breathing. When an animal sniffs, they intentionally move air in and out at a rapid pace in order to gain the most information about their surroundings. Anatomically, the inhaled air takes a controlled path that reduces the re-inhalation of air, and instead continues to bring new air up and into the nares to maximize function. Along with this pattern, animals use an organ that we humans do not. The **Jacobson's organ** or **vomeronasal organ** resides on both sides of the nasal passages just above the roof of the mouth in the region of the canine teeth (Figure 3.3). This highly specialized organ allows for smelling otherwise odorless chemicals like pheromones. More of the function of the olfactory system will be discussed in Chapter 16.

Anatomy of Hearing

Hearing or the **auditory sense** is a physical sense that allows sound waves to be transmitted into the ear and eventually turned into a nerve stimulus that can be sent to the brain for interpretation. The ear itself is divided into three regions: the **external** ear, the **middle ear**, and the **internal ear**. See Figure 3.4 for a diagram of the auditory anatomy.

The external ear is made of structures that collect sound waves and bring them into the middle ear. It is comprised of the **pinna**, or ear flap, the **external auditory canal**, or auditory tube, and the **tympanic membrane**, or the ear drum.

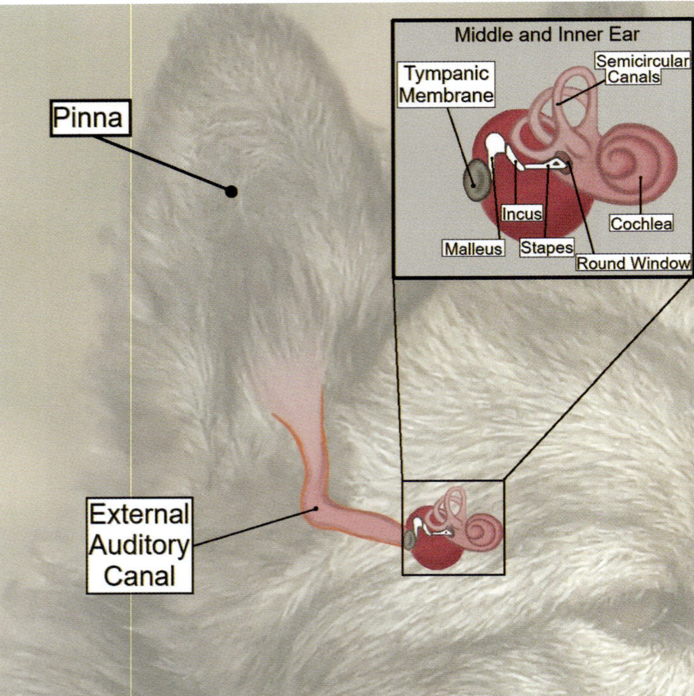

Figure 3.4 The external, middle, and inner ear. Note the placement of the ossicles to sit against the oval window. This is how vibrations from the ossicles will get translated into fluid movement within the middle and inner ear. These fluid waves will stimulate the nerves to send signals to the brain to perceive sound.

The pinna can look different on each animal due to species or breed differences. It can be positioned upright like in most cats and horses for example or be folded and down like in the Labrador Retriever. The external auditory canal is a tube that extends from the base of the pinna to the tympanic membrane. At the end of the external auditory canal lies the tympanic membrane or eardrum. The tympanic membrane is a thin sheet of tissue that separates the external and middle ear.

The middle ear is a hollow cavity that contains the **ossicles** and the **eustachian tube**. The ossicles are a series of three small bones called the **malleus, incus**, and **stapes**. The malleus is the first bone immediately behind the tympanic membrane, the incus is in the middle, and the last bone in the line is the stapes. The stapes sits against a part of the **cochlea** of the inner ear called the **oval window**. These bones are part of a system that helps translate sound waves into an audible stimulus for the brain. The eustachian tube is also found in the middle ear. This is a narrow tube that connects the hollow cavity of the middle ear to the **pharynx** or throat to help equalize pressure between the middle ear and the environment.

Deep to the middle ear is the inner ear, which has functions for hearing and equilibrium. Here we will focus on the anatomical parts that are used for hearing and move on to equilibrium next. The **cochlea** is a spiral-like cavity in the inner ear, shaped similarly to a snail shell, which has an **oval window** and a **round window** on it. The stapes from the middle ear sits against the oval window of the cochlea in the inner ear. Within the cochlea are channels of fluid and the **organ of Corti** which is the main receptor organ of hearing. The organ of Corti runs the length of the cochlea and has important components for the perception of sound. The components are **supporting cells, hair cells**, and the **tectorial membrane**. Supporting cells do as they are named and provide physical support for the hair cells. The hair cells are modified neurons that have microscopic hairlike projections that just barely touch the tectorial membrane. The tectorial membrane is a gelatinous shelf structure in the organ of Corti that helps produce sound in conjunction with the hair cells (Figure 3.5).

Anatomy of Equilibrium

Equilibrium also involves the inner ear and is a physical and mechanical sense of balance. We have discussed the cochlea in the inner ear for hearing, but also found in the inner ear are the **vestibule** and the **semicircular canals**, which control equilibrium. The vestibule is a portion of the inner ear attached to the cochlea. The semicircular canals are a set of three fluid-filled tubes that come off the vestibule at varying angles (Figure 3.4). Within the vestibule is a patch of specially modified sensory cells called the **macula**. The macula is organized somewhat similarly to the organ of Corti. It contains supporting cells and hair cells, as well as a gelatinous membrane. The gelatinous membrane of the macula has a special feature called **otoliths** which are like small stones in the gelatinous matrix. These serve to keep the gelatinous membrane weighted down so it can come into contact with the hairlike projections from the hair cells. The vestibule is responsible for the perception of linear motion (Figure 3.6).

The semicircular canals are fluid-filled tubes that sit at a right angle to one another with an area of enlargement in each tube at the end closest to the vestibule called the **ampullae**. The ampullae contains the **crista ampullaris** (Figure 3.7), another sensory organ pertaining to equilibrium. The crista ampullaris has similar anatomical structures to both the organ of Corti and the macula, featuring supporting cells, hair cells, and a gelatinous matrix called the **cupula**. Here the hair cells and their projections stick up into the cupula, which although gelatinous like in other structures, is not stationary or weighed down, but rather free floating in the liquid of the semicircular canals. The semicircular canals are responsible for the perception of rotary motion.

Anatomy of Vision

Vision allows animals to see their surroundings and the degree of precision varies among species. There are many anatomical parts related to forming the image, but only one specialized set of cells is used for detecting the image. The eyelids, **cornea, iris, retina, optic nerves**, and brain are all required to produce sight. The eyelids and eyelashes function to cover, protect, and help lubricate the eye. Lubrication comes from tears, made by the **lacrimal glands**, and a waxy product made in the **meibomian glands**. The inner side of the eyelids and the white of the eye are covered in a mucous membrane called the **conjunctiva**. There is also a "third eyelid" called the **nictitating membrane** which is found in the inner corner of the eye, or **medial canthus**. The eye itself is a globe with multiple layers, anatomical features, and different types of fluids. The eye has three tissue layers: the **fibrous layer**, the **vascular layer**, and the **nervous layer**.

The fibrous layer is the outermost layer and consists of the **cornea** and **sclera**. The cornea is the transparent window that admits light into the eye and overlays the **iris** and **lens**. The cornea is avascular, or without vessels, and is made of collagen fibers. Although there is no blood supply, there is a rich supply of pain receptors in the cornea. This means corneal injury can be extremely irritating or painful and should be addressed quickly. The other portion of the fibrous layer is the sclera, which is the "white" of the eye. This accounts for the majority of the fibrous layer and is also structured of collagen fibers (Figure 3.8).

The vascular layer, or the **uvea**, is deep to the fibrous layer and contains three main parts: the **choroid**, the **iris**, and the **ciliary body**. The choroid is pigmented and provides the retina with blood supply. In most animals, the choroid is pigmented with dark melanin, but it also forms the **tapetum lucidum** which is a highly reflective tissue that acts to help animals see in low light or dark conditions. The iris is a muscular diaphragm in the center of the front of the eye. When you

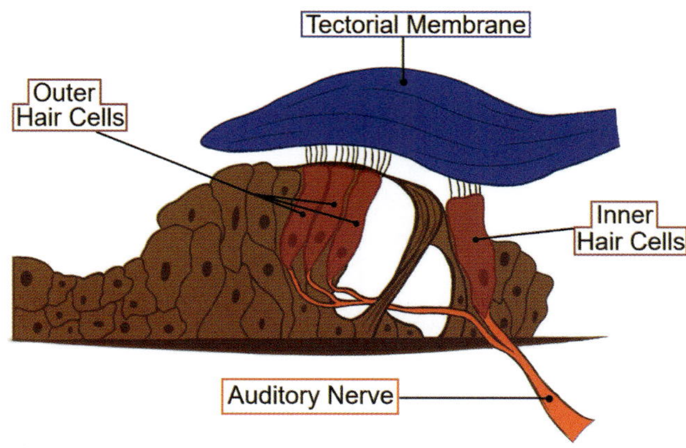

Figure 3.5 The organ of Corti. The gelatinous tectorial membrane will move when sound waves are transmitted into the ear, resulting in stimulation of the hair cells which will generate a signal to the central nervous system (CNS).

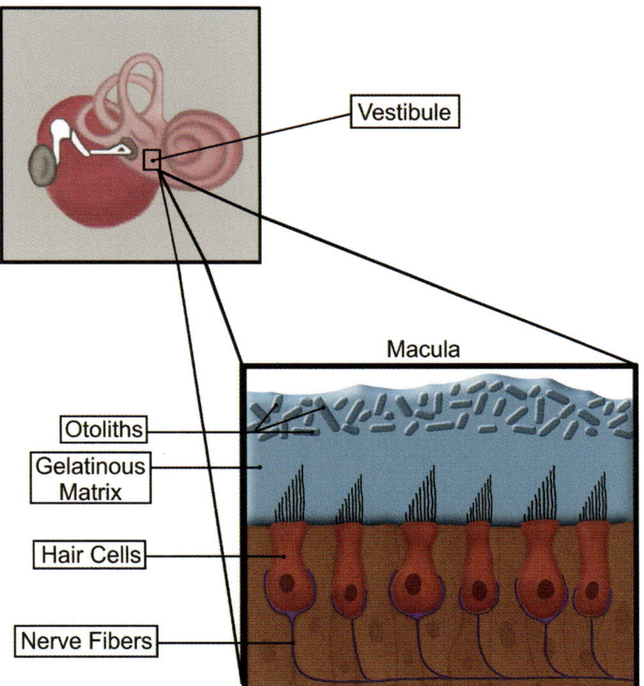

Figure 3.6 The Macula contains a gelatinous matrix similar to the tectorial membrane, but it is weighted down by small stones called otoliths.

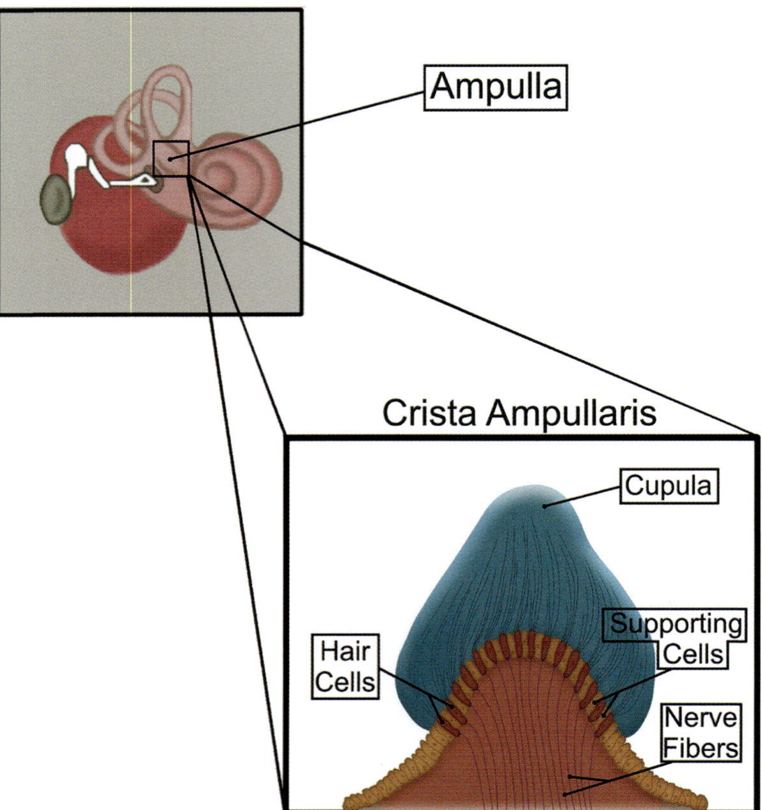

Figure 3.7 The crista ampullaris, or crista, has a gelatinous cupula that is free floating in fluid within the ampullae.

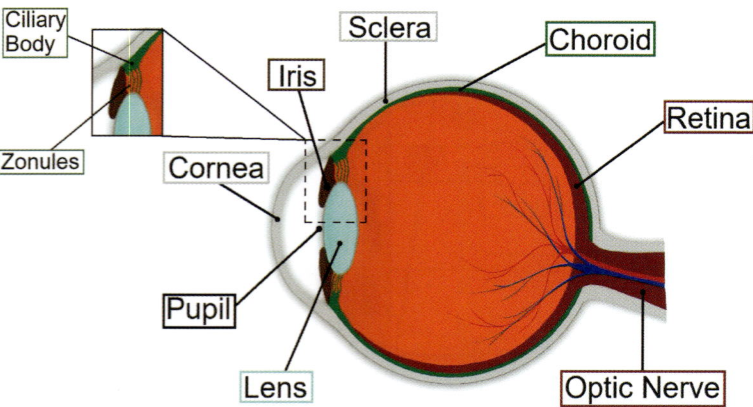

Figure 3.8 The anatomical features of the eye. The ciliary body is made of the ciliary muscles and suspensory ligaments called zonules which help to change the shape of the lens for near and far sight.

look at someone's eyes and say they are blue or brown, you are commenting on the pigments of the iris. The iris has two sets of muscles to help it open and close allowing more light or less light in, respectively. The opening at the center of the iris is the **pupil**. The ciliary body is directly behind the iris and is made of muscles, called ciliary muscles, and suspensory ligaments, called **zonules**. The ciliary muscles are attached to the zonules, which are attached to the **lens** of the eye. The lens is a round transparent structure that is elastic and biconvex (Figure 3.8).

The nervous layer of the eye is where the sensory receptors for vision are contained, called **photoreceptors**. The retina has multiple layers that all converge at the **optic disc** which leads to the **optic nerve**. The optic nerve is one of the twelve **cranial nerves** (see Appendix 2). The photoreceptors in the retina are either thin **rod-shaped** receptors or thick **cone-shaped** receptors (Figure 3.9). Rod receptors produce grey images and are light sensitive, while cone-shaped receptors are more sensitive to color and detail and do not perform well in low light. The **fundus** is also found in the retina. This is the caudal interior surface of the eye where the blood supply, retina, and optic disc can be viewed during a **fundic** examination.

Aside from the layers of the eye, there are also fluid-filled compartments within the eye that give it its distinct shape and help to nourish the tissue. The **aqueous compartment** is in the space in front of the lens of the eye. It is filled with a watery clear fluid called **aqueous humor**. The aqueous compartment can be subdivided into the **anterior chamber** of the aqueous compartment, encompassing the space in front of the iris, and the **posterior chamber** of the aqueous compartment, encompassing the space between the iris and the lens. The posterior chamber contains the **Canal of Schlemm** which is a small tube that helps to drain aqueous humor out of the eye and into the bloodstream. Caudal to the aqueous compartment is the **vitreous compartment**, which is the area behind the lens. The vitreous compartment is filled with **vitreous humor**, which is clear but gelatinous in texture (Figure 3.10).

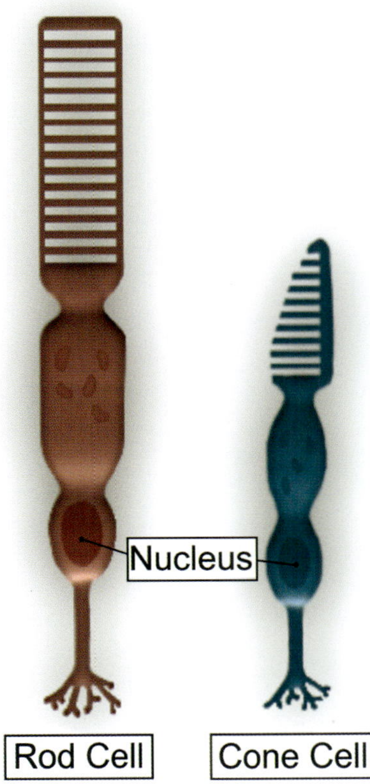

Figure 3.9 A representation of rod and cone photoreceptors from the retina. The rods help perceive grays and detail, while the cones help perceive colors.

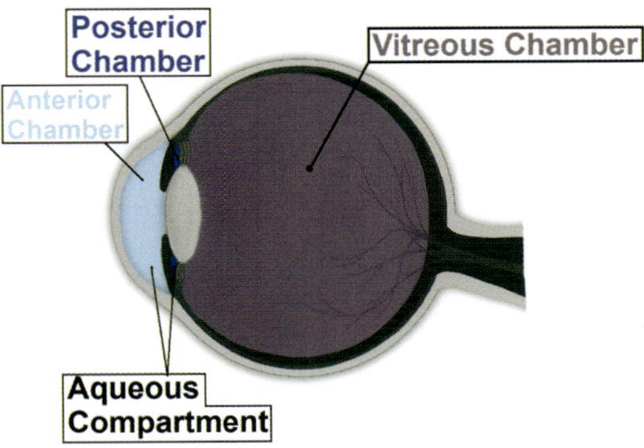

Figure 3.10 The chambers of the eye. Note that the aqueous compartment has two chambers separated by the iris.

Clinical Case Resolution: Roo

A physical exam is performed on Roo and reveals erythema and moderate ceruminous (waxy) and brown debris AS ([in the] left ear) with some small excoriations (scrapes/wounds from scratching) present. The left ear is also malodorous and sensitive to the touch. AD (the right ear) is normal with mild cerumen present. The remainder of the physical exam is normal.

It was noted that the ear was malodorous, which means the technician or doctor intentionally smelled the ear. Although we can see that the ear is irritated and full of debris, a thorough description sometimes involves more than just appearance. Ear infections caused by yeast often have a specific odor that many describe as bread-like or beer-like, while bacterial infections often have a more putrid or rotten smell.

A sample of the debris from the ear is collected on a cotton swab and prepared for microscopy. The external ear is gently cleaned, and an aural (ear) exam is performed on Roo using an otoscope. This allows visualization of the external auditory canal and tympanic membrane. Is it crucial to ascertain whether or not the tympanic membrane is intact, as it physically separates the external ear from the middle and inner ear. Roo does not have damage to her tympanic membrane.

Microscopy reveals a large number of Malassezia (a type of microscopic yeast, pictured in Figure 3.11) along with some inflammatory cells, and skin cells from the ear. This is a diagnosis of Otitis Externa, or an infection of the external ear. Roo will be prescribed the appropriate antifungal medication to put into the ear to resolve this issue.

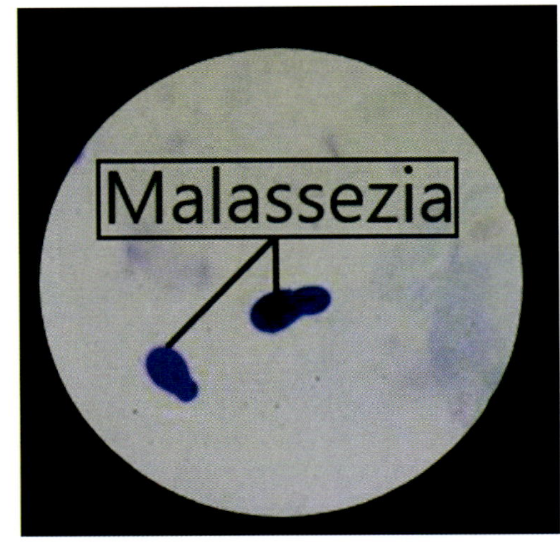

Figure 3.11 *The microscope results from an ear cytology on our patient, Roo, showing Malassezia.*

Clinical Case Critical Thinking

Use all of Roo's case details to think about the following questions.

1) *It was mentioned that an aural exam was performed with an otoscope. Why do you think it is so important to ensure the tympanic membrane is intact before moving forward?*
2) *What part of the case or plan might change if we find that the tympanic membrane is not intact?*
3) *Is there any part of the clinical case history or patient signalment (patient description) that may have predisposed her to this ear infection? Can any of these things be prevented in the future?*

Review Questions

1 Which of the following is NOT a general sense?
  A Touch
  B Temperature
  C Pain
  D Equilibrium

2 True or False: Proprioception does not involve any stretch receptors.
  A True
  B False

3 Where can the organ of Corti be found?
  A Eustachian tube
  B Ossicles
  C Cochlea
  D Tympanum

4 Which of the following is responsible for rotary motion?
  A Semicircular canals
  B Vestibule
  C Cochlea
  D Perilymph

5 An animal presents with a corneal ulcer (an injury on the cornea). What symptoms might this animal be experiencing?

6 Which portion of the eye contains pigment?
  A Ciliary body
  B Lens
  C Iris
  D Optic disc

7 The ciliary body is behind the iris and contains suspensory ligaments to the iris. These are called __________________________.

8 Which photoreceptors will produce a coarse grey image?

9 What is the specialized organ that is used to identify and perceive "odorless" chemicals like pheromones?

10 What are the names of the three ossicles?

4

Skeletal Anatomy

> **Clinical Case: Unnamed Puppy, Male Intact, 3 Days Old**
>
> *A newborn puppy is brought into the hospital. He has been having difficulty nursing and seems to have milk running out of his nose right after a meal. He sometimes coughs while nursing. The remainder of the litter appears thriftier and has no issues latching or feeding.*

Introduction

The study of the skeleton is the study of the framework of the animal's body. Some animals have an **exoskeleton**, where the structural framework is the outermost layer, while some have an **endoskeleton**, where the structural framework lies internally. **Invertebrates**, or animals without a backbone or spinal column, such as insects, may have an external skeleton. **Vertebrates**, or animals with a backbone, can also have a variety of skeletal structures; for example, the skeleton of the dogfish shark is mostly cartilage rather than bone.

This discussion will concentrate on vertebrates, specifically mammalian skeletons, which are mostly composed of bones. While there are small interspecies differences, the general features are the same.

Vocabulary

There are some important terms that are used in skeletal anatomy across a variety of bones. These are some, but not all, of the more common terms you may see.

Crest – a long, narrow ridge or line, often where muscles or connective tissue are connected.
Eminence – a small projection or bump of bone.
Foramen – an opening or hole that typically allows for blood supply, nerves, or other structures to pass through.
Fossa – a depression, hollow, or dip in the bone.
Fovea – a small indent or pit generally found on the end of the bone.
Meatus – a short canal or channel that opens to another part of the body.
Process – a large projection or bump of bone.
Spine – a sharp, slender projection of the bone.
Tubercle or Tuberosity – a projection or bump with a roughened surface.

Bone Categories

Bones can be categorized by a physical description and are broken down into the following groups: **long bones, short bones, flat bones, irregular bones**, and **sesamoid bones** (Figure 4.1).

Anatomy and Physiology for Veterinary Technicians and Nurses: A Clinical Approach, Second Edition. Lori Asprea.
© 2026 John Wiley & Sons, Inc. Published 2026 by John Wiley & Sons, Inc.
Companion website: www.wiley.com/go/asprea/anatomy_vettech2e

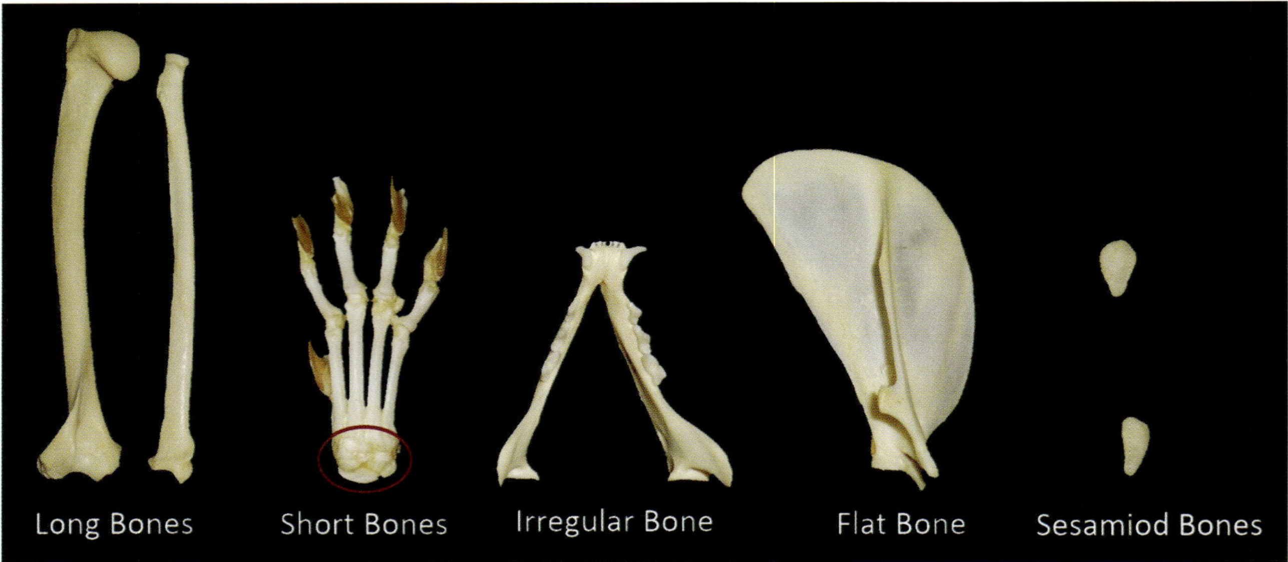

Figure 4.1 Types of bones. The sesamoid bones shown here are the patellae, which are located in the patellar tendon. The short bones are a circle in the carpus of the thoracic paw (shown intact above it).

Long bones have cylindrical bodies, with a round or plateau-like end. The term long bone refers to the shape of the bone, not necessarily the size. These bones are longer than they are wide. The rounded area at the proximal end is referred to as the **head**, and at the distal end is generally referred to as a **condyle**. Condyles usually come in pairs and are generally described as medial or lateral. It is clear that it is not sufficient to say "the lateral condyle," as that can refer to a number of locations. It is always necessary to reference the landmark to the specific bone, as in "the lateral condyle of the humerus." It is also worth noting that not all bones adhere to this rule, as the proximal end of the tibia has a medial and lateral condyle rather than a head (see Figures 4.2 and 4.8).

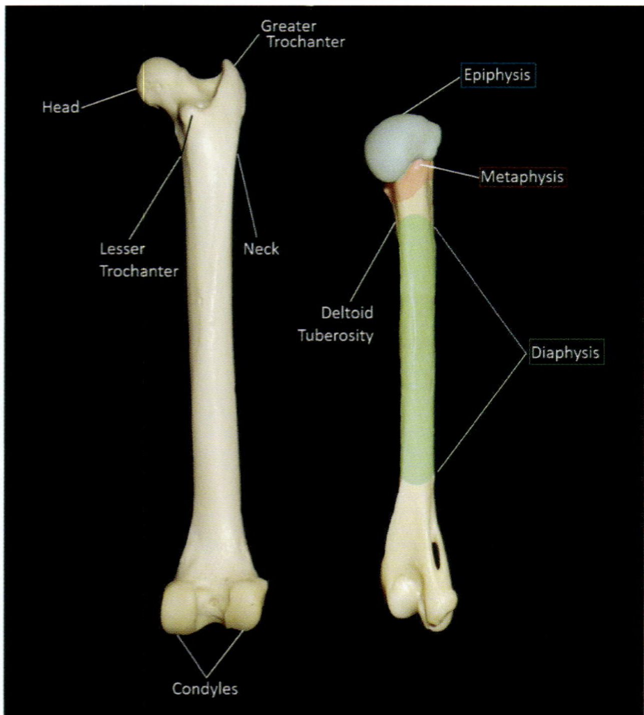

Figure 4.2 Features of long bones. The femur is on the left and the humerus on the right.

The shaft of the bone is referred to as the **diaphysis**. The proximal and distal surfaces are referred to as the **epiphysis**. The relatively short area between the epiphysis and the diaphysis of the bone is the **metaphysis**. These different areas have distinct growth patterns. In fact, there is a cartilaginous plate that separates the metaphysis from the epiphysis, which is known as the physis or **epiphyseal plate**. This plate **ossifies**, or becomes bony, as the animal ages.

The superficial diaphysis and metaphysis are covered by a fibrous tissue called **periosteum**. This covering contains blood vessels and nerve fibers. The vessels enter a pinpoint opening into the diaphysis called a **nutrient foramen**. The diaphysis has an interior tunnel that runs through it called a **medullary cavity**, which houses the **bone marrow**. The lining of the medullary cavity is called the **endosteum**, which is similar to the periosteum in that it is a layer of tissue with blood vessels.

Short bones are bones that are shorter than they are wide or equal in length to their width and are often cuboidal in shape. Short bones are confined to very distinct areas in the body, particularly the carpus and tarsus (Figure 4.1).

Flat bones, unlike short and long bones, are a bit of a misnomer. Flat bones are not necessarily cylindrical in nature, earning their name, but are not dimensionally flat. They are often thin and curved bones, for example, many bones that make up the skull are considered flat bones. They are often used as protection for organs and serve as attachment points for muscles.

Irregular bones are bones with no easily defined shape (i.e., not long or short or flat). These bones tend to have complex shapes with many projections, like the **vertebrae** in the spinal column.

Sesamoid bones are small, rounded bones that earn their name from their sesame seed-like appearance. Do not be fooled into thinking that sesamoid bones are minuscule, though, they are relative to the size of the animal. A sesamoid bone in a horse is larger than a cat's entire paw.

The Skeleton

Now that we are familiar with the categories of bone, we can approach the skeleton as a whole. The skeleton is traditionally divided into two parts: the **axial skeleton** and the **appendicular skeleton**. The axial skeleton is considered to be the skull and vertebral column, including the caudal (tail) vertebrae. Some experts also consider the ribs and sternum to be part of the axial skeleton. Everything else, the thoracic and pelvic limbs, is considered the appendicular skeleton. All the bones of the skeleton are grown and maintained by special cells and hormones, which is discussed in Chapter 17.

The Appendicular Skeleton

The Thoracic Limb

The thoracic limb, or forelimb, is made up of the **scapula, humerus, radius, ulna, carpus, metacarpals, and phalanges**. Conventionally, the scapula, or shoulder blade, is considered to be a part of the limb because it is connected via the shoulder joint to the leg. The scapula forms the **scapulohumeral joint**, or shoulder, in association with the humerus. The scapula is considered a flat bone as it is not cylindrical or irregular but does have some additional geometry. The lateral surface of the scapula has a long, thin projection called the **spine of the scapula** (see Figure 4.3). It should be palpable on examination of the living animal. The shallow depressions dorsal and ventral to the spine of the scapula are the **supraspinous** and **infraspinous fossae**, respectively. The ventral-most part of the spine of the scapula is a process called the **acromion**, which is important as a muscle attachment. The fossa on the distal end of the scapula, into which the head of the humerus fits, is called the **glenoid fossa**. A species-specific process exists, called the **suprahamate** process, and it protrudes ventrally off the spine of the scapula. It is only present in felines and rabbits. It is noteworthy that the scapula in cats and dogs is not directly attached to the rest of the skeleton; the only thing that holds it in place is muscle. Among other things, it means that it is easier to amputate the thoracic than the pelvic limb (such as in cases of malignancy), as no bony connections need to be severed.

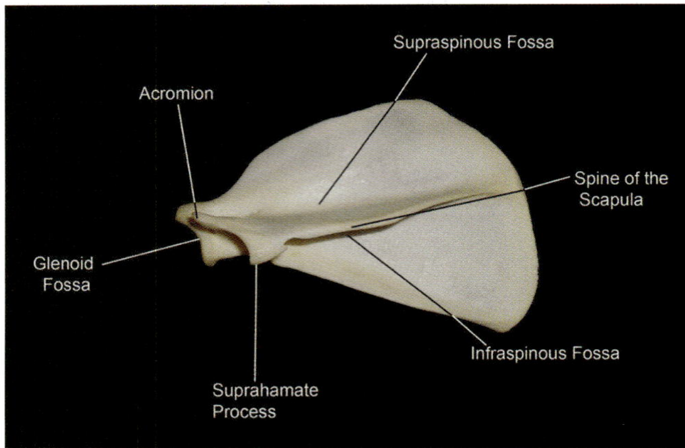

Figure 4.3 Landmarks of the scapula.

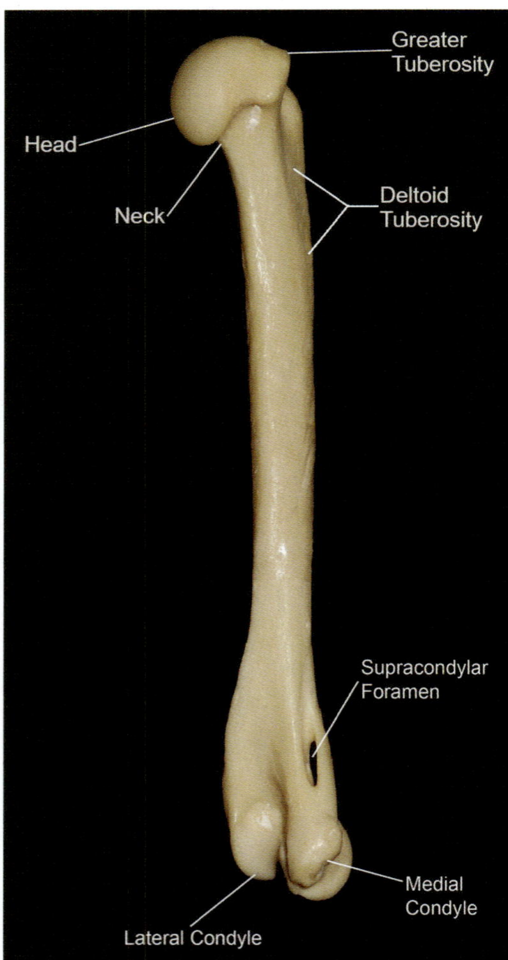

Figure 4.4 The humerus. Note that cats have a foramen to the medial side of the bone, called the supracondylar foramen, as pictured here; in dogs, this opening is in the center, between the condyles. It is called the supratrochlear foramen.

Immediately distal to the scapula is a long bone called the **humerus**. The proximal end of the humerus has the **head of the humerus**, which is a distinctly rounded end and is paired with the **greater tuberosity** and then narrows at the **neck** at its proximal boundary. The humerus has a structure called the **deltoid tuberosity** on its medial surface, which is the attachment for the deltoid muscle. The distal humerus has two condyles, a **lateral condyle** and a **medial condyle**. In dogs, there is a **trochlear foramen** between the condyles. In cats, the equivalent is the **supracondylar foramen**, which is on the medial surface of the bone and proximal to the condyles rather than between them (Figure 4.4).

The humerus meets up with two long bones – the **radius** and **ulna** – at a joint that is referred to as the **radiohumeral joint** and is commonly called the elbow. The radius crosses over the cranial surface of the ulna from the medial to the lateral side, where the ulna is situated so that it points slightly medially. The proximal ulna has a number of specific features of importance (see Figure 4.5). The **olecranon** is the part that projects caudally (or caudodorsally, depending on the position of the limb) and is clearly palpable when examining the limb during an office visit. Going distally, there is a C-shaped structure called the **trochlear notch**. The proximal tip of it is called the **coronoid process**, and the distal tip is called the **anconeal process**. This notch is where the distal end of the humerus fits into the joint. At the very distal end of the medial ulna is a bony projection called the **styloid process of the ulna**. The **head of the radius** has a plateau shape with a central dip at the very proximal end called the **articular fovea**. At the distal end, like the ulna, is the **styloid process of the radius** (Figure 4.5).

Distal to the elbow, radius, and ulna is the **carpus**, which is made of a series of seven short bones called the **carpal bones**. The two most proximal bones of the carpus are named the **radial bone** and the **ulnar bone**, as the radius and ulna meet these bones in the joint, respectively. Distal to the carpal bones is a series of long bones called the **metacarpus**, made of **metacarpal bones**. There is one metacarpal bone for each digit. It is important to note that the metacarpals, and for that matter the digits, are numbered from the medial to the lateral side. In other words, the lateral-most digit (the pinky) in the dog and cat is number 5. The dewclaw, which does not normally come in contact with the ground, is number one and is counted regardless of if it is present or not (Figure 4.6).

Caudal to the metacarpals are the **metacarpophalangeal joints**, which are the joints between the metacarpal bones and the proximal phalangeal bones. Within these joints are small sesamoid bones, which help reduce tension on the tendons and ligaments of the paw. The **phalanges**, or digits, are made of three bones per digit in dogs and cats (usually only two in the dewclaw). The bones of the digits are

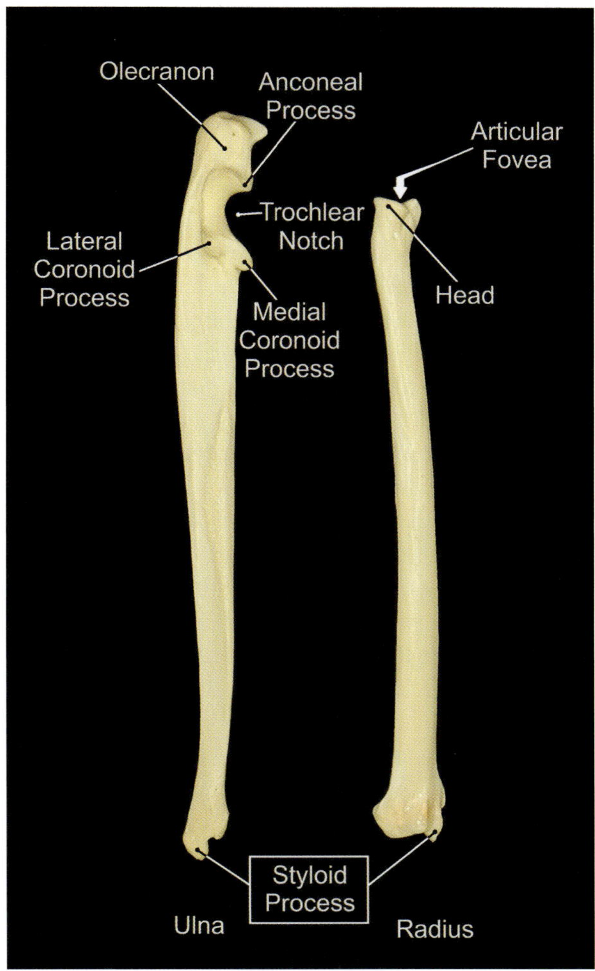

Figure 4.5 The radius and ulna. In normal anatomy, these two bones sit snugly together and slightly cross over one another.

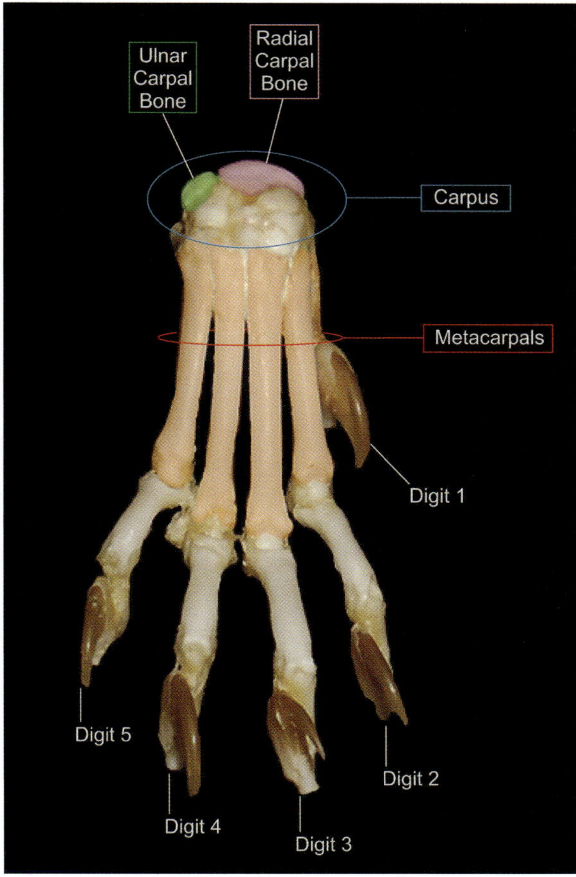

Figure 4.6 The carpal bones, metacarpals, and the thoracic limb paw, or the manus. The digits of the paw are counted from medial to lateral using numbers 1–5. Number 1 is the dewclaw and is counted even when not present, such as in the hind limb, making the lateral-most toe always digit 5.

called the **proximal phalanges, middle phalanges**, and **distal phalanges**. These can also be referred to as in the singular **phalanx** (i.e., the middle phalanx) or, more frequently in clinical practice, abbreviated as **P1, P2**, and **P3**, where P1 is the proximal phalanx, P2 is the middle phalanx, and P3 is the distal phalanx. The distal part of P3 has a shallow fossa with a collar referred to as the **ungual crest**. It is here that the claw attaches to the digit (Figure 4.6).

The Pelvic Limb

Unlike the thoracic limb, the joint where the pelvic limb connects to the body does, in turn, connect to the rest of the skeleton. As a result, the pelvic limb is considered to begin at the proximal-most long bone, which is the **femur**. The pelvic limb is also comprised of the **patella, tibia, fibula, tarsus, metatarsals**, and **phalanges**. The femur is the longest bone in the dog and cat skeleton. The proximal end is distinguished by a large bulbous head, which fits into the **coxofemoral** (hip) joint. It also has a prominent feature called the **greater trochanter** on the lateral surface of the proximal end, which should be readily palpable on physical examination of the living animal. There is also a flattened area on the proximal end of the bone called the **patellar surface**. The distal end of the femur has a **lateral condyle**, a **medial condyle**, and an **intercondylar fossa** between the two (Figure 4.7).

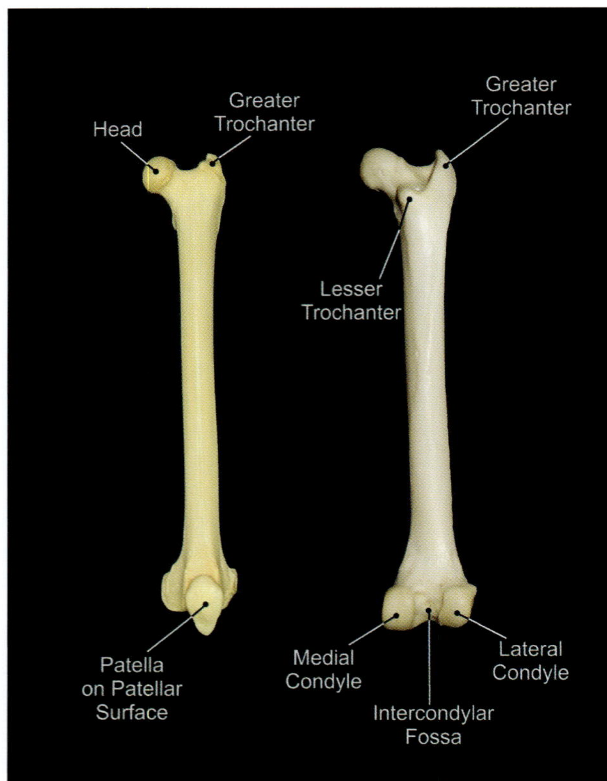

Figure 4.7 Features of the femur in two views.

The joint that is between the femur and the next most distal bone is the **stifle joint**; although the joint is properly called the **femorotibial joint**, the term stifle is universally used. It is incorrect to refer to this joint as the knee, as the knee in equines is actually the common name for the carpus, and confusion could easily result. The stifle joint has a sesamoid bone called the **patella** or kneecap. This is the largest sesamoid bone in the body and is encapsulated in soft tissue in life. It sits on the patellar surface of the femur on the proximal end and ends in the joint toward the next series of long bones, the **tibia** and **fibula**.

The **tibia** and **fibula** are the long bones distal to the stifle (Figure 4.8). The tibia has a plateau or flattened proximal end that has a **medial condyle** and a **lateral condyle**. In between the two condyles is a peak called the **intercondylar eminence**. On its cranial surface, it has a projection called the **tibial tuberosity**. These landmarks are important in discussing surgery of the stifle joint, particularly involving cruciate ligament disorders. At the distal end of the tibia is the **medial malleolus**, which meets the tarsal joint. The **fibula** is a thin, long bone that runs parallel to the tibia with a small nondescript **head** at the proximal end and a **lateral malleolus** at the distal end, paired with the medial malleolus of the tibia. In equines and ruminants, this bone is actually fused to the tibia and is incomplete in its length. In dogs and cats, it ends along with the tibia at the next joint, the **tarsus**.

The tarsus is made of a series of short and irregular bones, two of which are of note: **the talus**, which is rounded, and the other is **the calcaneus**, which is rectangular. The calcaneus is particularly important as the distal attachment for the **gastrocnemius muscle**, called the **calcanean tendon**; in humans, this is known as the Achilles tendon. Distal to the tarsus are the **metatarsal bones**, which are an analog of the metacarpal bones discussed above. Distal to the metatarsals are the phalanges, each containing three bones per digit, with the exception of the dewclaw, which is generally absent in the pelvic limb of the feline (Figure 4.9).

The Pelvis

The **pelvis** is known as the **os coxae**, and although it appears to be one large bone, it is actually composed of three flat bones that are fused during fetal development (Figure 4.10). The pelvis is considered part of the appendicular skeleton.

The cranial-most section is known as the **ilium**. The cranial part of the ilium sweeps dorsally and is called the **wing of the ilium**. A dorsocranial section of the wing is called the **iliac crest** and is important as an area from which we take bone marrow samples in dogs. In cats, the bone is too thin, and the head of the humerus is used more often for this.

The **ischium** is the section caudal and ventral to the ilium. It is a relatively short section but is important because it accommodates a fossa known as the **acetabulum** (Figure 4.11). This area is where the head of the femur sits, forming the coxofemoral joint. Fracture of the ischium, therefore, is often associated with hip joint problems. It should be noted that the acetabulum contains overlapping sections of the ilium, ischium, and pubis. Abnormalities of the acetabulum or of the head of the femur are part of hip dysplasia, which is a common orthopedic problem in large-breed dogs.

The caudal part of the pelvis is the **pubic bone** or **pubis**. The pubis and the ischium together make up the borders of the **obturator foramen**, a large opening that is an important landmark.

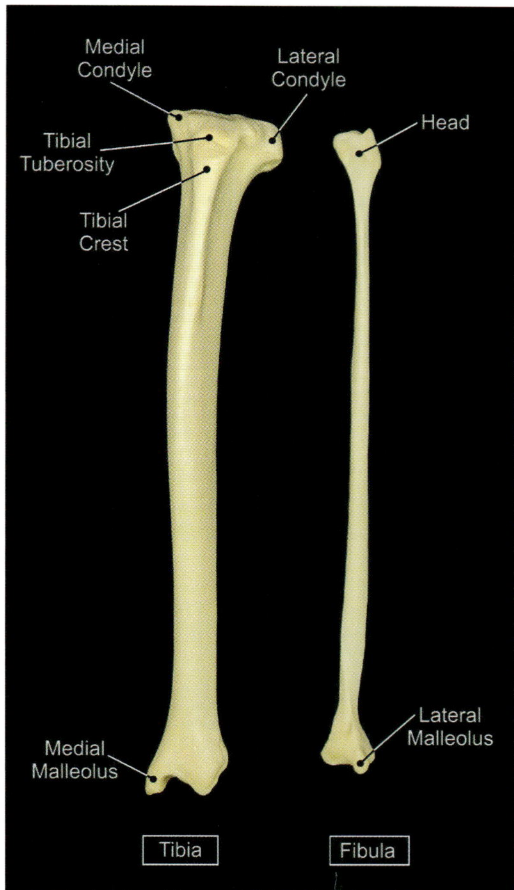

Figure 4.8 The tibia and fibula. In the living animal, these two bones are aligned tightly together with the fibula on the lateral aspect.

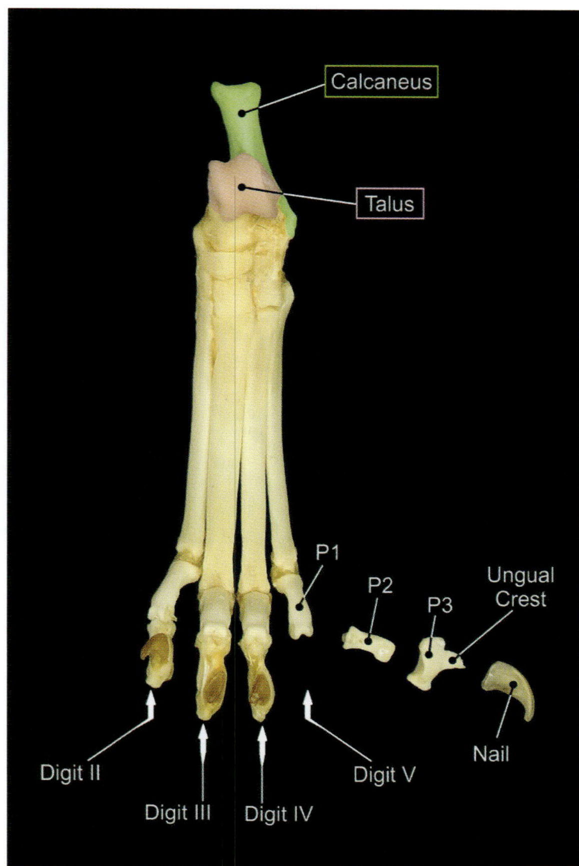

Figure 4.9 The bones of the tarsus and pelvic limb paw, or the pes. Each phalange is broken down into three bones: the proximal phalanx (P1), the middle phalanx (P2), and the distal phalanx (P3). The nail is seated on the ungual crest.

Figure 4.10 The bones of the pelvis.

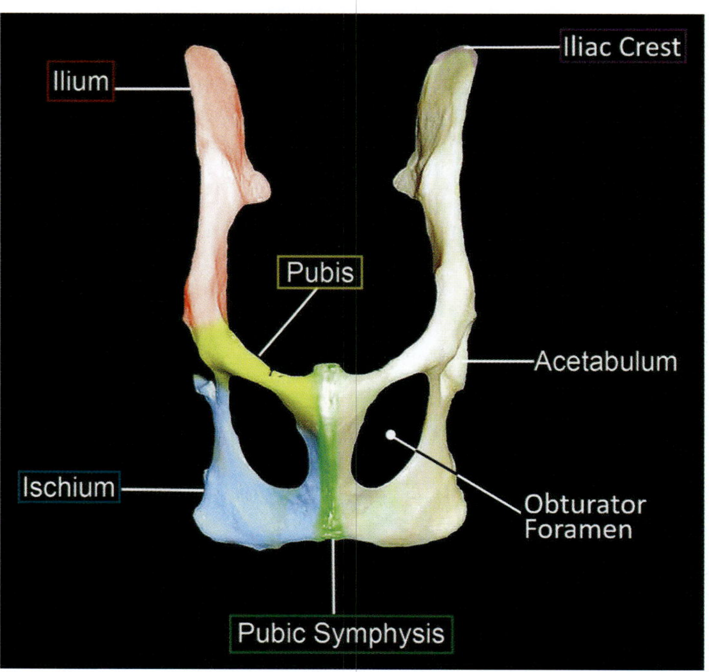

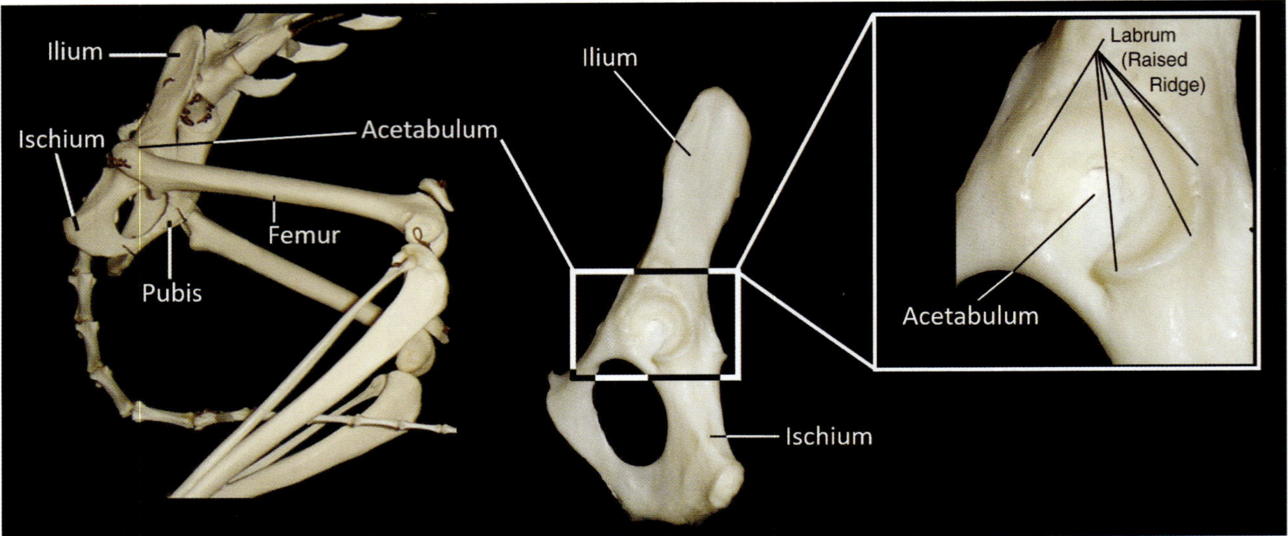

Figure 4.11 View of the pelvis with acetabulum magnified to reveal the labrum.

The Axial Skeleton

The Skull

The skull is composed mostly of flat bones. The cranium is the part of the skull that contains the brain. Most of the bones on the skull are paired, meaning there is one of each bone for the left and the right side that usually fuse together with visible joint lines called **sutures** to become one solid structure during fetal development. Occasionally, when the dorsal plates of the skull have not completely come together at birth, there is a small spot on the dorsal cranium that is left with no bony covering. This is called a **fontanel**. It should close shortly after birth. It can allow significant damage to the brain by traumatic injury if it remains open.

The jaw is composed of a single bone on each side ventrally, called the **mandible**. These two sides are joined together at the center rostral-most point called the **mandibular symphysis**. The mandible has a dorsoventral projection at its caudal end called the **ramus of the mandible**, and it is the only part of the mandible that does not have teeth. The mandible also has notable foramina called **mental foramen** on the lateral distal aspect (Figure 4.12). The dorsal jaw is made of two paired bones that fuse together during development but is generally referred to by one name, the **maxilla**. Technically, the maxilla is the part that encompasses the lateral surface of the dorsal jaw. The rostral point of the upper (maxillary) jaw is composed of a small bone called the **incisive bone**, which holds the small teeth known as incisors.

The bone that is deep to the soft tissue that forms the roof of the mouth is the **palatine bone**. It too is composed of two bones from the left and the right sides that meet at the midline during fetal development. If these bones do not meet, the animal is born with a gap in the roof of the mouth, and milk or other ingested material can travel up into the nasal cavity and out the nose. This gap is referred to as a **cleft palate** and can usually be remediated surgically.

The dorsal-most part of the cranium is referred to as the **parietal bones**. Ventral and lateral to the parietal bone are the **temporal bones**. Caudal to the parietal bone are the **occipital bone** and **occipital crest**, and rostral to it are the **frontal bones** (Figure 4.13).

On the rostrum are the **zygomatic arches**, the **nasal bones**, and **incisive bones**, as well as the **lacrimal bones**. The zygomatic arch is the bone ventral to the eye socket or orbit; in humans, it is called the cheekbone. Technically, the zygomatic arch is made from the zygomatic bone (which forms the rostral part of the arch) and a part of the temporal bone projecting to become its caudal section. The nasal bone consists of small bones on either side of the nasal passage. The lacrimal bones are small bones forming the ventromedial surface of the orbit. All these bones are paired. The **nasal septum** is the wall that divides the nasal passages into right and left. The bone at the caudal nasal passages is called the **ethmoid bone**. It forms the rostral wall of the skull.

Figure 4.12 The mandible with mandibular symphysis highlighted. The mandibular symphysis is where the left and the right sides of the mandible are joined.

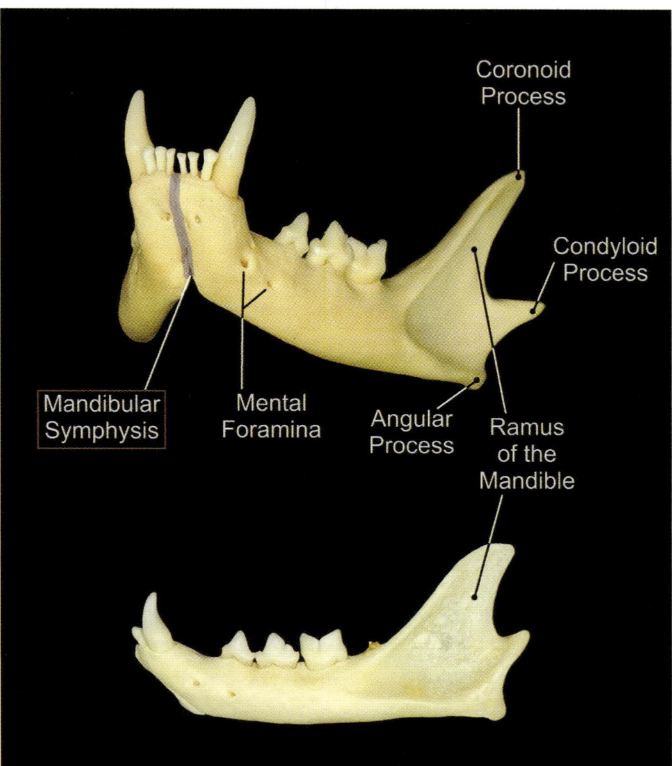

Figure 4.13 The bones of the lateral view of the skull as seen on a feline.

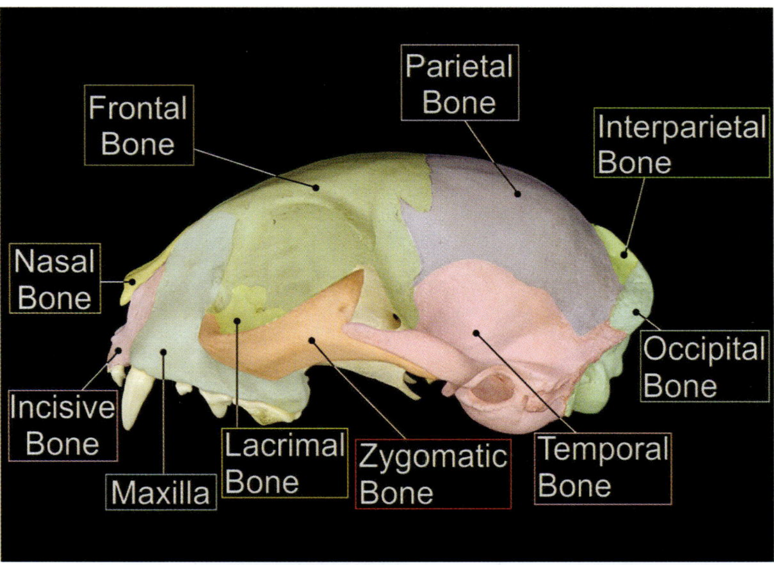

Note that the rostral part of the septum is cartilage, and only the caudal part is composed of bone. It is for this reason that a nose will appear incomplete when looking at a skull. The cartilaginous part does not survive the process of preserving the bone. The lateral orbit in dogs and cats also is not completely bony. There is a small area, which appears as a gap in the preserved skull, whereas in the living animal there is a ligament. This is in contrast to equines, which do have a completely bony orbit.

The temporal bone has a feature of interest called **tympanic bulla**. It is a cuplike ventral projection on either side of the skull that houses the middle part of the ear. It should be full of air, with the exception of three tiny bones called **ossicles**, which are an important part of the process of hearing. The ossicles are the smallest bones in the body of dogs and cats (and humans). The opening into the bulla is at the medial border called the **external auditory meatus** (Figure 4.14). As with

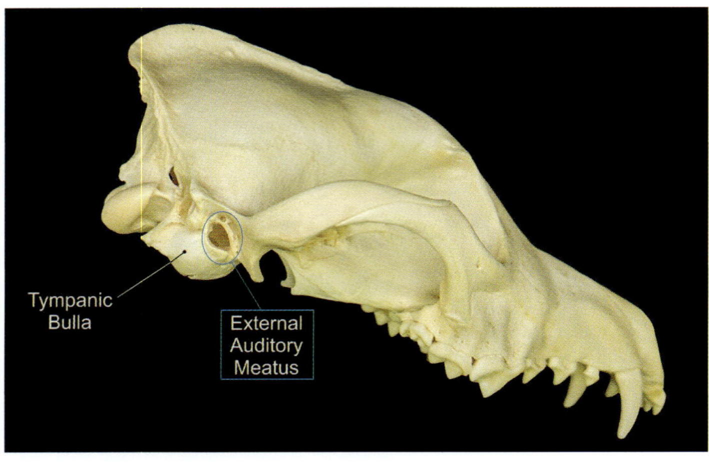

Figure 4.14 The external auditory meatus on the canine skull.

the nasal septum, the ear canal is mainly cartilaginous. The ear canal is composed of bone only in its medial portion; the area from its entrance is composed of cartilage.

On the ventral surface of the cranium is the **palatine bone**, which forms the upper border of the oral cavity or the "hard palate." Cleft palate is the condition mentioned earlier where the two plates that form this bone do not meet. This is a condition that can be genetic or caused by abnormal growth prior to birth. It can cause severe problems with eating and breathing. The **choanae** are openings seen on the ventral skull that serve as openings for the pathway of air through the respiratory tract from the nose and into the **pharynx** or throat. Choanae should not be confused with **nasal conchae** or **turbinates**, which are fine bony scrollwork in the nasal passages, visible from a rostral or bisected view. The **sphenoid** is another bone visible on the ventral skull, important in supporting the braincase (Figure 4.15).

A caudal view of the skull reveals the **occipital bone**. Here there are two bony projections called the **occipital condyles**, which are an important site for muscle attachment and lie on either side of the large central opening known as the **foramen magnum**. The foramen magnum is the opening for the spinal cord to enter the skull and meet the brainstem. Slightly rostral to this, there are two prominences known as the **jugular foramen** where the jugular veins exit (see Figures 4.15 and 4.16).

It should be noted that certain breeds of dogs and cats have a "flat" appearance to the face. These animals are referred to as **brachycephalic**, referring to the arch from which the planes of the face form during fetal development (see Figure 4.17). Bulldogs and Persian cats are brachycephalic. As a result of the short nasal and oral cavities, among other things, these animals are at greater risk for respiratory problems when under sedation, and special measures are usually undertaken to afford them more oxygen.

On the other hand, a cat or dog with a very long muzzle is said to be **dolichocephalic**. The Siamese cat and Borzoi are good examples of these animals. Animals with a medium-length snout are referred to as **mesocephalic**; this includes the tabby cat and the beagle.

The Ribs and Sternum

The ribs are a series of flat bones that attach to the spinal column and descend ventrally. The distal part of the rib is composed of cartilage. In an animal with a normal body condition, the ribs should not be easily visible but should be readily palpable. The ribcage is made of rib bones and **costal cartilage**. Where the rib bones and cartilage meet is known as the **costochondral joint** (Figure 4.18).

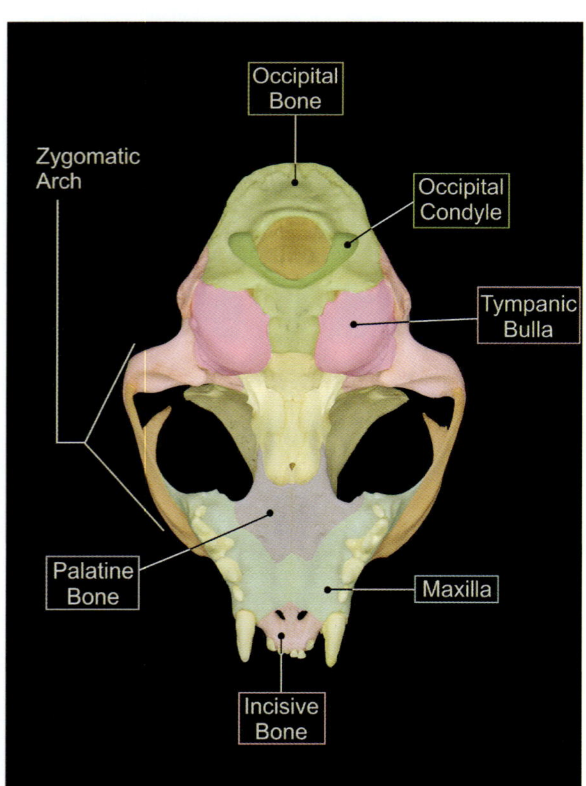

Figure 4.15 The bones of the ventral view of the skull as seen on a feline.

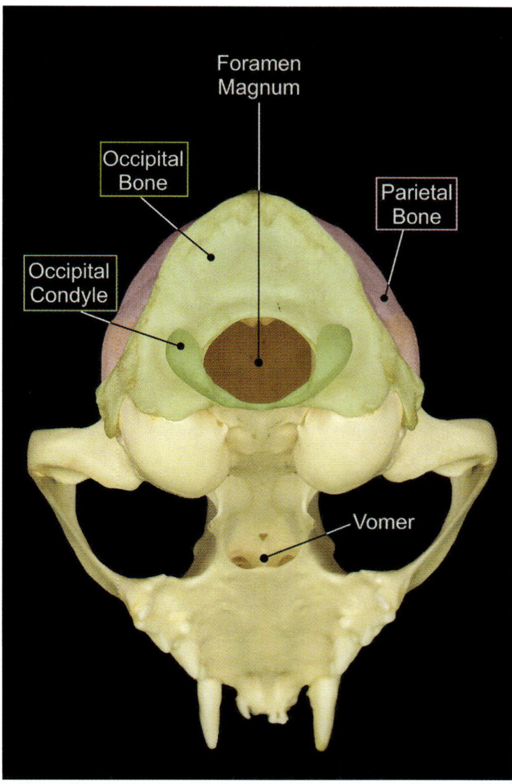

Figure 4.16   A caudal view of the skull showing the foramen magnum where the spinal cord enters to meet the brainstem.

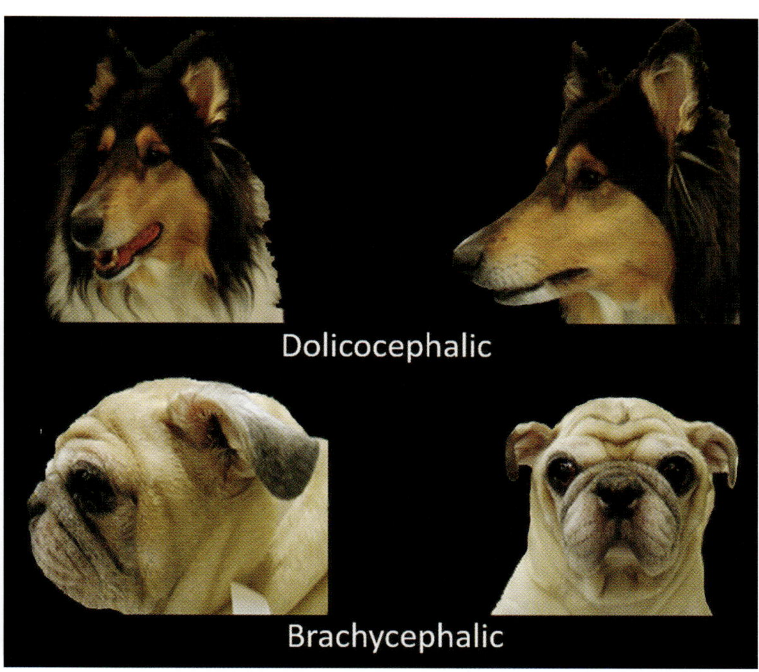

Figure 4.17   The shape of the skull has an effect on everything from how the animal's teeth look to how they breathe; a brachycephalic dog has a much shorter nasal passage and oral cavity and can have respiratory problems severe enough to require surgical correction of those structures.

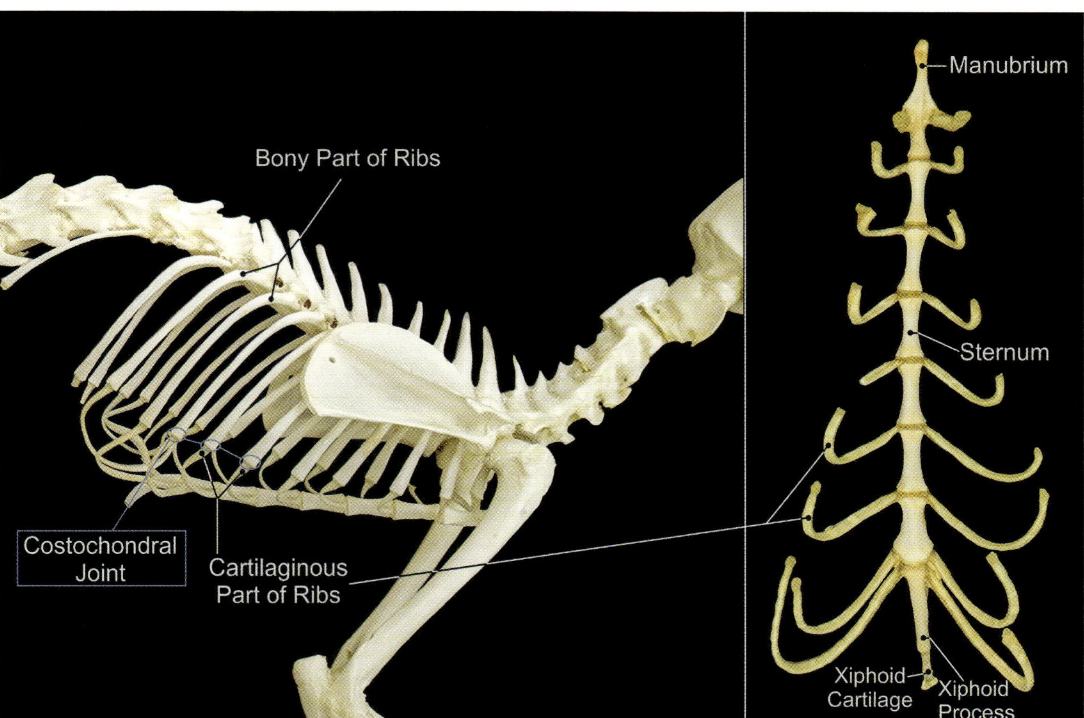

Figure 4.18   The ribcage with a subset of the sternum. Note the preservation of the ribcage cartilage yields misshapen rib cartilage. In life, these would all line up perfectly with their matching rib and form the costochondral joint.

The **sternebrae**, or bones of the **sternum**, are irregular bones that run along the ventral surface of the thorax. The cranial-most point of the sternum is called the **manubrium**, and the caudal-most the **xiphoid**. This last is an important landmark as most abdominal surgeries have an instruction to prepare the surgical area in some relation to the xiphoid. Note that in primates, the sternum is a single piece of bone.

The Vertebrae

The **vertebrae** are a series of irregular bones which make up the spinal column (see Figures 4.18 and 4.19). Note that the word spine can refer to a number of things: a feature of some bones like the scapula and vertebrae, the long, thick bundle of nerves known as the spinal cord, or the series of vertebrae that make up the **spinal column**. When referring to the chain of vertebrae, the spinal column is the most correct term.

The vertebrae are divided into five main sections: **the cervical vertebrae** in the neck area, **thoracic vertebrae** dorsal to the thoracic cavity, **lumbar vertebrae** dorsal to the abdominal cavity, **sacral vertebrae** dorsal to the pelvis, and **caudal vertebrae** representing the tail. In cats and dogs, there are 7 cervical vertebrae, 13 thoracic vertebrae, 7 lumbar vertebrae, 3 sacral vertebrae, and a variable number of caudal vertebrae. A good piece of trivia is that the giraffe has the same number of cervical vertebrae as the dog; they are just larger in scale. In fact, all mammals except the manatee and her relatives have seven cervical vertebrae.

The vertebrae are known only by capital letter and number with three exceptions, which have actual names. Other vertebrae are labeled by their section of the vertebral column and their position along the chain. For example, the atlas is also known as C1, indicating that it is the first cervical vertebra. A radiographic report may indicate that there is a fracture at T3, meaning the third thoracic vertebra or an injury spanning from T10–L1 or from the tenth thoracic vertebra to the first lumbar vertebra.

Most vertebrae, with the exception of a few special bones, have the same anatomical features but look different from one to the next. These anatomical features are the **spinous process, transverse process, articular process, lamina, body**, and **vertebral foramen** (Figure 4.20). The **spinous process** is a bony projection on the dorsal aspect of each vertebra and can be very pronounced, as seen in the thoracic vertebrae, or more subtle, as seen in the lumbar vertebrae. The **transverse process** is another bony projection but can be found on the lateral aspects of the vertebrae. Similar to the spinous process, its appearance can differ depending on which vertebra one is observing. It can be prominent, as seen in the lumbar

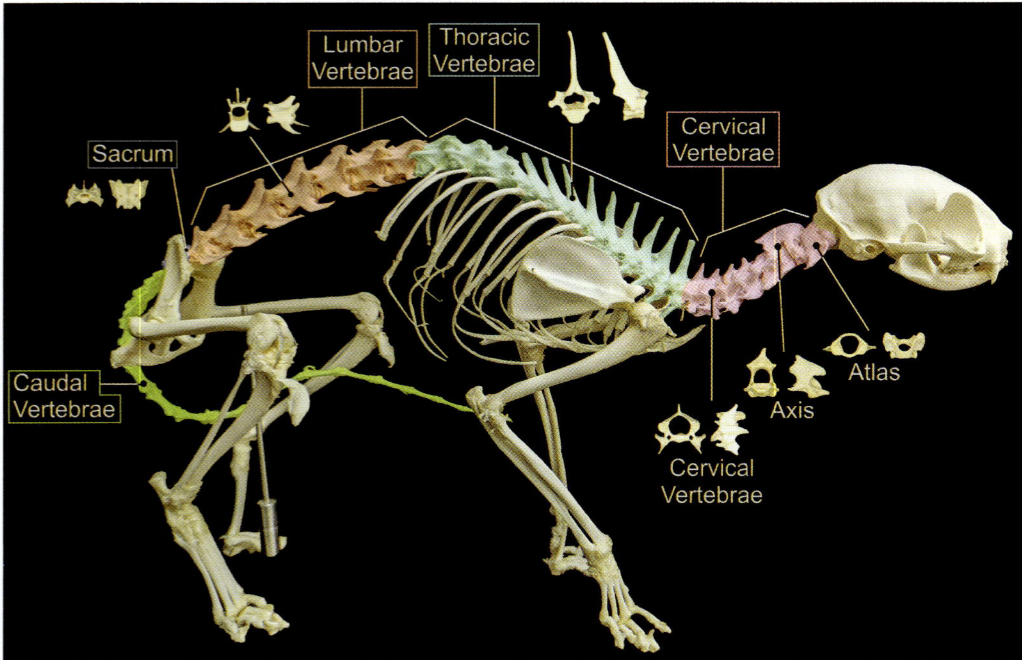

Figure 4.19 The vertebrae as viewed on the whole animal as well as lateral and caudal views of each category. Note the first two vertebrae, atlas and axis, are strikingly different than the rest.

Figure 4.20 The parts of the vertebrae. Each vertebrae contains a spinous process, lamina, vertebral foramen, transverse process, and body, however different types of vertebrae have more pronounced or subtle projections. Pictured above is a cervical vertebra.

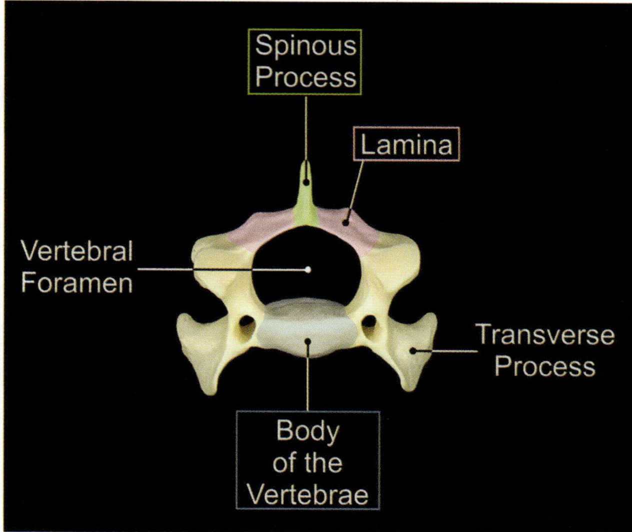

vertebrae, or more subtle, as seen in the thoracic vertebrae. The **articular processes** are slightly flattened areas where one bone of the vertebral column meets the next, forming a joint. The **vertebral foramen** is a hole that runs through each vertebra, which accommodates the tissue of the spinal cord. The roof of this opening is formed by the **lamina** at the dorsal aspect and the **body of the vertebrae** at the ventral aspect.

The Named Vertebrae

The cranial-most vertebra is known as the **atlas,** named for the mythical man who held up the world, just as the atlas helps support the skull. The bone directly caudal to the atlas is the **axis**. The other named vertebra, **the anticlinal vertebra**, will be discussed in a moment.

The atlas has two lateral projections called **the wings of the atlas**. The axis has a small projection that sits in the vertebral foramen of the atlas called the **dens** (Figure 4.21). Abnormality of this structure, particularly if it is absent or foreshortened, is associated with a neurologically based difficulty with ambulation. The axis also has a large dorsal projection called the **spinous process**, which is present on most vertebrae but absent on the atlas. The remainder of the **cervical vertebrae** have small to moderate spinous and transverse processes with a somewhat flattened ventral body.

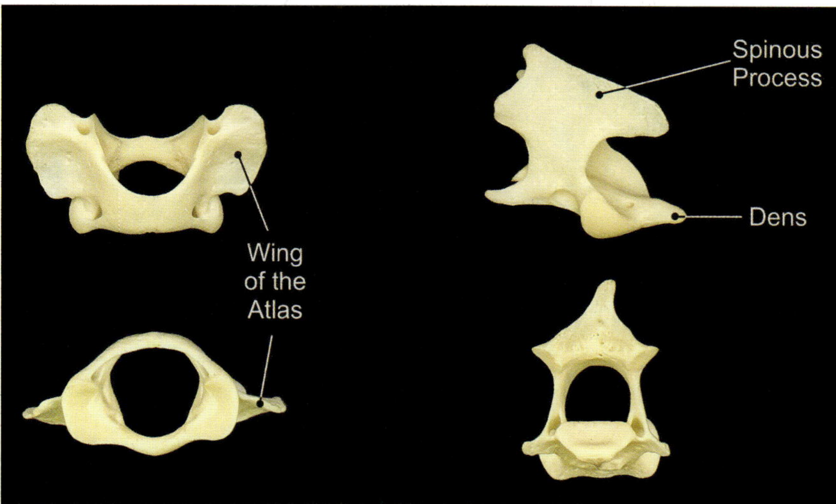

Figure 4.21 The atlas, or cervical vertebrae 1 (C1), and the axis, or cervical vertebrae 2 (C2). The atlas is the cranial-most of the vertebrae, followed by the axis. One way to remember it is that, just as "t" comes before "x," the atlas comes before the axis. Note the dens, which is congenitally absent in some dogs.

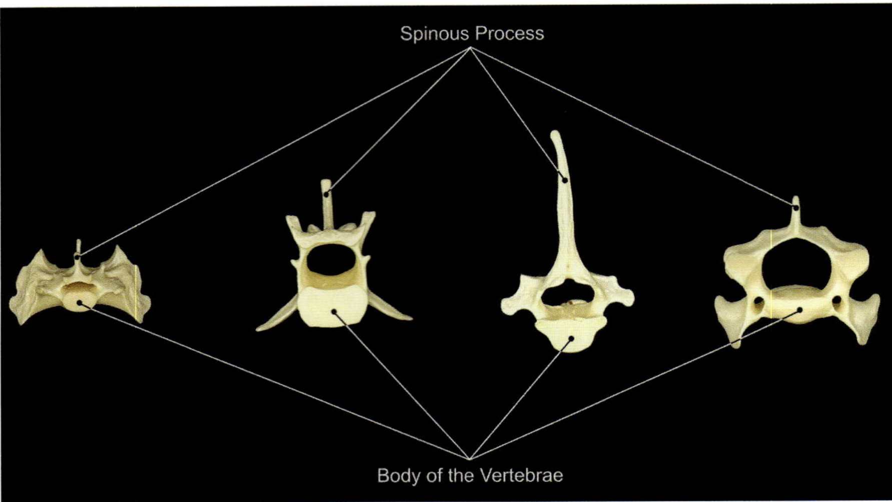

Figure 4.22   A comparison of the anatomical features of each type of vertebrae.

The **thoracic vertebrae** are distinguished by their large spinous processes. It is in the thoracic spinal column that the anticlinal vertebra is found. It will be noted that the spinous processes of the thoracic vertebrae point caudally, up until the anticlinal vertebra in most dogs and cats. At the anticlinal vertebra, the somewhat smaller spinous process points cranially. It is, therefore, called the anticlinal vertebra as it inclines in the opposite direction, and it is important because it is a good landmark when looking at radiographs. The anticlinal vertebra is usually T11 in most dogs and cats but can be T10 in some smaller dogs. The ventral body of the thoracic vertebrae is more pronounced and rounded than that of the cervical and lumbar vertebrae (Figure 4.22).

The **lumbar vertebrae** have short spinous processes. They do, however, have long transverse processes, which have the appearance of wings, making them easy to identify.

The **sacral vertebrae** in dogs and cats are fused together and are referred to collectively as the **sacrum**. There are three bones that have no space between them and have both very short spinous and transverse processes.

The **caudal vertebrae** make up the tail of the animal. Most "tail-less" animals actually have at least one or two caudal vertebrae. As dogs and cats have tails of different lengths, there is a variable number of caudal vertebrae in most species and in different breeds of each species.

Equines

There are a few notes about the skeletal features of equines that are important (see Figure 4.23). There is only one digit on each leg, which results in an altered anatomy than previously discussed. It is fascinating that an animal weighing around or even more than 500 kg depends on one digit on each leg.

The thoracic limb of the equine is analogous to the canine and feline until the level of the carpus. Anatomically, the pelvis and femur remain similar to that of the cat and dog, aside from being significantly larger and with some more prominent areas. The tibia is similar, but the fibula, as discussed earlier, is significantly smaller and often fused to the tibia. The distal end of the tibia meets the tarsal joint. Distal to the carpus or tarsus in each limb is a single metacarpal/metatarsal bone. This is metacarpal/metatarsal bone number three and is referred to as the **cannon bone** in common terms. There are vestigial remnants of the second and third metacarpal/metatarsals, which are short, thin projections on either side of the proximal metacarpal/metatarsal. These are commonly referred to as the **"splints," or splint bones** in common terms.

The three bones of the single phalange are still named the proximal, middle, and third phalanx (P1, P2, and P3) but can also go by common names. The proximal phalanx is commonly called the **long pastern**, the middle phalanx is commonly called the **short pastern**, and the distal phalanx is commonly called the **coffin bone**. The coffin bone is encased in the hoof. Repeated stress on the limb (or other causes, such as nutritional issues) can cause laminitis or inflammation of the layers of the hoof. The swelling can be associated with a change in the angle of the coffin bone to the point where it actually tilts straight down. Basically, the horse is standing on the point of the "toe." As might be imagined, this is extremely painful and can be very difficult to treat.

In the horse, a particularly important sesamoid bone is the **navicular bone**, which sits just caudally to P3. It serves an important function in relation to tendons and ligaments in the area. As such, it can cause severe problems if the area is inflamed.

Bovines

In contrast to equines, each bovine limb has two digits (see Figure 4.24). The space between the digits is known as the **interdigital cleft**. In the living animal, there is a cutaneous gland that produces a pheromone in that area.

Bird Bones

Avians have a special bone structure (see Figure 4.25). Unlike the popular conception, bird bones are not hollow. However, they are **pneumatized**, except for the skull; that is, they have many hollowed-out areas, like the recesses of a sponge. This decreases the overall weight of the animal, assisting its ability to fly. Some of the concave areas are connected to the air sacs, which do the job of pulling air into the body. As a result of this, bone fractures can also cause respiratory complications.

The entire avian structure is adapted to flight, which causes a multitude of skeletal changes from the aforementioned mammalian skeletons. Some of the vertebrae are fused together to support flight, and the caudal vertebrae are called the **pygostyle**, which is used for tailfeather attachment. In non-flighted birds, the sternum is flattened, whereas in flighted birds, it is more pronounced forming a **keel**. Birds do not have a typical "thoracic limb" but instead, a wing. The shoulder is formed to support flight via the **pectoral girdle**, which is made of three bones: **the scapulae, furcula**, or **the clavicle** (some might know this as the wishbone), and **the coracoid bone**. These attach to the humerus which leads to the radius and ulna, then to a fused **carpometacarpus**, then phalanges. In the legs, the femur is similar to previously discussed; however, the tibia and fibula are fused to create the **tibiotarsus**, which is followed by another fusion of bones called the **tarsometatarsus**, then phalanges.

The Bone That Isn't

In humans, the clavicle is a bone that connects the sternum to the scapula. In cats, the clavicle is vestigial, a small, thin, sticklike structure that serves no particular purpose. It is important to know about, as it might appear to be a bone chip when viewing a radiograph. Note that there are species, such as rabbits, rodents, and birds as mentioned above, that do have a clavicle.

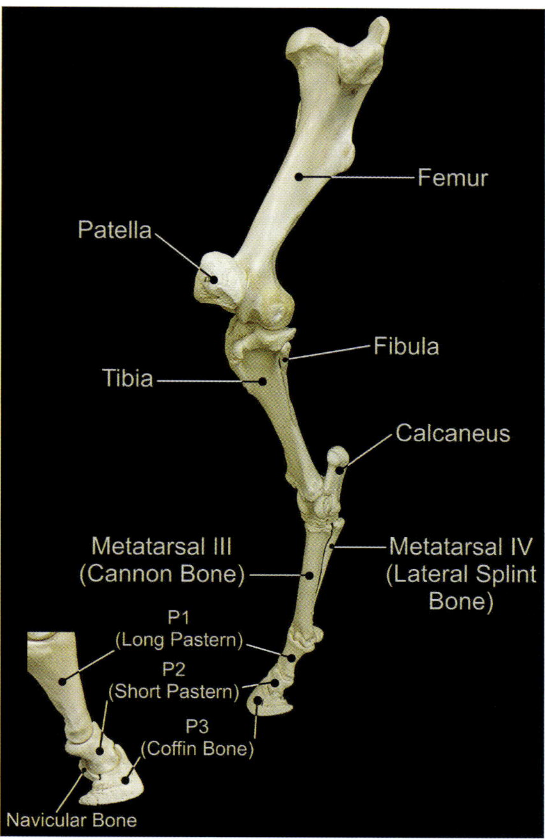

Figure 4.23 The equine lower limb. The caudal-most bone, distal to the navicular, is phalanx 3, also known as the coffin bone. The short bone proximal to it is the short pastern, and the one proximal to it is the long pastern. The navicular bone has an important role to play in joint movement.

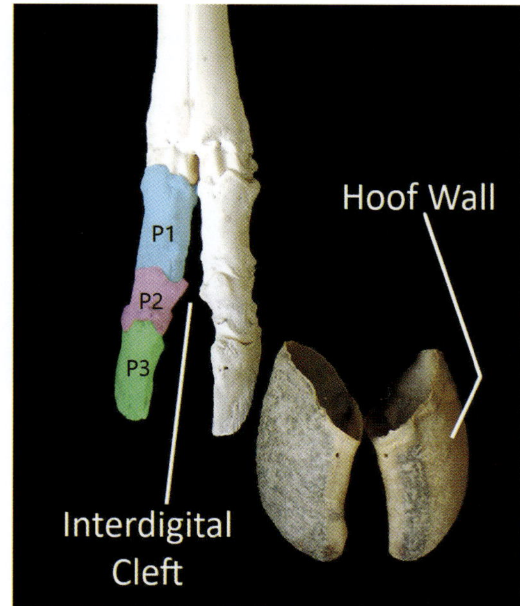

Figure 4.24 The bovine limb has two digits, each with the same three phalangeal bones as the dog and cat. The hoof is also in two parts, joined at the interdigital cleft. The wall of the hoof is indicated.

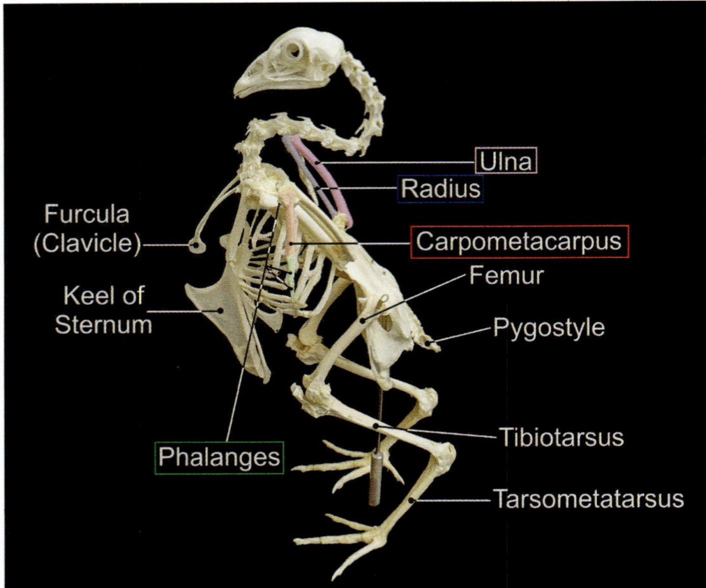

Figure 4.25 The avian skeleton. Note the fused bones as well as the prominent sternum (keel) present, which serves as an attachment point for the powerful pectoral muscles needed for flight.

Clinical Case: Unnamed Puppy, 3 Days Old

Examination of the puppy's oral cavity revealed that the plates of the maxillary and palatine bones never came together in the appropriate suture joints to form the hard palate (Figure 4.26). The space between them allows food to travel up into the nasal cavity. Food can thus either come out of the nose or up into the airway, causing coughing or sneezing. This can cause food to be aspirated into the lungs, which can cause severe respiratory disease. This problem was readily fixed surgically, and the puppy developed normally thereafter

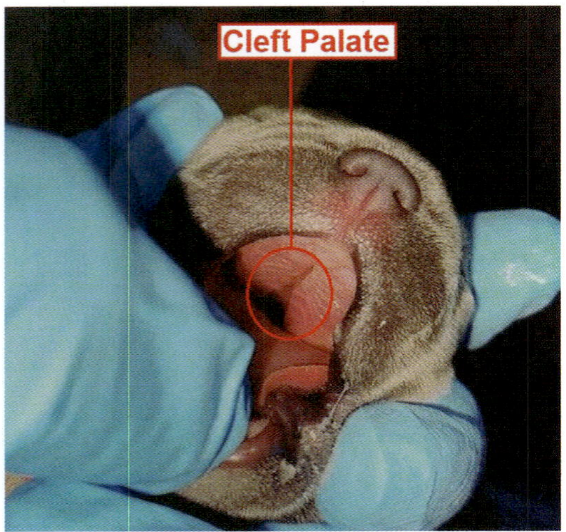

Figure 4.26 *The view inside the mouth of the puppy. Notice that the distal most area shows the failure of the palatine bones to form, resulting in a cleft palate.*

Review Questions

1 What category of bone is a vertebra?
   A Flat bone
   B Long bone
   C Irregular bone
   D Short bone

2 What is the proper name of the shaft of a long bone?

3 Where would you find short bones in the feline skeleton?
   A The vertebral column
   B The knee
   C The tail
   D The tarsus
   E All of the above

4 What is the tissue covering the outside of the bone?

5 How many phalangeal bones are there in each digit?

6 What is the common name for the third metatarsal in the equine?
   A Splint bone
   B Cannon bone
   C Hock
   D Stifle

7 What is the name of the cranial-most vertebra?
   A Atlas
   B Axis
   C Anticlinal vertebra
   D Sacrum

8 What type of bone is the patella?
   A Long bone
   B Short bone
   C Irregular bone
   D Sesamoid bone

9 How many digits can be found on each bovine foot?

10 Which of the following belong uniquely to the avian species?
   A The cannon bone
   B The interdigital cleft
   C The tarsometatarsus
   D The splint bone

5

Joint Anatomy

> **Clinical Case: Turtle, a 7-Year-Old Male Neutered Domestic Short Hair Cat**
>
> *Turtle is presented to the emergency room after the owners found him on the ground outside of their apartment building last night. The owners live on the fourth floor and the only way Turtle could have gotten down is falling out of the window. The owners report they were cleaning and left the window and screen open. As per the owner, Turtle seemed fine except he will not eat his food and has been drooling excessively since they found him. It appears as though he cannot completely close his mouth.*

Introduction

The study of joints is called arthrology. Joints are junctions between distinct bones or other tissue. They are an articulation, a point where things intersect. In the limbs, these connections allow certain types of movement. In other parts of the body, a joint may be a remnant of an embryonic structure or may delineate a border.

Movement

There are many different types of joint movement. We use terms to describe these movements. Some of the more common terms are as follows:

Abduction – Movement away from the midline of the body.
Adduction – Movement toward the midline of the body.
Circumduction – Movement of the appendage in a circular manner from a stationary axis point.
Extension – A bending movement that increases the angle of the joint (Figure 5.1).
Flexion – A bending movement that decreases the angle of the joint (Figure 5.1).

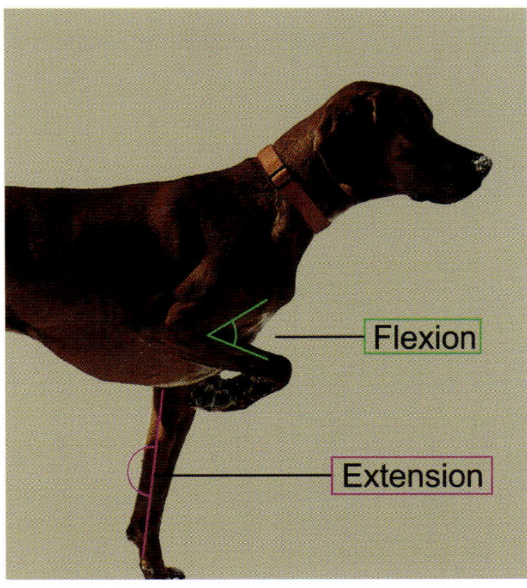

Figure 5.1 A canine in a point position showing both flexion and extension of the front limbs.

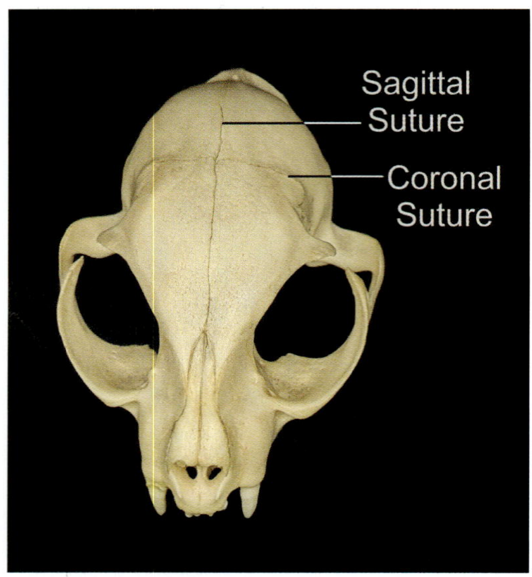

Figure 5.2 The named suture joints of the skull.

Joint Types

Along with terms used to describe movement, there are also terms to describe the type of joint. There are three main categories of joints in the body: **fibrous joints**, **cartilaginous joints**, and **synovial joints**.

Fibrous Joints

Fibrous joints are the least mobile of all the joints. We traditionally think of joints as being something very moveable, but remember a joint is just a term used to describe where bones and soft tissue are meeting together. Fibrous joints are made of very dense collagen connective tissue and can be further broken down into three types: **suture joints**, **syndesmosis joints**, and **gomphosis joints**.

Sutures are joints that are fibrous and completely immovable. These joints describe where two bones are fused together. This is seen in the skull, where many bony plates come together through suture joints to form a unified skull. The sutures on the skull are visible to the naked eye, and many of these joints are visible between the bony plates. There are two landmark sutures on the skull called the **coronal suture** and the **sagittal suture** (Figure 5.2). The coronal suture is a transverse joint that runs across the whole skull from right to left, in between the left and right frontal bones and the left and right parietal bones. The sagittal suture runs down the length of the skull from rostral to caudal and divides the left from the right.

Syndesmosis is another type of fibrous joint that is very slightly moveable. These joints are between two adjacent bones that become connected with a strong fibrous membrane. This can be seen between the radius and ulna in the antebrachium (Figure 5.3). These two long bones are joined together along their length with a syndesmosis. It allows for the radius and ulna to move as one with stability but still maintains some ability for the two bones to move slightly around one another and their surrounding joints.

The **gomphosis** joint is the third type of fibrous joint where the root of a tooth is attached to its bony socket (Figure 5.3). This joint allows for a small amount of movement, as the teeth must be able to ever so slightly move within the mouth to prevent damage.

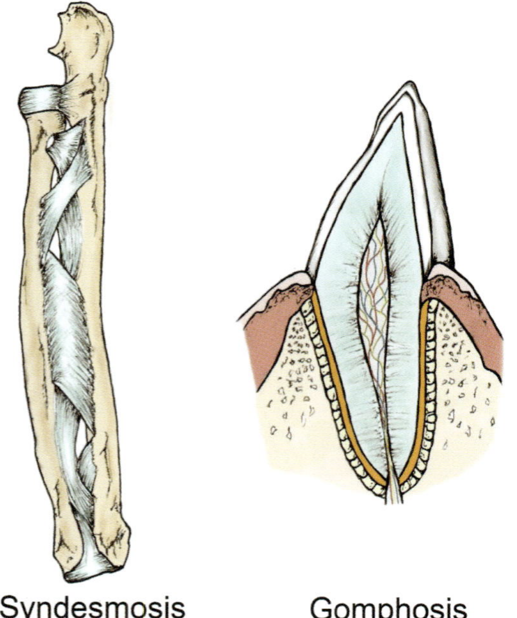

Figure 5.3 The syndesmosis joint between the radius and ulna of the forelimb and the gomphosis joint between the tooth and jaw.

Cartilaginous Joints

Cartilaginous joints are comprised mostly of cartilage. There are three main types of cartilage in the body: **hyaline cartilage**, **fibrocartilage**, and **elastic cartilage**. Hyaline cartilage is the most common cartilage in the body, comprised of collagen, and can be found lining joints, supporting soft tissue structures, and at the ends of bones forming joints, where it is called **articular cartilage**. Fibrocartilage is a dense connective tissue that is the strongest type of cartilage in the body and the least flexible of the three. It is used in holding joints together, cushioning from impact and supporting muscles, ligaments, and tendons in the body. Elastic cartilage is, as it sounds, flexible. It is used to provide shape and structure but can be easily bent and bounce back to its original shape. A good example of elastic cartilage is the pinna.

Cartilaginous joints utilize both hyaline cartilage and fibrocartilage. There are two types of cartilaginous joints to discuss. The first is the **primary cartilaginous joint**, also known as **synchondrosis**. This is a stable and unmovable joint made of hyaline cartilage and is found between **ossification centers** where bones are growing. This area of cartilage is referred to as the **growth plate** and will eventually **ossify or** become hard and bony. The next type of cartilaginous joint is the **secondary cartilaginous joint**, also known as a **symphysis**. A symphysis uses hyaline cartilage and fibrocartilage and is usually found joining bones at the midline. These joints have more movement than other joints described so far, but it is still limited. Symphysis joints can be found in a number of places, for example, in the mandible at the mandibular symphysis, in the pelvis at the pubic symphysis, and in between each of the vertebrae as intervertebral discs (Figure 5.4).

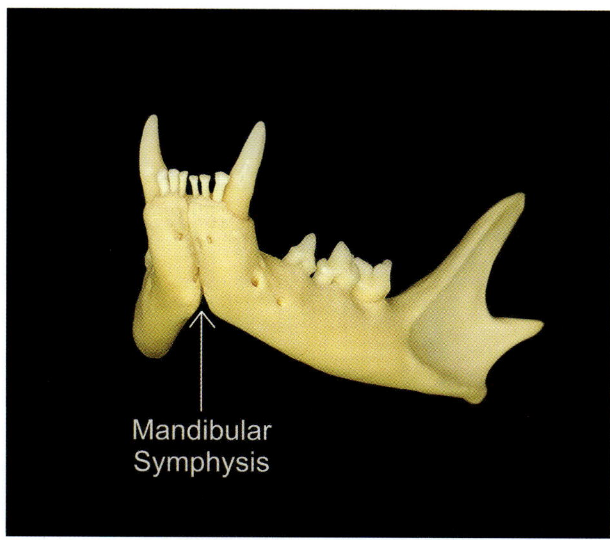

Figure 5.4 The mandibular symphysis, an example of a symphysis joint.

Synovial Joints

Where a primary cartilaginous joint is called synchondrosis, a synovial joint is also known as diarthrosis. A synovial joint exists between two or more adjoining bones and contains many different components. These are the most mobile of joints and may be what people traditionally think of when they hear the word joint. All synovial joints contain the following three features: **synovial cavity, joint capsule,** and **articular cartilage** (Figure 5.5). The synovial cavity is the space surrounding the bones in the joint and is filled with **synovial fluid**. The joint capsule is the fibrous capsule around the joint that is continuous with the periosteum. To understand what we mean when we say continuous, consider the following: If you paint an entire room white, including the ceiling and floors, it creates a layer of paint covering every surface. The paint doesn't stop even though it goes from the wall to the ceiling—it is continuous. Similarly, the joint capsule is continuous with the periosteum of the adjoining bones. The periosteum is the outermost layer of bone. This means that the joint capsule is fused, or one, with the periosteum, creating a layer of tissue that changes but remains connected in one sheet from the periosteum of the proximal bone, becoming the joint capsule, then joining back into the periosteum of the distal bone(s). The articular cartilage, as discussed earlier, is a hyaline cartilage that covers the ends of the bones in the joint.

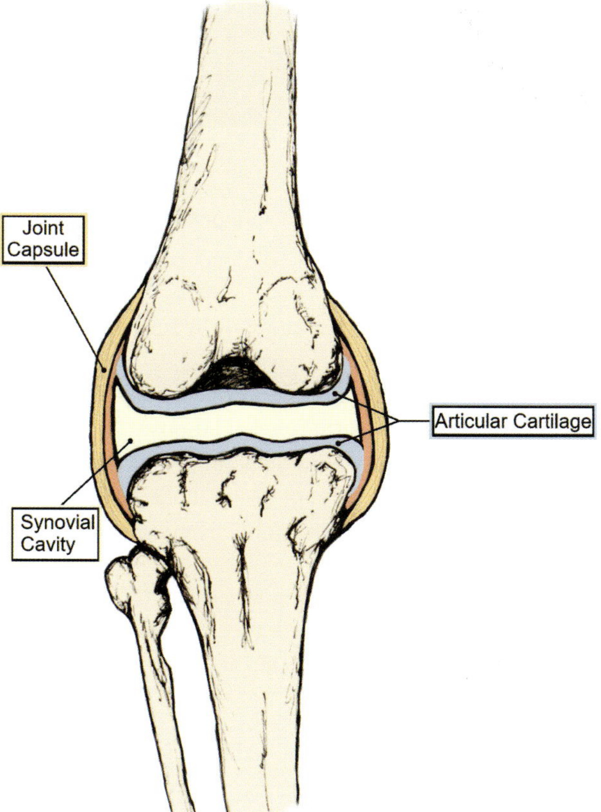

Figure 5.5 An example of the components of a synovial joint, all of which contain a joint capsule, articular cartilage, and a synovial cavity. Synovial joints may also contain other components, as discussed in the text.

Table 5.1 Examples of synovial joints, their locations and movement descriptions.

Synovial joint name	Location example	Description
Condyloid or ellipsoidal	Femorotibial joint (stifle)	A modified ball and socket joint that allows movement in two axes that are perpendicular to one another.
Hinge	Metacarpophalangeal joint (fetlock of equine)	Acts as a hinge, allowing flexion and extension in one plane.
Pivot	Atlantoaxial joint	One bone rotates around a point of the other bone.
Plane	Carpal bones in carpus	Multi-axial sliding or gliding motions.
Saddle	Distal interphalangeal joint	One convex surface and one concave surface meet.
Spheroidal	Acetabulofemoral joint (hip joint)	Ball and socket joint, allows for all movement except gliding.

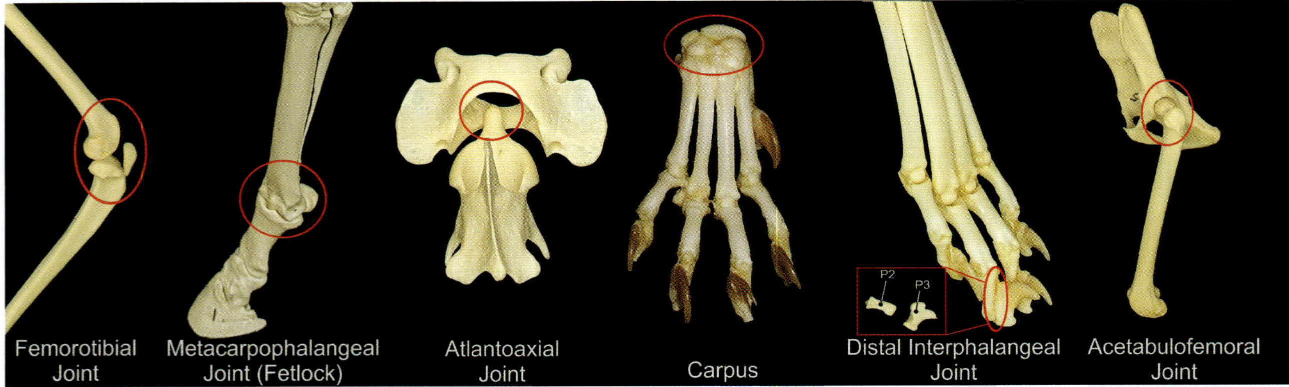

Figure 5.6 Examples of synovial joints. From left to right: the condyloid or ellipsoidal joint example of the femorotibial joint, the hinge joint example of the equine fetlock, the pivot joint example of the atlantoaxial joint, the plane joint example of the carpus, the saddle joint example of the distal interphalangeal joint, and the spheroidal joint example of the acetabulofemoral joint.

Synovial joint may also contain or be functionally involved with any of the following items:

Articular discs – pads of fibrocartilage between bones in a joint, also called **menisci**, that provide spacing and stability.
Articular fat pads – gatherings of adipose tissue that help protect the articular cartilage.
Bursae – fluid-filled sac-like structures that reduce friction.
Ligaments – a tough band of tissue that connects bone to bone.
Tendons – a tough band of connective tissue that connects muscle to bone.

Synovial joints are also categorized into different types depending on their movement (Table 5.1). A table of these joints can be found below, along with an example of each.

See Figure 5.6 for examples of these joints.

The Skull

The skull has several kinds of joints. The sutures of the skull have been discussed, as has the mandibular symphysis. Within the middle ear (between the tympanic membrane and the cochlea) are three small bones known as the ossicles. The connection between them is ligamentous, but since they allow for slight movement, they may be considered fibrous joints. The ramus of the mandible meets the temporal bone of the skull at a point called the **temporomandibular joint** or (TMJ). This is a synovial joint and has a single meniscus between the ramus and the skull. The TMJ also has a ligament associated with it (Figure 5.7).

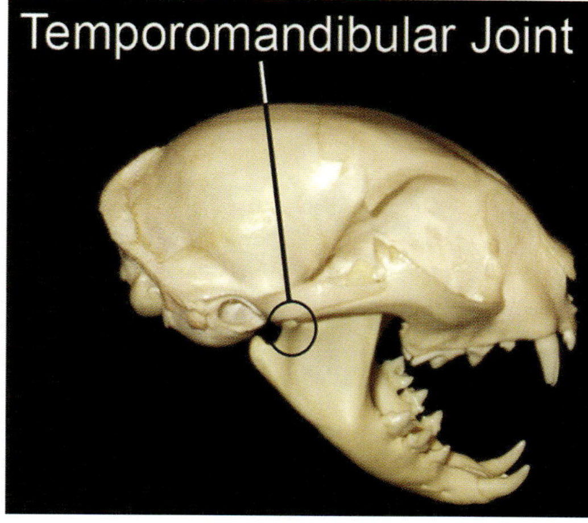

Figure 5.7 The temporomandibular joint (TMJ), a synovial joint in the skull.

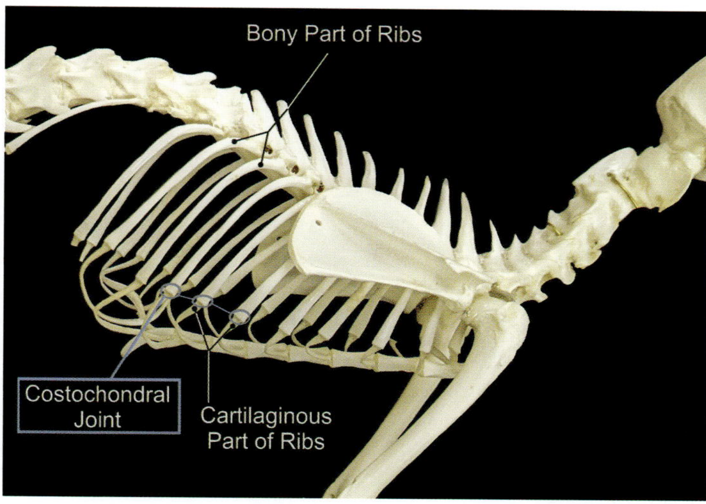

Figure 5.8 The costochondral joint, a fibrous joint in the ribcage.

The Ribs and Vertebral Column

Moving caudally, the atlantooccipital and the atlantoaxial joints are synovial joints. The former allows dorsoventral movement, and the latter side-to-side movement, of the skull. There are ligaments that help connect the dens to the skull and to the spinal column. The costovertebral joints are "ball-and-socket" synovial joints where the ribs meet the vertebrae. Note that there is another joint distal to this along the rib, the costochondral joint. This is a fibrous joint connecting the bony and the cartilaginous portions of the rib (Figure 5.8).

The Pelvis and The Hip

The pelvis has several joints. The **sacroiliac** joint is a relatively immobile joint that connects the sacrum and the ilium. The pubic symphysis was mentioned earlier. Also of note is the **sacrotuberous ligament**, which runs from the sacrum to the ischiatic tuberosity. It is immobile and thus not really associated with a joint but is a stabilizing structure.

The **coxofemoral joint** is commonly known as the hip. The head of the femur is nested in the acetabulum. This is a synovial joint and has the most range of movement of all the joints involving the limbs. There is a small ligament, the ligament of the femoral head, that helps stabilize the femur within the joint space. An abnormal shape of the head of the femur, and/or a shallow or angled acetabulum, is a cause of lameness. The condition is known as **hip dysplasia** and is unfortunately common in many dogs, particularly larger breeds.

The Shoulder and Thoracic Limb

The shoulder, or the **scapulohumeral joint**, involves the intersection of the glenoid fossa of the scapula and the head of the humerus. It is a synovial joint. A congenital condition in some dogs called **osteochondritis dissecans** often affects the shoulder joint, resulting in a chip of bone or cartilage to break off in the joint. The elbow (**humeroradioulnar joint**) involves the condylar intersection with the trochlear notch of the ulna. It too is a synovial joint. There are collateral ligaments (ligaments at the lateral and medial sides of the joint) associated with this joint, preventing excessive lateral movement of the antebrachium relative to the brachium.

The carpus has three sets of joints that are collectively known as the carpal joint. The **antebrachiocarpal joint** is the proximal most one, the space between the antebrachium and the proximal carpal bones. The middle carpal joint is between the proximal and middle rows of bones. The distal-most of these joints is the **carpometacarpal joint**. Of the three, this one has the least movement.

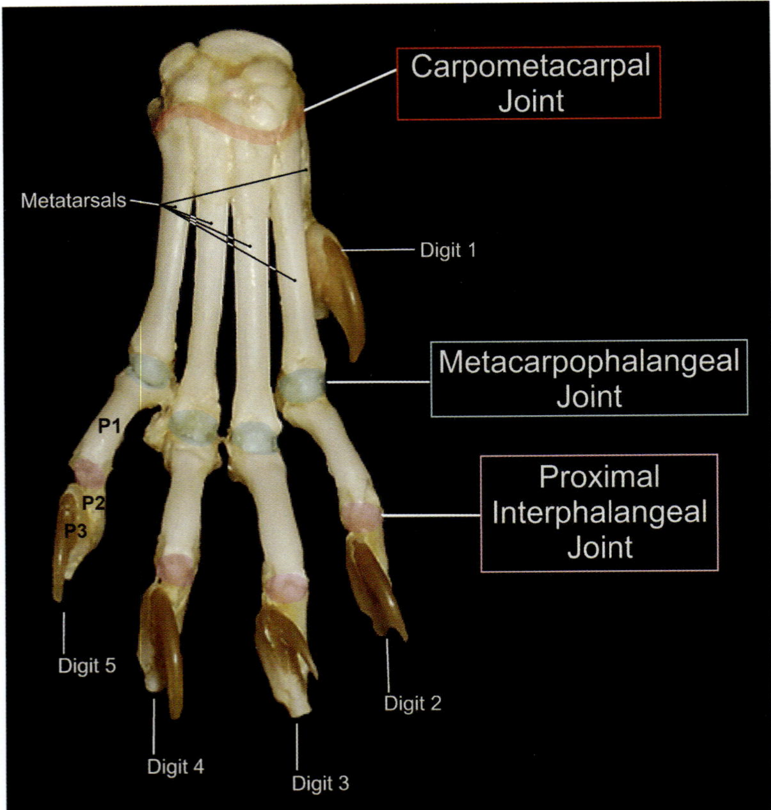

Figure 5.9 The joints and bones of the manus.

The digits have three bones, as we discussed earlier. The joints associated with the digits are the **metacarpophalangeal**, **proximal interphalangeal**, and **distal interphalangeal**. Respectively, these are the joints between the metacarpals and proximal phalangeal bones (P1), the proximal and middle phalangeal bones (P1 and P2), and the middle and distal phalangeal bones (P2 and P3). The interphalangeal joints are synovial joints (Figure 5.9). Note that in equines, these three joints are commonly known as the fetlock, the long pastern, and the short pastern. There is only one of each phalangeal bone in each leg. The metacarpal/metatarsal bone of consequence is the third; metacarpal/metatarsal bones two and four are also known as the "splint bones." They serve no function and are adhered to metacarpal/metatarsal three. Refer back to Chapter 4, Figure 4.23 for equine anatomy.

The Pelvic Limb

Perhaps the most intricate of the synovial joints in the mammal is the **femorotibial joint**, commonly known as the stifle. This joint includes a medial and lateral meniscus, a medial and lateral collateral ligament, and is supported by a patellar ligament. The patellar ligament is actually a part of the patellar tendon; the ligament provides further support by connecting the patella and the tibial tuberosity. While the stifle has a major role in weight-bearing and locomotion in all mammals, larger animals such as equines and ruminants have a particularly large ratio of body surface to limb surface. This puts even more strain on the stifle. These animals have three patellar ligaments, which assist in weight-bearing.

Two major ligaments of the stifle are the **cranial** and **caudal cruciate ligaments**. In dogs, damage to the cranial cruciate is a common cause of stifle-related lameness. The cranial cruciate ligament runs from the caudolateral femur to the cranial tibia. If this ligament does not function correctly, the tibia can slide forward of the femur; testing for this abnormal movement, known as the drawer test, is a part of any canine or feline lameness examination. The caudal cruciate ligament runs from the craniomedial femur to the caudal tibia.

The joints of the tarsus and the distal limb are analogous to those in the thoracic limb. The difference is mostly in the names of the bones and in the use of the root "tarso" (as in the tarsometatarsal joint).

Clinical Case Resolution: Turtle

Turtle is given a full physical examination which reveals multiple broken nails and what appears to be a mouth injury. The remainder of the examination seems unremarkable, and the doctor and technician come up with a plan to collect diagnostic imaging on Turtle.

*Turtle is given mild sedation and pain medication, and a series of **radiographs** (X-ray images) are collected. Radiographs of the skull reveal a mandibular symphysis fracture, while radiographs of the thorax, abdomen, and pelvis with hind limbs show no significant findings.*

Turtle is diagnosed with a mandibular symphysis fracture, which requires surgical repair. Turtle is scheduled to have reconstructive surgery the next day with a board-certified dentist and should make a full recovery.

Clinical Case Critical Thinking

1) *Why do you think Turtle was given sedation and pain medications to take radiographs and complete an oral examination?*
2) *Did Turtle break any bones?*
3) *Why do you think Turtle had multiple broken nails?*
4) *What might be difficult for Turtle while he recovers with his surgical repair? How might we make it easier?*
5) *What education, if any, can you provide the client regarding this situation?*

Review Questions

1 Which of the following terms means to move the limb away from the midline of the body?
  A Abduct
  B Adduct
  C Flexion
  D Extension

2 How many main categories of joints are there?
  A 1
  B 2
  C 3
  D 4
  E 5

3 Which category of joints is most mobile?
  A Fibrous joints
  B Cartilaginous joints
  C Synovial Joints
  D Synarthroses

4 Where can we find suture joints?
  A The knee
  B The elbow
  C The spine
  D The skull

5 What type of cartilage makes up the flexible pinna?
  A Elastic
  B Hyaline
  C Fibrocartilage
  D Hyaline and elastic
  E Elastic and fibrocartilage

6 True or False: A diarthrosis must contain bursae.

  A True

  B False

7 Which type of joint allows for flexion and extension in a single plane?

  A Condyloid

  B Hinge

  C Pivot

  D Spheroidal

8 Which joint has the most movement but doesn't allow for gliding?

  A Pivot

  B Plane

  C Saddle

  D Spheroidal

9 True or False: The joint capsule is continuous with the endosteum.

  A True

  B False

10 What type of joint is the growth plate?

  A Suture joint

  B Synchondrosis

  C Symphysis

  D Saddle joint

  E Spheroidal joint

6

Muscle Anatomy

> **Clinical Case: Belle, An 8-Year-Old Female Spayed German Short Haired Pointer**
>
> *Belle comes into the clinic for what the owner describes as a "broken tail." The owner reports that they were camping with Belle over the last few days and the day after hiking and swimming, Belle's tail seemed to stop working. They noted that it is hanging down and she cannot wag it properly and that she seems very hesitant when attempting to sit and lay down.*

Introduction

This section will introduce the various muscles and muscle groups that make up the bulk of the mammalian body. The reader is encouraged to use some of the online resources that accompany this text to help the visualization of these structures. Appendix 1 contains tips on proper dissection of muscle tissue, while Appendix 3 has specific information about some of the muscle insertions and origins.

There are three main types of muscle: **skeletal muscle, smooth muscle**, and **cardiac muscle**. Cardiac muscle is only found in the heart and is often put into a separate category because the heart muscle has some components that look like skeletal muscle and some like smooth muscle. As will be discussed in the physiology section, smooth muscles function without the animal having to consciously think about moving them. The heart too moves in this fashion, but its structure has enough skeletal characteristics that a compromise category was created. This chapter will primarily focus on skeletal muscle anatomy and some smooth muscle anatomy. Cardiac muscle anatomy can be found in Chapter 10.

Cellular Anatomy

Each of the muscle groups mentioned above differ not only in their function and gross anatomy, but their differences start even at the cellular level (Figure 6.1). **Skeletal muscle cells** are narrow and long and can be up to several centimeters in some locations. Because of this, they are referred to as "**muscle fibers**," so it is important to remember that a single muscle fiber is the same as saying a single skeletal muscle cell. The cell itself is made of many thin protein filaments called **myofibrils**. Each of the cells has multiple nuclei and a variety of important organelles, including **mitochondria**, the **sarcoplasmic reticulum**, and the **transverse tubules**. Mitochondria create energy for cells in the form of adenosine triphosphate (ATP), while the sarcoplasmic reticulum stores calcium ions and the transverse tubules act as a highway for muscle signals to travel. The outermost layer of each cell is called the **sarcolemma**, which is responsible for muscle signal transmission and cell regulation. Figure 6.2 is an illustration of a muscle cell and shows the above-mentioned component. On a more microscopic level, each muscle cell has **contractile units** called **sarcomeres**, as seen in Figure 6.3. The organization of these sarcomeres in the cell, and then the cells organized together, creates a striped or **striated** appearance, which looks different from smooth muscle tissue. These organelles and their functions, as well as the mechanics behind sarcomeres and muscle contractions, will be more heavily discussed in Chapter 19.

Anatomy and Physiology for Veterinary Technicians and Nurses: A Clinical Approach, Second Edition. Lori Asprea.
© 2026 John Wiley & Sons, Inc. Published 2026 by John Wiley & Sons, Inc.
Companion website: www.wiley.com/go/asprea/anatomy_vettech2e

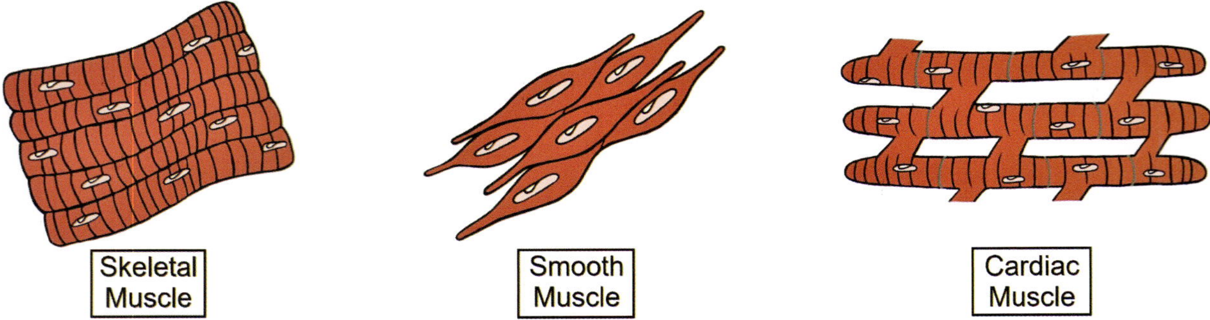

Figure 6.1 A comparison of the three different types of muscle cells: skeletal, smooth, and cardiac. Note the intercalated discs in cardiac muscle represented by gray bars in between each cell.

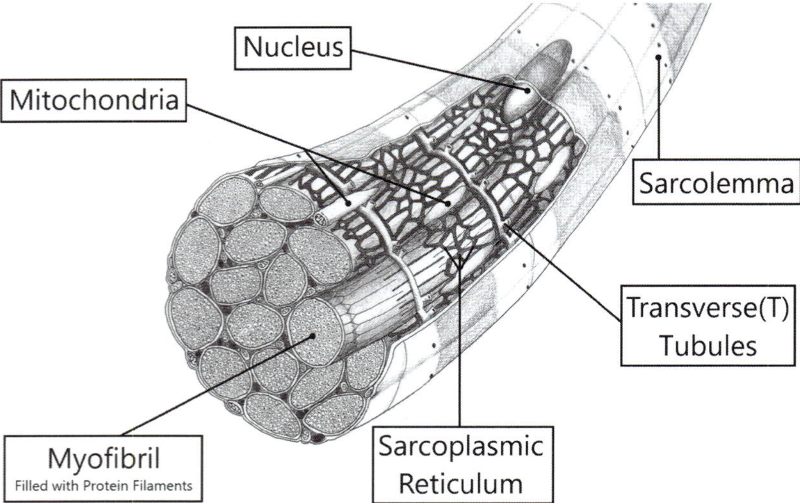

Figure 6.2 The skeletal muscle cell with organelles.

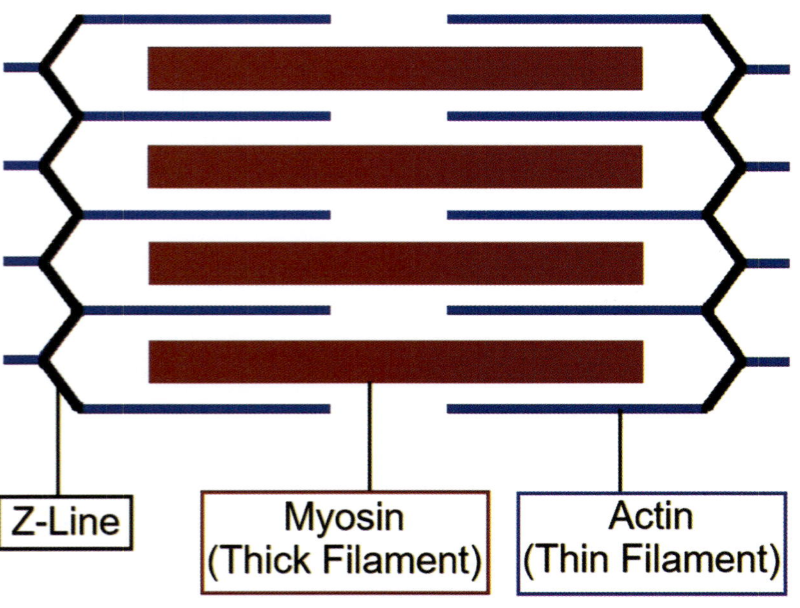

Figure 6.3 A single sarcomere in the relaxed state.

Smooth muscle cells have many of the same organelles as skeletal muscle cells but do differ anatomically. They are comparably shorter than skeletal muscle cells, and each cell only contains one nucleus. They have the ability to contract, just like skeletal muscle cells, but the elements that allow them to contract are organized differently. They appear like a net on the cell which tightens down when contraction occurs instead of in rows like the skeletal muscle cell. The net of contractile units is anchored down with structures called **dense bodies** (Figure 6.4). This organization paired with the tapered ends of each cell results in the smooth appearance this muscle is named for.

Cardiac muscle cells share characteristics from skeletal and smooth muscle, but also have unique characteristics which earn them their own category, and chapter (see Chapter 10).

Skeletal Muscle

Skeletal muscle does the major work of locomotion and strength maneuvers. Skeletal muscle is striated, and is controlled by the conscious mind, and thus can also be called **striated voluntary muscle**. Skeletal muscle is composed of many muscle fibers, each of which is a single cell, as discussed above. Each cell is covered in a layer of connective tissue called **endomysium**. Bundles of fibers are grouped together and called **fasciculi** (single, fasciculus). The fasciculi are bound together and surrounded by a connective tissue called **perimysium**. Bundles of fasciculi are grouped together and encased by a connective tissue sheath called the **epimysium**, which is the part immediately seen when looking at the muscle during dissection (see Figure 6.5). The part the epimysium encircles is referred to as the **belly** of the muscle. The belly is known as a "head" when there is more than one next to each other and working together. For example, the biceps muscle is composed of two heads, or muscle bellies, which function as a unit.

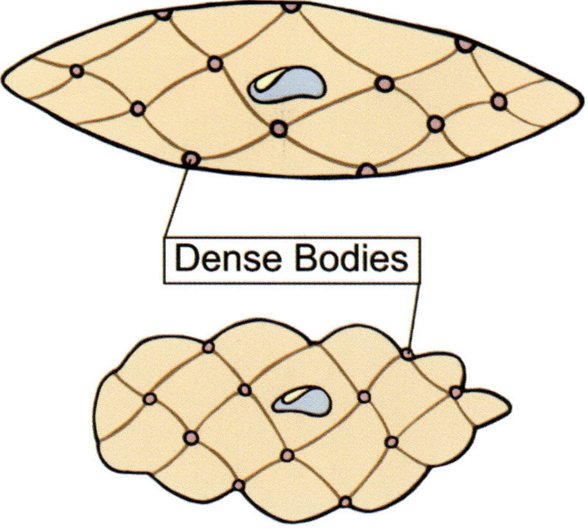

Figure 6.4 The smooth muscle cell relaxed and contracted. Note that the behavior of the contractile units is different in smooth muscle and actin and myosin are organized across the cell, creating a net pattern. The anchors are the dense bodies.

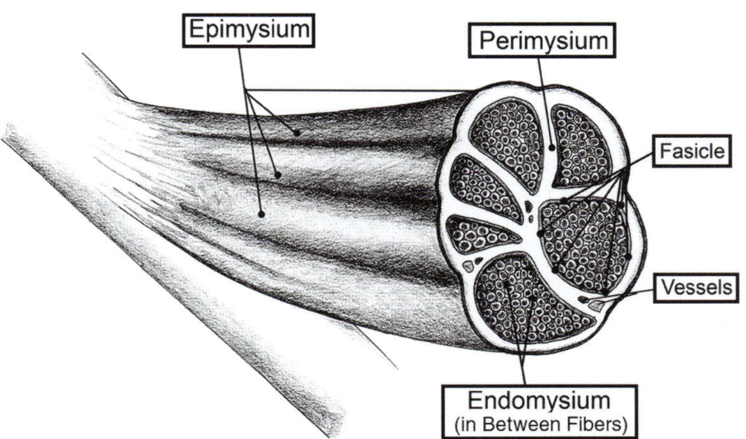

Figure 6.5 The structure of a muscle and fascicles.

The **origin** of any muscle or muscle group is defined as the proximal-most, cranial-most, or central-most connection of a muscle or tendon to the body, and the **insertion** is the connection distal-most, caudal-most, or furthest away from the median plane of the body. There are some exceptions to this, which we will discuss below. In most cases, the origin is the more fixed point of the muscle, and the insertion is the area where the greatest movement occurs.

The various connective tissue sheets converge at either end of many skeletal muscles to form **tendons**. They are dense, regular fibrous tissue. Tendons are composed mostly of **collagen**, a tough protein. They are present at the insertion and origin of the muscle. Tendons usually connect the muscle to the bone. Some tendons are short and flat; others are long and thin. Sometimes, one muscle connects directly to another by way of fibrous material that is not formed as a tendon. This connection is a special type of joint called **aponeurosis**. The **linea alba** ("white line") is the best known of these and will be discussed later; it connects two of the superficial muscles of the abdomen.

Muscles are supplied by arteries, veins, nerve fibers, and lymphatic vessels. The latter runs through the loose connective tissue called **fascia** surrounding the muscle fibers. Tendons, on the other hand, are poorly vascularized, if at all. Among other things, this means that they do not heal well when injured as the inflammatory cells of the blood cannot reach them.

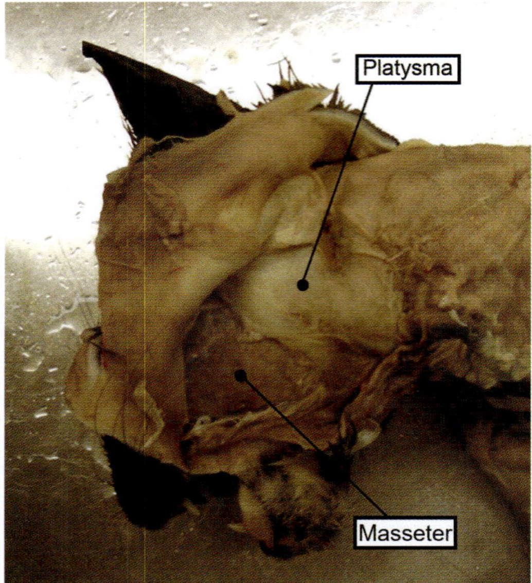

Figure 6.6 The platysma is a superficial muscle encompassing most of the head. The masseter, one of the powerful muscles of chewing, is deep to it.

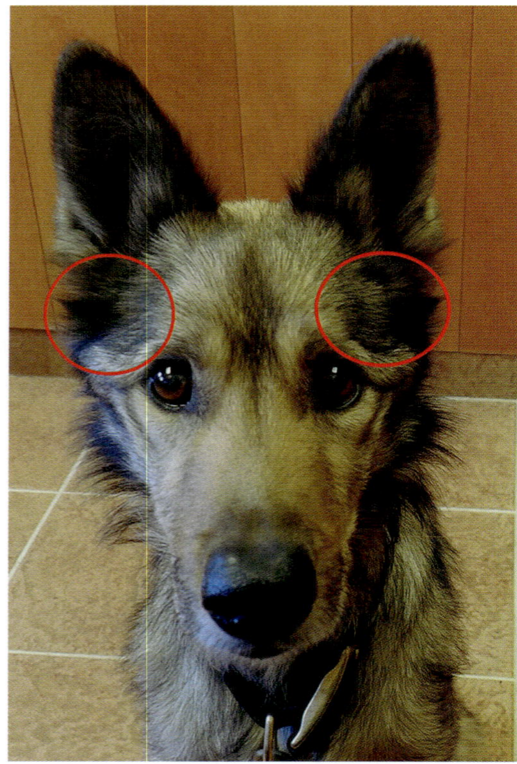

Figure 6.7 Muscle atrophy in the temporalis muscle of a dog with chronic disease. Notice the indentations where the muscle has wasted away.

We can characterize skeletal muscles as either **superficial**, or nearer to the surface of the body, or **deep**, or nearer to the internal surface of the body. We will take a regional approach to the study of anatomy, starting with the head. In each case, we will describe the superficial muscles first and then work to the deeper layers. The following muscles are skeletal unless otherwise noted.

The Head and Neck

The superficial layer of muscle on the head is called the **platysma** (see Figure 6.6). It is a very thin layer and can be difficult to separate from the dermis. Running from the zygomatic arch to the mandible is the **masseter muscle**. This is a massive muscle that is crucial to chewing and moving the jaw. Running from the parietal and frontal bones to the mandible is the **temporalis muscle**. It lies somewhat dorsal to the masseter. Certain neurological diseases can cause the lateral surfaces of the head to have a concave appearance, caused by the atrophy of the temporalis (Figure 6.7).

The **orbicularis oculi** are muscle fibers that surround the eye, and **orbicularis oris** are those surrounding the mouth. **Digastricus** is a large muscle forming the floor of the oral cavity, important in opening the mouth. The **tongue** is a large muscle composed of several sections. The muscles of the tongue are the **styloglossus, genioglossus**, and **hyoglossus**. They function as one muscle. The **buccinator** on each side runs from the maxilla to the mandible and is equivalent to the interior oral ("cheek") muscle.

The **preauricular** muscles are those rostral to the pinna and assist in moving the pinna to pinpoint sounds in various locations. In mammals that depend to a great extent on hearing, these muscles are crucial to survival.

The superficial muscles of the neck include the **brachiocephalicus** (broken down to mean "arm head"; the word "brachi" refers to the arm and "ceph" refers to the head), which runs from the mastoid process of the temporal bone toward the scapula. Another superficial muscle of the neck is the **sternocephalicus**, which runs to the sternum from the mastoid bone. **Trapezius** goes from the neck to the thoracic vertebrae, running along the dorsal and lateral surface of the thorax.

The Thorax

There are scattered areas of muscle tissue around the subcutaneous layer of the skin along the thorax and abdomen. They have fascicles running in a cranial-caudal direction. They are involved in the fasciculation ("twitching") of the skin, which dogs and cats engage in when they are stimulated. The particular muscles involved in this movement are called the **panniculus muscles**.

Superficial muscles of the ventral thorax are identified in Figures 6.8 and 6.9. These muscles include the **superficial and deep pectorals**. The name deep pectoral is misleading as it is in fact a superficial muscle and can also be called **pectoralis minor**. The superficial pectoral can also be referred to as **pectoralis major**. The pectorals are present on the ventral thorax and run from the sternum to the proximal thoracic limb. The superficial pectoral is cranial to the deep pectoral. Both have some fibers that run in a "V" shape. In the dog and cat, these muscles are rather thin.

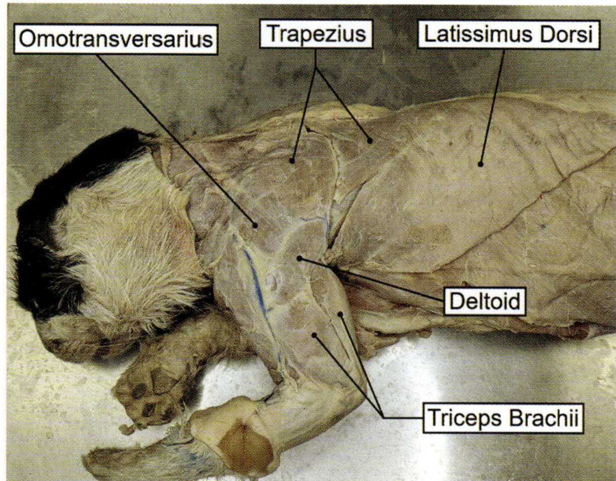

Figure 6.8 The superficial muscles of the lateral thorax.

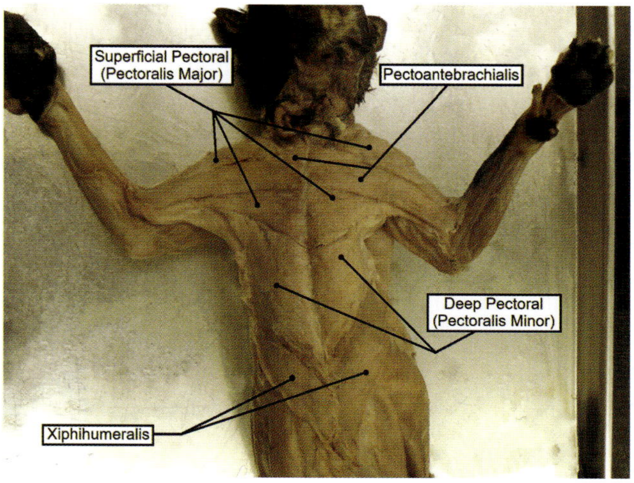

Figure 6.9 The pectoral muscles and xiphihumeralis.

In avians, the pectorals are an important part of the ability to fly and are very thick and powerful. There is a band of muscle in between two bellies of the pectoralis major called the **pectoantebrachialis**. At the caudal-most point of the pectorals is another muscle called **xiphihumeralis**.

Another superficial muscle is the **deltoid**, which runs from the spine of the scapula to the deltoid tuberosity of the humerus. Near the deltoid is the **omotransversarius** muscle, which is associated with the shoulder. The **latissimus dorsi** runs from the thoracolumbar spine to the humerus. It is one of the rare muscles where the origin is caudal to the insertion. It is a large but thin muscle and needs to be carefully pulled away from the trunk in order to observe the muscles deep to it; use blunt dissection to separate it rather than a scalpel.

Deeper muscles of the thorax are included in Figure 6.10. Deep to the trapezius muscle lie the **supraspinatus** and the **infraspinatus**. These are thick muscles that fill the fossae

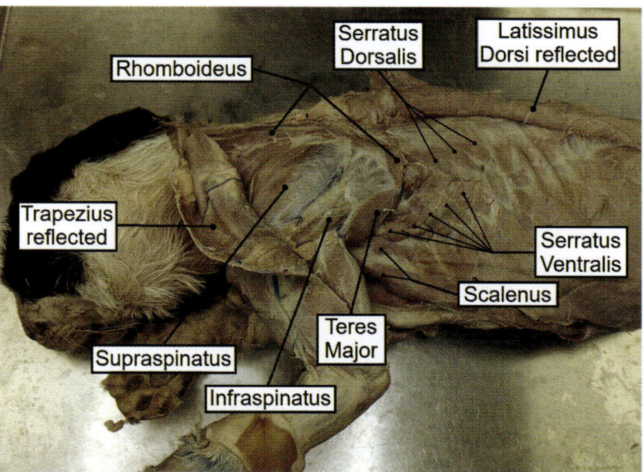

Figure 6.10 The deep thoracic muscles. Latissimus dorsi and trapezius are reflected.

on either lateral surface of the spine or the scapula. Also, found deep in the trapezius is the **rhomboideus** muscle, which is one of the muscular components that attaches the thoracic limb to the body. Ventral to the infraspinatus muscle is **teres major**. Other muscles of the deep thorax include the **internal and external intercostals**, which are deep to the serratus ventralis and are important in breathing. The externals are superficial to the internals. Lastly, there is the **scalenus muscle**, which extends from the dorsal neck of the animal to the cervical vertebrae. The scalenus is also involved in respiration.

The **serratus muscle** is actually a series of sections. The largest parts are the **serratus dorsalis** and the **serratus ventralis**. Dorsalis rides along the dorsum of the thorax and ventralis along the lateral surface. Ventralis is just deep to the latissimus dorsi. The lateral section of the serratus ventralis is arranged in bands of tissue that form flat sections running at an angle. It is from this "serrated" appearance that the muscle draws its name. This muscle helps to form the sling that holds the scapula to the body wall.

A term that has some clinical significance is "**thoracic girdle**." The term girdle implies encircling the body. The thoracic girdle includes the latissimus dorsi, trapezius, serratus ventralis, and the pectoral muscles. They are all involved in connecting the thoracic limb to the trunk and function as a joint during movements such as shifting weight from one leg to the other. These muscles are the only things that attach the thoracic limb to the body as there are no bony attachments. In contrast to the thoracic girdle, the **pelvic girdle** refers to the bone only; that is, the pelvic limbs are connected to the rest of the skeleton by a direct joint between the femur and the pelvis.

The Dorsum

Some muscles of the dorsum deserve special mention. The group of muscles known as **epaxial** muscles run dorsally to the transverse processes of some of the vertebrae, including particularly the lumbar vertebrae. This group includes the muscles **iliocostal, longissimus** (which has four sections), and **transversospinalis**. These muscles are important because they assist in respiration. They are often the site of intramuscular injections. They must be handled gently in conducting any kind of spinal surgery, such as laminectomy. They are particularly sensitive to significant weight loss and will show mild atrophy early in the process of losing weight. This atrophy will be particularly noticeable if the weight loss is long-standing or dramatic. As such, these muscles give a good informal clue as to the state of health of the animal. They lie just underneath the **epaxial aponeurosis**. The **hypaxial muscles** are deep to the epaxials. They include the **major psoas** and **minor psoas** and the **iliacus**. They help flex the spinal column and move the pelvic limbs. Due to their location, they are also referred to as **sublumbar muscles**.

The Abdomen

Superficial muscles of the abdomen include the **external abdominal oblique** muscles. Just deep to the external abdominal oblique is the **internal abdominal oblique**. Their fibers are oriented at an angle to each other, with the striations flowing in opposite directions. They are found on the ventral and lateral abdomen. The internal abdominal oblique is deep to the external abdominal oblique. They meet at the ventral abdominal midline at the **linea alba**, a thick fibrous line described above as aponeurosis. The linea alba is a convenient place to make an incision when doing abdominal surgery, if for no other reason than that it is easy to see and allows the surgeon to avoid cutting into the muscle of the body wall. Ovariohysterectomies (spays) are always begun at the linea alba in dogs and cats. The internal abdominal oblique at its caudal-most part becomes the **cremaster muscle in males**. This muscle plays an important part in reproductive activities (Figure 6.11).

Deeper abdominal muscles include the **rectus abdominis**, running cranially to caudally down the center of the abdomen, and the **transverse abdominis**, which follows a course from one lateral surface to the other. The rectus abdominus is covered by a sheath, which can be used to place sutures to anchor the skin and body wall during abdominal surgery (Figure 6.12).

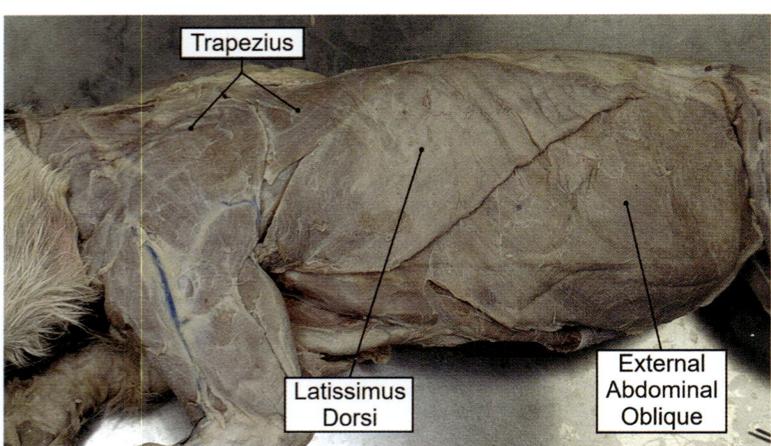

Figure 6.11 The superficial muscles of the abdomen.

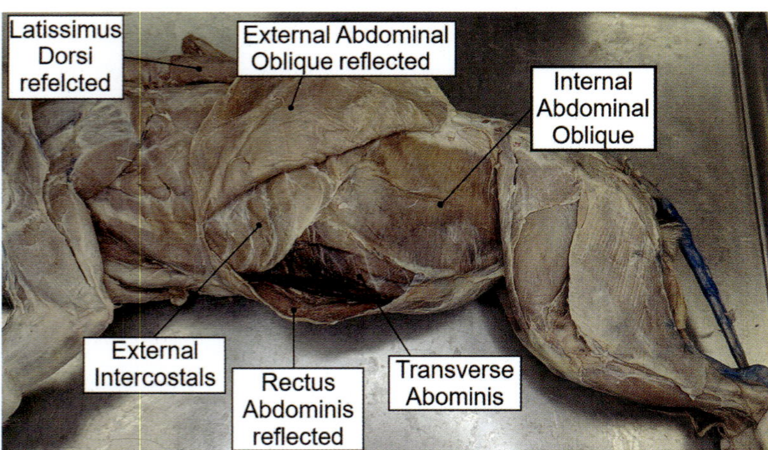

Figure 6.12 The deep abdominal muscles with latissimus dorsi and external abdominal oblique reflected. Rectus abdominus runs in a straight line with cranial to caudal striations along the linea alba and is reflected here.

The Pelvis

The **medial gluteal** and **superficial gluteal** muscles run from the pelvis to the femur. The medial gluteal muscle is cranial to the superficial gluteal muscle. There is a deep gluteal muscle as well. Interestingly, despite its sizable rump, the ruminant does not have superficial gluteal muscles.

Other muscles of the pelvis include the **internal and external obturators**, which cover the **obturator foramen**. The **gemelli** (from the Greek word for twins) help connect the pelvis and the femur as does the **quadratus femoris**.

The **perineum** refers to the area under the tail and lateral to the anus. It also includes the anus. The anus itself actually has two sphincter muscles – an **external anal sphincter** and an **internal anal sphincter**. The external anal sphincter is composed of skeletal muscle and is a voluntary muscle. The internal anal sphincter is composed of smooth or involuntary muscle.

The **coccygeus** is a muscle that goes from the ischium to the tail. The **levator ani** also goes from the pelvis to the perineum. It slings around the rectum and is important in the process of defecation. In any surgery involving the anus or the anal glands, it is crucial not to sever this muscle. If it is disrupted, the animal may become incontinent. The coccygeus and levator ani are both muscles used in raising the tail.

The Limbs

We now come to a discussion of the limbs. Muscles of the limbs are often described as extrinsic or intrinsic. Extrinsic muscles are those that connect the limb to the body. Intrinsic muscles have both their origin and their insertion on the limb itself.

The Thoracic Limb

Extrinsic muscles of the thoracic limb include the **brachiocephalicus, trapezius, omotransversarius, latissimus dorsi, deltoid**, and **superficial pectoral**. **Triceps brachii** and **biceps brachii** originate on the scapula and insert on the olecranon or radius, respectively. The tendon of origin of the biceps brachii is important in flexing the shoulder. As mentioned, the scapula is considered to be a part of the thoracic limb in that the scapula does not have any bony attachment to the rest of the skeleton. **Teres major** and **teres minor** are deep muscles involved in the flexion of the shoulder joint (Figure 6.8).

Deeper muscles of the brachium include **brachialis** and **anconeus**. These muscles are involved in flexion and extension of the elbow, respectively.

The muscles of the dorsolateral antebrachium are almost all involved in the extension of the limb, particularly relating to the paw and digits. Going clockwise toward the lateral surface, these muscles include the **brachioradialis, extensor carpi radialis, common digital extensor, lateral digital extensor**, and **extensor carpi ulnaris**. The **supinator muscle** is deep to these (Figure 6.13).

The caudal surface of the antebrachium includes the **flexor carpi radialis, the flexor carpi ulnaris** (which has two heads), and the **superficial digital flexor**. The deeper muscles include the **deep digital flexor, pronator teres**, and **pronator quadratus**. The deep digital flexor has three heads. All of these muscles are flexors. Reference to the interosseous "muscle" actually indicates ligaments that run from the metacarpals to the digits. In horses, they form a thick bundle called the **suspensory ligament**, which is important in the **stay apparatus**.

The stay apparatus is a vital part of locomotion in horses and cows. Actually, the stay apparatus has to do with the animal at rest. The large amount of weight that these large animals put on their relatively thin legs would ordinarily cause significant fatigue and possibly injury. In order to give the muscles and joints of the limb time to rest, the ligaments, tendons, and muscles are constructed in such a way that weight is distributed over three limbs at any one time in the standing animal. The "free" limb does not bear weight and usually remains in a flexed position with the tip of the hoof on the ground. Periodically, the animal will shift his weight to give another limb a rest. The result is that the wear and tear on the limbs is considerably less. The combination of muscles, ligaments, and tendons that allow this shifting of weight is called the stay apparatus.

Carnivores, some omnivores, and pigs are the only animals that can **supinate** (turn the

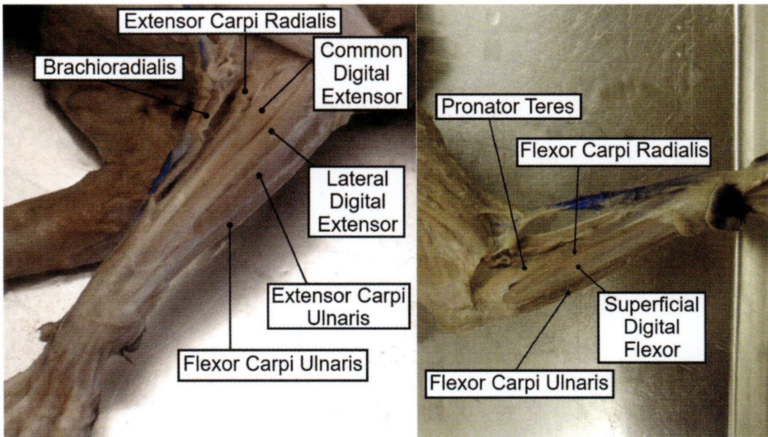

Figure 6.13 Muscles of the antebrachium.

palmar/plantar surface upward) and **pronate** (the reverse of supinate) the distal extremity. Herbivores generally cannot. The latter do not have the pronator muscles, and their radius and ulna are fused.

The Pelvic Limb

The muscles of the pelvic limb are generally quite large and very powerful. Most mammals use the pelvic limbs to accelerate movement, while the muscles of the thoracic limbs are more involved in supporting the heavier structure of the head. The muscles of the pelvic limb can be seen in Figures 6.14–6.16.

The middle, deep, and superficial gluteals all connect the pelvis and the proximal thigh and are found on the dorsolateral surface of the limb. Lateral muscles of the pelvic limb include the **biceps femoris**, a very large muscle running all the way from the pelvis to the tarsus. The **tensor fasciae latae** runs from the pelvis to the stifle. However, only the proximal section of it looks like a muscle; the rest of it is composed of fascia, which has a silvery appearance. To see the deeper muscles, cut through the fascia, not the proximal part of the muscle. **Semitendinosus** is a muscle of the lateral and caudal surface of the limb. It is not recommended to use this muscle for injection as it is just superficial and caudal to the **ischiatic (sciatic) nerve**. If an injection is made into this muscle, and the sciatic nerve is punctured, it might render the limb useless. The risk is significantly greater with smaller dogs and cats as the distance to the nerve is even shorter. Deep to the biceps femoris muscle is the **vastus lateralis**. As the name implies, it too is a large, powerful muscle.

The superficial medial thigh includes muscles such as **gracilis** and **sartorius**, with the former medial to the latter. These muscles extend to the stifle. Sartorius has two heads in dogs and one in cats. **Semimembranosus** extends from

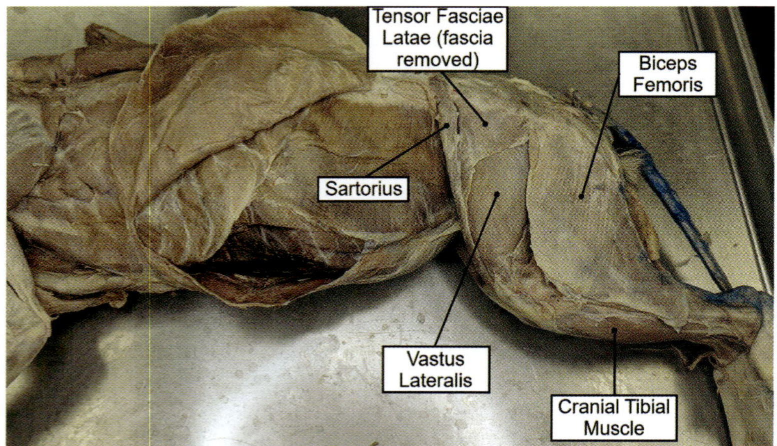

Figure 6.14 Superficial muscles of the lateral pelvic limb.

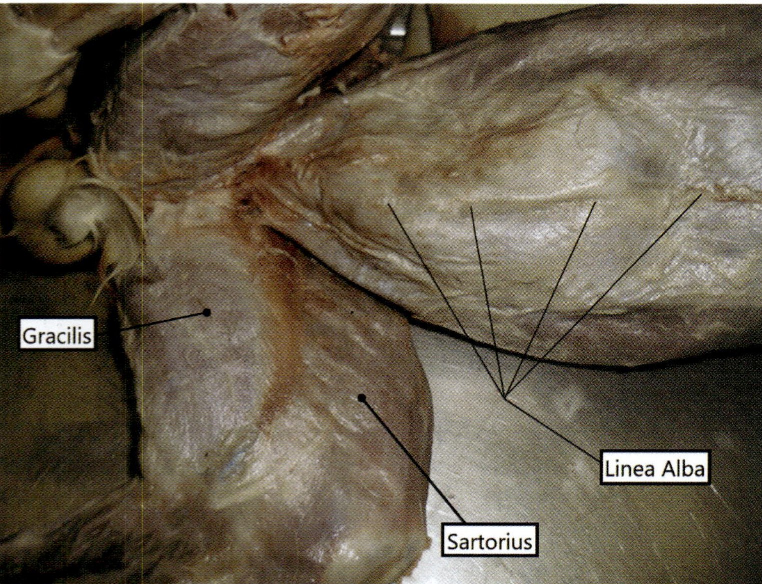

Figure 6.15 Superficial muscles of the medial pelvic limb.

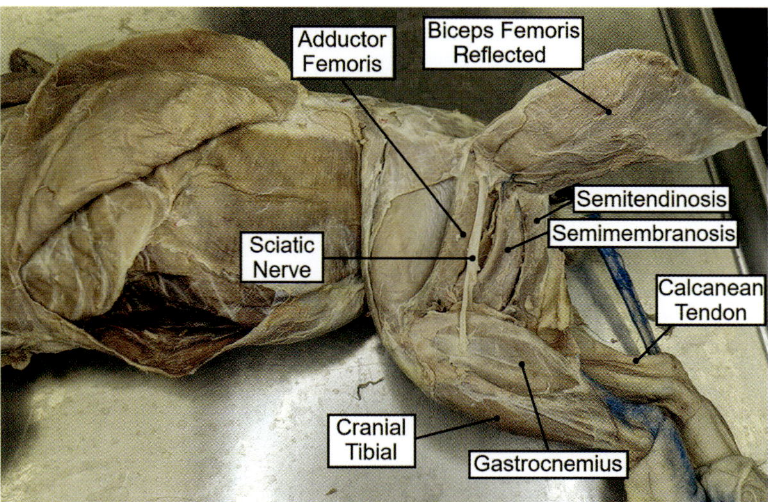

Figure 6.16 Deep muscles of the lateral pelvic limb.

the ischiatic tuberosity to the femur and the tibia by way of two heads. The muscle runs medial to semitendinosus and wraps around the cranial section of the proximal thigh. The cranial portion of this muscle is often used for injections, particularly in cats. On occasion, the epaxial muscles are used for this purpose as well.

The **quadriceps** muscle, comprised of four heads: vastus lateralis, **rectus femoris, vastus medialis**, and **vastus intermedius**, runs both superficially and deeply in the thigh. All four join to form one very thick tendon that inserts into the tibial tuberosity. The tendon of insertion of the quadriceps is also called the **patellar tendon**. Contained within it is the patella itself. In horses and ruminants, there are three patellar ligaments associated with this tendon. The ability of the animal to use them to stabilize the patella in one position or another is another important part of the stay apparatus.

The **crus** (the area from the stifle to the tarsus) contains the long and lateral digital extensors on its cranial surface and the **gastrocnemius** muscle on the caudal surface. The **cranial tibial muscle** is a superficial muscle of the cranial crus. The gastrocnemius has two bellies and is equivalent to the human calf muscle. The tendon of insertion of the gastrocnemius muscle ends at the calcaneus and is thus known as the **calcanean tendon**. It is the equivalent of the human Achilles tendon and is extremely thick

Smooth Muscle

This chapter has not yet dealt with the subject of smooth muscles. These muscles are found throughout the body, for example, in the eyes, forming the walls of some internal organs, the walls of vessels, and the airways. They are mostly triggered by the autonomic nervous system and will be discussed in conjunction with it. Since the autonomic nervous system controls smooth muscle, that means that it cannot be consciously controlled like skeletal muscle. An animal can control skeletal muscle movement in its limbs but cannot control the smooth muscle movement of the gastrointestinal tract or eyes. In general, smooth muscle does not appear to have the striations of skeletal muscle.

Smooth muscle is generally organized in one of two ways: **single-unit** and **multiunit**. This is related to the amount of nerve signals to the tissue. In single-unit smooth muscle, the cells are connected to each other forming one large sheet of muscle that contracts together. The signal travels across the expanse of cells, making them function as one. This type of smooth muscle can be found in the walls of hollow organs and as such is also referred to as **visceral smooth muscle**. This includes locations like the bladder, intestines, and uterus. If you consider **peristalsis**, or the wave-like contractions of the gastrointestinal tract, this is a great example of single-unit smooth muscle in action. There are many individual muscle cells, but they act as a single sheet of tissue, contracting in a wave-like pattern to move digesta, or processed food, forward.

Multiunit smooth muscle differs anatomically in the way it is innervated and arranged. Multiunit smooth muscle is not arranged in large sheets and does not function as one piece of tissue. Where in single-unit smooth muscle, the signal from the nerves is communicated through all the cells to act as one, in multiunit, the signal is confined to the individual area that was stimulated and thus has many more nerves bringing in signals. This anatomy allows for much finer and more detailed movements. This can be found in the airways, some vessels, and the **ciliary muscles** of the eye that control the iris opening and closing in response to light.

Clinical Case Resolution: Belle

Belle is given a full physical exam which is almost completely normal aside from the obvious injury to her tail. She has full range of motion in all four limbs and does not appear to be painful upon palpation of any joint or her spine. When observing the tail, it extends out from the body for several centimeters then sharply drops straight down to the floor (Figure 6.17).

Belle is diagnosed with acute caudal myopathy, which is a strain or sprain of the muscles used for tail movement, like the coccygeus. This goes by many other names like Limber Tail and Swimmers Tail and is more common in sporting and hunting dogs that are very active. This can happen to dogs that suddenly overuse their tail or have sudden exposure to cold weather or water. Belle is diagnosed on signalment, exam, and history alone, and no further diagnostics are needed at this time. Radiographs (X-ray images) can be considered in some cases to assess for any other injuries.

Belle is sent home with instructions to rest, particularly her tail, and a prescription for nonsteroidal anti-inflammatory drugs (NSAIDs). Within 3 days, the owners report that Belle seems back to normal and will continue resting and watching her for the rest of the week.

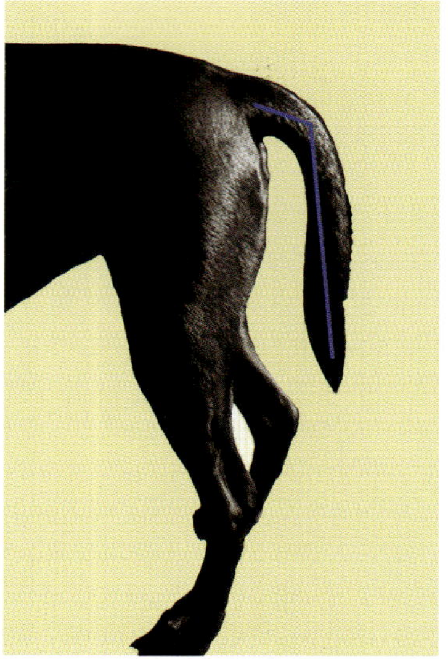

Figure 6.17 Belle's tail with the characteristic extension and sharp droop downward seen in this condition.

Clinical Case Critical Thinking

1) *Is there anything in Belle's signalment that may have helped lead to our diagnosis?*
2) *Break down the diagnosis "Acute caudal myopathy" using the vocabulary you have learned.*
3) *The owners reported that Belle seemed hesitant to sit and lay down. Why might this be? What other activities might be difficult for Belle while she is healing from her injury?*

Review Questions

1 Which muscle type is under conscious control?
  A Smooth muscle
  B Skeletal muscle
  C Cardiac muscle

2 What is the name of the white line on the abdomen?

3 Which of the following muscles can be found on the lateral thorax?
  A Internal abdominal oblique
  B Gracilis
  C Latissimus dorsi
  D Brachioradialis

4 Which of the following muscles can be found deep in the trapezius?
  A Supraspinatus
  B Brachiocephalicus
  C Rhomboideus
  D Sartorius
  E A and B
  F A and C

5   What is the difference between control of skeletal muscle and smooth muscle?

6   What is another name for the deep pectoral muscle?

7   Which of the following muscles is involved in the thoracic girdle?
   A Serratus ventralis
   B Semitendinosus
   C Biceps femoris
   D Gastrocnemius

8   Name any two of the antebrachium muscles on the lateral surface.

9   Name the muscle that is part muscle belly, part thick fascia.

10   Name one location you can find multiunit smooth muscle.

7

Anatomy of the Nervous System

> **Clinical Case: Petey 12-Week-Old Male Intact Domestic Long Hair Feline**
>
> *Petey is brought into the clinic because the owners say that Petey seems to not be able to walk appropriately. The owners found Petey and two presumed litter mates approximately 2 weeks ago. When the kittens were found, they were malnourished and weak and had a flea infestation. The owners decided to take all three kittens home to foster and nurse back to health. Petey appeared particularly weak and uncoordinated and despite adequate nutrition and care, he still seems to be ambulating abnormally. The owners jokingly refer to him as "drunk" when he walks or runs. They note he has a great appetite and energy otherwise but has an issue getting into the litterbox. The owners report this has not gotten any better or worse since they took him in.*

Introduction

This chapter will cover some of the major anatomical structures associated with the system of nerve fibers running throughout the body of an animal. At the end of this book is a guide (Appendix 2) that provides a mnemonic device for remembering the names of the 12 cranial nerves. Material regarding the function of the nerves will be covered in the nerve physiology chapter.

The Neuron

A **neuron** is a single cell and is also referred to as a nerve fiber (see Figure 7.1). The neuron is the functioning unit of the nervous system. The body of the nerve cell is referred to as a **soma**. Small fibers that branch from the soma and each other are referred to as **dendrites**. The long extension from the soma toward another neuron is called an **axon**, which comes to rounded ends called **terminal boutons** or **synaptic bulbs**. The space between the distal end of the axon and either another neuron or a final receptor is called a **synapse**. It is from the terminal bouton that **neurotransmitters** are sent across the synapse to stimulate the next neuron in the sequence. Neurotransmitters are chemicals crucial to neurological function and will also be discussed in Chapter 20.

Nerves in the brain or the spinal cord are referred to as part of the **central nervous system** (CNS). Other nerves are considered **peripheral nerves**, meaning that they directly branch from the central nervous system. All nerves do not necessarily end or begin in the brain; peripheral nerves can arise and/or return directly from or to the spinal cord, particularly those nerves involved in reflex or autonomic responses.

Nerves are either considered **myelinated** or **unmyelinated**. Myelin is a layer of proteins and lipids that wrap around the axon, creating the **myelin sheath**. Myelin is formed by **glial cells** called **oligodendrocytes** in the central nervous system and **Schwann** cells in the peripheral nervous system. The spaces in between the myelin sheath are the **nodes of Ranvier**. If nerve tissue in the central nervous system is myelinated, it will appear white and is thus called **white matter**. If it is unmyelinated tissue, it is called **gray matter**. Generally, the axon is myelinated and the soma is unmyelinated, resulting in white matter being bundles of axons and gray matter being bundles of soma and dendrites.

Anatomy and Physiology for Veterinary Technicians and Nurses: A Clinical Approach, Second Edition. Lori Asprea.
© 2026 John Wiley & Sons, Inc. Published 2026 by John Wiley & Sons, Inc.
Companion website: www.wiley.com/go/asprea/anatomy_vettech2e

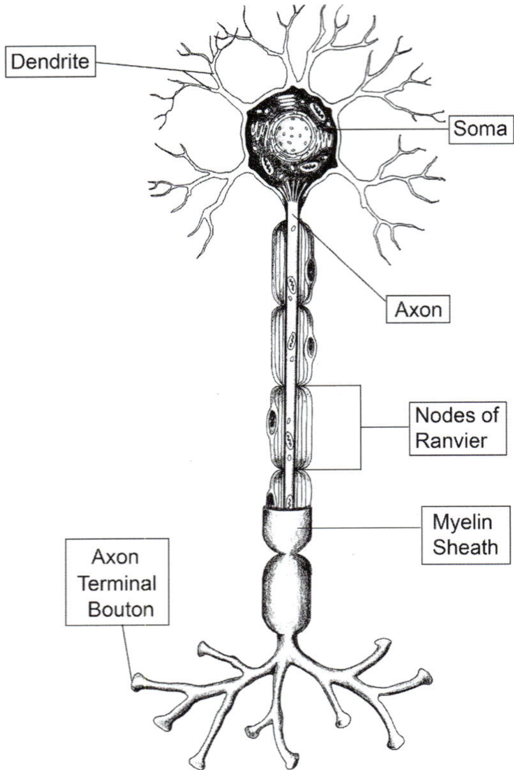

Figure 7.1 The neuron with myelin sheath.

A bundle of nerve fibers that arise from a common origin in the central nervous system is known as a **fascicle**. The major fasciculi have specific names. Not all fasciculi, and certainly not all nerve fibers, have names. Most major nerves derive their names from their location. Some, particularly those associated with the brain stem, are named for their function. When the layperson refers to a nerve, they are referring to a fascicle.

Some basic vocabulary: A collection of nerve cell bodies within the brain is referred to as a **nucleus**. A "nucleus" that occurs outside the brain is known as a **ganglion**. Some of these are readily seen on dissection and appear as a small white or beige swelling with a number of nerves radiating out from them. Many ganglia are associated with the autonomic nervous system.

The Synapse

The synapse (Figure 7.2) is the space between two communication neurons or a neuron communicating with a tissue. Information travels from the dendrites through the soma and axon and ends at the terminal boutons. The terminal bouton is the **presynaptic** neuron or the neuron before the synapse. The tissue or nerve after the synapse is called **postsynaptic**, which receives information from the presynaptic neuron. Information travels from the terminal bouton to the postsynaptic tissue (either another neuron or other tissue like muscle) by way of neurotransmitters. Neurotransmitters are chemical messengers stored in the terminal boutons in **vesicles**, which are like storage packages. The synapse is a physical space, which means the neurons don't actually touch the tissue receiving information on a microscopic level. The postsynaptic tissue has receptors on it that are specific to select neurotransmitters.

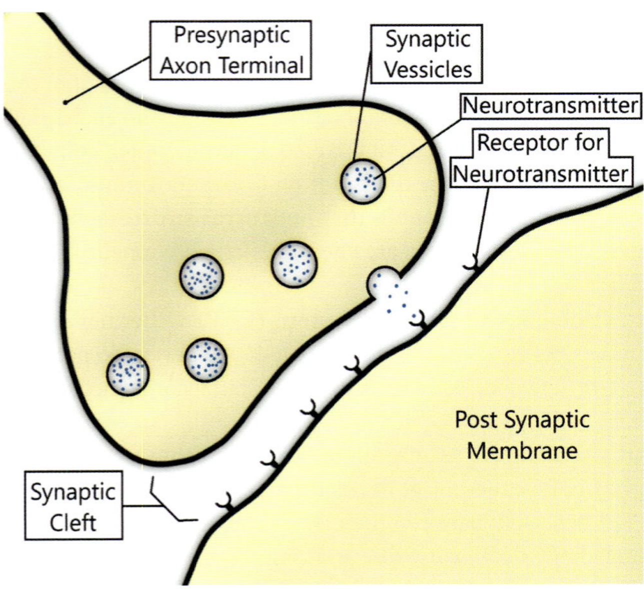

Figure 7.2 The synapse. A presynaptic axon terminal communicates with a postsynaptic membrane. The postsynaptic membrane can be that of another neuron or any tissue.

The Meninges

Surrounding the brain and spinal tissue is a set of connective tissues called the **meninges**. The outermost layer is called the **dura mater**; it is essentially fused to the skull in most mammalian species, where it covers the brain, just as the periosteum is fused to the bone. Deep to the dura mater is the **subdural space**, deep to which is the delicate weblike layer, the **arachnoid membrane**. The space deep to it, the **subarachnoid space**, is where the cerebrospinal fluid circulates around the brain and spinal cord. The innermost layer, which sits directly on the brain or spinal cord, is called the **pia mater**. These layers make up a complex network of blood vessels and **cerebrospinal fluid** that supply nutrients and oxygen to the superficial layers of the brain and spinal cord.

The Brain

An expansion of the subarachnoid space, called the **cisterna magna**, is an area near the transition of the cerebellum into the medulla oblongata. It is from this space that we sample cerebrospinal fluid to check for certain diseases; the common name of this procedure is a cervical or cisternal spinal tap. The animal should be in lateral recumbency, with its nose at a 90° angle to the spinal column; in other words, you should be facing the dorsal neck, with the spinal column as straight as possible and the space as accessible as possible. The placement of the sampling needle should be on the midline, between the occipital condyles (cranially) and the wings of the atlas (caudally). As might be imagined, serious damage can be inflicted if the needle penetrates the spinal cord, so the animal must be under general anesthesia. Another space for sampling cerebrospinal fluid can also be utilized by sampling from an area between two of the distal lumbar vertebrae; the exact location depends to some extent on the size of the animal.

The surface of the mammalian brain is composed of a series of folds (Figure 7.3). The folds are called **gyri** (singular: gyrus), and the valleys between them are **sulci** (singular: sulcus). The gyri help increase the surface area of the brain and allow for more brain function. Avians have a smoother brain surface, which we associate with the capacity for fewer complex or integrative thought processes. Animals without a true brain, such as sea stars, are not believed to have any higher brain function and presumably do not interpret stimuli but merely react reflexively.

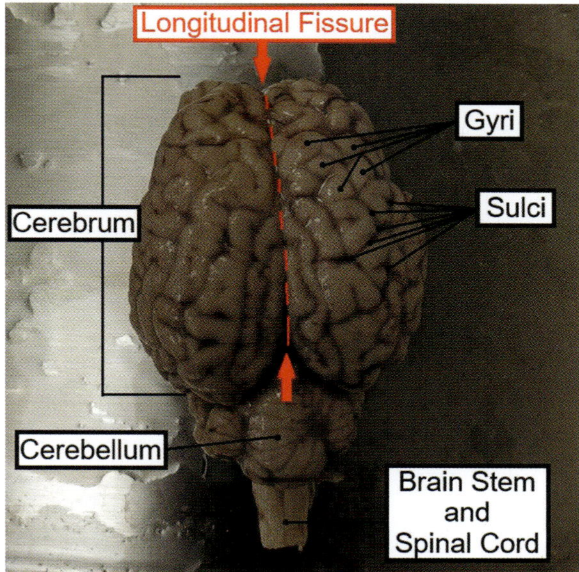

Figure 7.3 The sections of the brain: cerebrum, cerebellum, and brainstem. Also shown are the peaks and valleys, or gyri and sulci, as well as the longitudinal fissure that divides the right and left half of the cerebrum.

The brain is comprised of a few main sections. The **cerebrum** is the largest section of the brain and is comprised of several lobes that are demarcated by their location relative to the skull. The **cerebellum** is caudal to the cerebrum and is smaller comparatively. The **brainstem** is the lower extension of the brain and connects to the spinal cord. Included in the brainstem are the **midbrain, pons**, and **medulla oblongata**. The **diencephalon** is situated in between the two halves of the cerebrum and rostral to the midbrain and is sometimes referred to as the "in between brain." Within the brain are **ventricles**, areas that act as reservoirs for cerebrospinal fluid. They are numbered and drain different areas of the brain, depending on their location. As the brain is critical for survival, it is protected in a number of ways. The bony and soft tissues of the skull, along with the cerebrospinal fluid, help to protect the brain from trauma. Along with this, gross anatomical protection is a cellular level of protection called the **blood–brain barrier**.

The Cerebrum

The cerebrum is separated into **cerebral cortex** and **corpus callosum**. The cerebral cortex is the more superficial portion of the cerebrum and is gray matter. It is here that we find the gyri and sulci. The cerebral cortex is divided down the center into two hemispheres and is comprised of lobes called the **frontal lobe, parietal lobe, temporal lobe**, and **occipital lobe**. Each of these lobes is paired with one on the left and right of the brain. There is no clear boundary of each lobe when looking at the superficial brain surface. The deep sulcus that divides the right and left hemispheres is called the **longitudinal fissure** (Figure 7.4). A small protuberance at the rostral cerebrum is the **olfactory bulb**, which is involved in the sense of smell.

The two gray matter cerebral cortex hemispheres of the brain are connected by a "C-shaped" band of white matter called the **corpus callosum**. The corpus callosum allows the two hemispheres of the cerebral cortex to communicate with one another. It is located at the very center of the cerebrum.

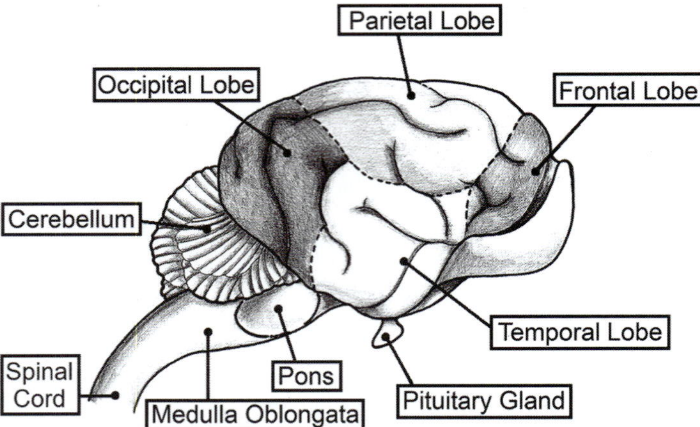

Figure 7.4 The lobes of the brain.

The Cerebellum

Caudal to the cerebrum is a rounded structure known as the **cerebellum**. This is the second largest portion of the mammalian brain. Similar to the cerebrum, the cortex is gray matter. Making a longitudinal incision in this area will reveal a pattern that resembles the branches of a tree. These structures are collectively referred to as the **arbor vitae** (tree of life) and are the white matter tracts within this part of the brain. This area of the brain is responsible for the coordination of movement. Some animals are born with a malformation of the cerebellum in which the tissue is smaller than normal or not completely developed. This is known as **cerebellar hypoplasia**, and it causes a wobbly gait, poor balance, and difficulty maneuvering in the environment.

The Brainstem

The brain stem is caudoventral to the cerebellum and tapers at its caudal point to become the spinal cord. The brainstem is the most primitive part of the brain and lacks the distinct gray and white matter layering seen in the cerebrum and cerebellum. As mentioned earlier, the brainstem contains the midbrain, pons, and medulla oblongata. The midbrain is sometimes referred to as the mesencephalon, and it is a complex structure that helps control many functions, such as hearing and movement. The pons is found on the ventral portion of the brainstem and protrudes slightly. It is the origin site for some of the cranial nerves, which will be discussed later. The pons helps to control many functions like chewing and focusing vision. Its name reflects the Latin root word meaning bridge, as the pons serves to bridge the midbrain and the medulla oblongata. The medulla oblongata, although fairly small in size relative to the cerebrum, is vital for life. It is the caudal-most portion of the brain and connects the brain to the spinal cord. It is here that we find the control center that regulates breathing and heart rate, among other important tasks (Figure 7.5).

Diencephalon

The diencephalon or "in-between" brain is situated in between the rostral hemispheres of the cerebrum. It contains one of the main ventricles of the brain as well as some critically important structures like the **thalamus** and **hypothalamus**. The thalamus is like a relay station for regulating sensory and motor information and delivering the information to the cerebral cortex. The hypothalamus oversees regulating many factors of homeostasis like temperature, appetite, and growth, among many others, which will be discussed in later chapters. It is also responsible for communication between the nervous system and the endocrine system. The diencephalon acts as a passageway between the primitive brainstem and the cerebrum.

The Blood–Brain Barrier

The blood–brain barrier is one of the many features to protect the brain. The blood–brain barrier (occasionally abbreviated as BBB) acts as a functional barrier separating the blood supply in the brain from the nervous tissue itself. In a normal vessel

Figure 7.5 The bisected brain.

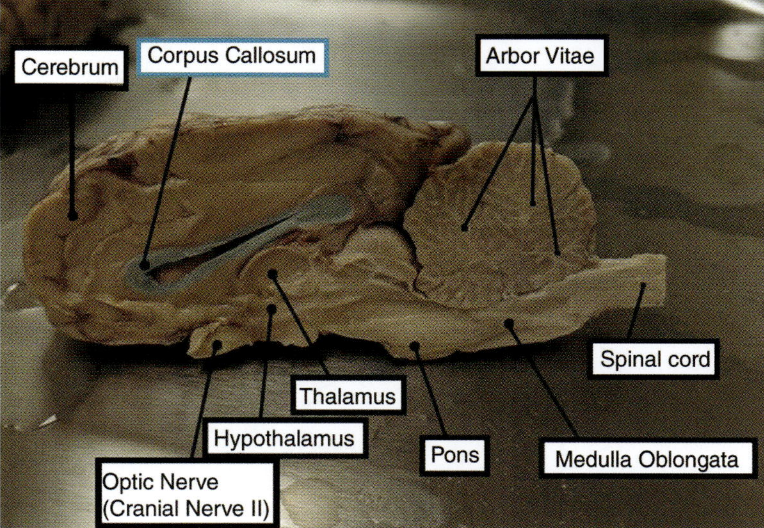

(vein or artery) wall, there are microscopic holes or **fenestrations** for chemicals to pass through to the surrounding tissue. In the brain, the vessel walls have no fenestrations, which is one step in the blood–brain barrier's protection. Because these spaces don't exist, it makes it very challenging for anything to exit the blood vessels and enter the nervous tissue of the brain. The second step of the blood–brain barrier is specialized glial cells called **astrocytes** (Figure 7.6). These cells wrap around the vessels in the brain to form an additional wall of protection with very narrow openings. The blood–brain barrier is extraordinarily effective, blocking 100% of large molecular drugs and only allowing about 2% of small molecular drugs through and into the brain tissue.

Cranial Nerves

The cranial nerves are nerve cell bundles, each of which serves one or more specific functions. Their names are associated with their target (the part of the body they aim toward) or their function. See Table 7.1 for their names and numbers; note that we use Roman numerals to denote the numbers.

    Cranial nerve I, the **olfactory nerve**, emerges from the olfactory bulbs of the cerebrum and runs near the nasal cavity. The **optic nerve, cranial nerve II**, arises on the ventral surface of the brain to the retina of each eye. The area where some of the nerve fibers from each eye cross to the opposite side of the brain is called the **optic chiasm**, which can be seen on the ventral surface of the brain. The remainder of the cranial nerves originate from the brainstem. **Cranial nerves III and IV**, or the **oculomotor nerve** and **trochlear** nerve, arise from the midbrain. The **trigeminal nerve (cranial nerve V)** originates from the pons and is the largest of the cranial nerves. **Cranial nerves VI to XII** arise from the medulla oblongata area. (Figure 7.7) Among this set is **Cranial nerve X**, or the **vagus nerve**. The vagus nerve is sometimes called "the wanderer" as it travels almost the entire length of the body and is the mediator of the autonomic nervous system (see Figure 7.8). We will discuss this at greater length in the physiology section.

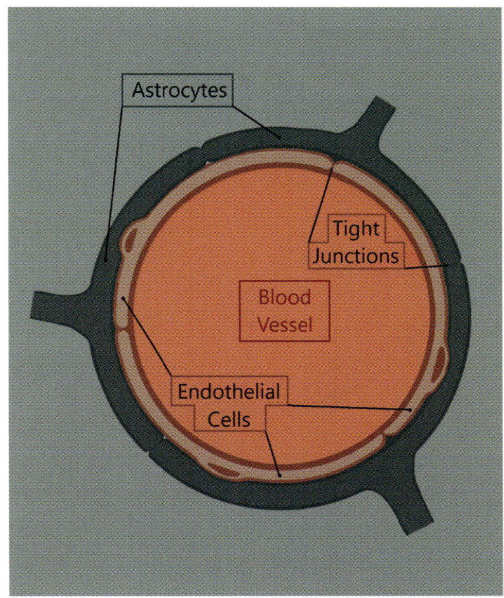

Figure 7.6 The blood–brain barrier. Note the tight junctions between the epithelial cells forming the vessel as well as between the astrocytes surrounding it.

Table 7.1 The Cranial Nerves.

I: Olfactory	VII: Facial
II: Optic	VIII: Vestibulocochlear
III: Oculomotor	IX: Glossopharyngeal
IV: Trochlear	X: Vagus
V: Trigeminal	XI: Spinal accessory
VI: Abducens	XII: Hypoglossal

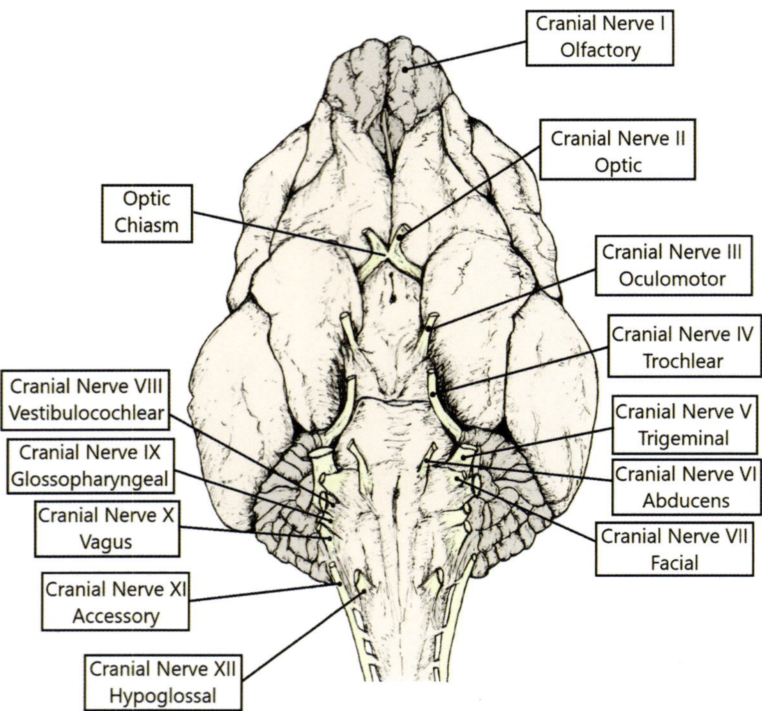

Figure 7.7 The cranial nerves as they emerge from the ventral side of the brain.

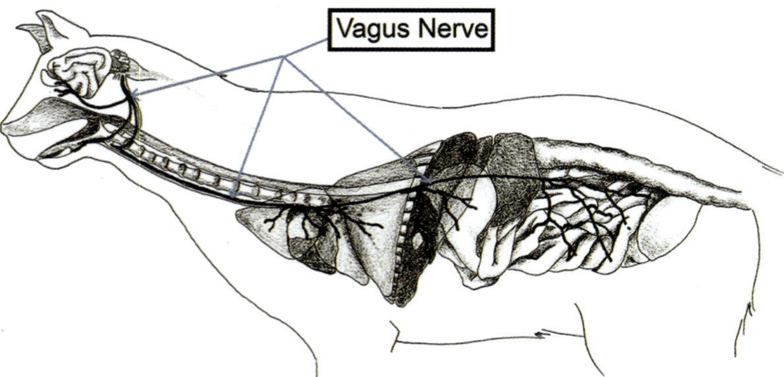

Figure 7.8 The vagus nerve (from the Latin root word for "wanderer") is the longest nerve of the body. It is cranial nerve X and is one of the major carriers of information for the autonomic nervous system.

The Spinal Cord

The brain stem narrows as it runs caudally, but it widens again slightly at the medulla oblongata as it approaches the **foramen magnum**. The spinal cord has meninges similar to the brain, with one exception. Superficial to the dura, between the dura mater and the wall of the spinal canal, is a space called the **epidural space**. The epidural space is an area in which local anesthetic is often injected prior to surgical procedures in the area.

The body of the spinal cord consists of white matter on the superficial surface with a gray matter core. This is the opposite of brain structure, in which the gray matter is on the outside and white matter is deep to it. On the transverse section of the spinal cord, the gray matter is shaped like a butterfly. Nerves enter and exit the spinal cord as a trunk called the dorsal or ventral root. There is one on each side, in the dorsal or ventral area of the cord. See Figure 20.2 for a schematic drawing of a section of the spinal cord. There is a channel that runs through the whole spinal cord called the **central canal**, which is filled with cerebrospinal fluid and connects with the cerebrospinal fluid-filled ventricles of the brain.

The spinal cord does not go all the way through the body to the end of the tail. In the area of the sacrum, the spinal cord fans out into a series of smaller nerves. This area is known as the **cauda equina**—literally, horse's tail—which it resembles. Peripheral nerves radiate out from this area.

Peripheral Nervous System

The peripheral nervous system is the series of nerves outside of the brain and coming off the spinal cord, with the exception of the cranial nerves. Although the cranial nerves originate from different areas of the brain, they are considered part of the peripheral nervous system since they innervate and help control body parts outside of the brain. The peripheral nervous system works to connect the central nervous system to the limbs and organs, serving as a relay between the CNS and the body.

A **plexus** is an interlacing series of multiple nerve fiber junctions (not neuronal bodies, which is what distinguishes it from a ganglion). There is a **cervical plexus** that involves many of the nerves supplying the neck and diaphragm. There is also the **brachial plexus**, a large area of nerves serving the thoracic limb. It is easily seen in the area of the axilla (where the thoracic limb meets the body) once the surrounding musculature is reflected. Another major plexus is the **lumbar plexus**.

Nerves supplying the head include many of the cranial nerves; one-third of them have some specific function related to the eye. The trigeminal nerve runs in part along the mandible. The **auriculopalpebral nerve** is a branch of the facial nerve (cranial nerve VII) and courses in an area around the rostral pinna and the eyes. It is a convenient place to deliver analgesic medication when doing eye surgery.

In the thoracic limb, there are a few nerves of major importance. The **radial nerve** runs along the lateral surface all the way to the paw. This nerve is the one that is responsible for the pain response when blood is taken from the thoracic limb (usually from the cephalic vein). The **median nerve** runs along the medial surface, dividing into medial and lateral branches at the paw. A tourniquet that is too tight may compress either of these nerves to the point where damage occurs. In this case, given that these nerves affect the entire limb, significant lameness will result. The **ulnar nerve** also runs along the medial surface of the antebrachium toward the paw.

The pelvic limb has several major nerves. The **femoral nerve** arises directly from the spinal cord and supplies much of the medial femoral area. The **saphenous nerve** arises from the cranial femoral nerve and continues to run distally to the tarsus.

The **ischiatic** or **sciatic nerve** is very thick and is easily located deep to the muscles biceps femoris and semitendinosus (see Figure 7.9). It innervates much of the pelvic limb. It is very important to avoid impinging on this nerve when giving an

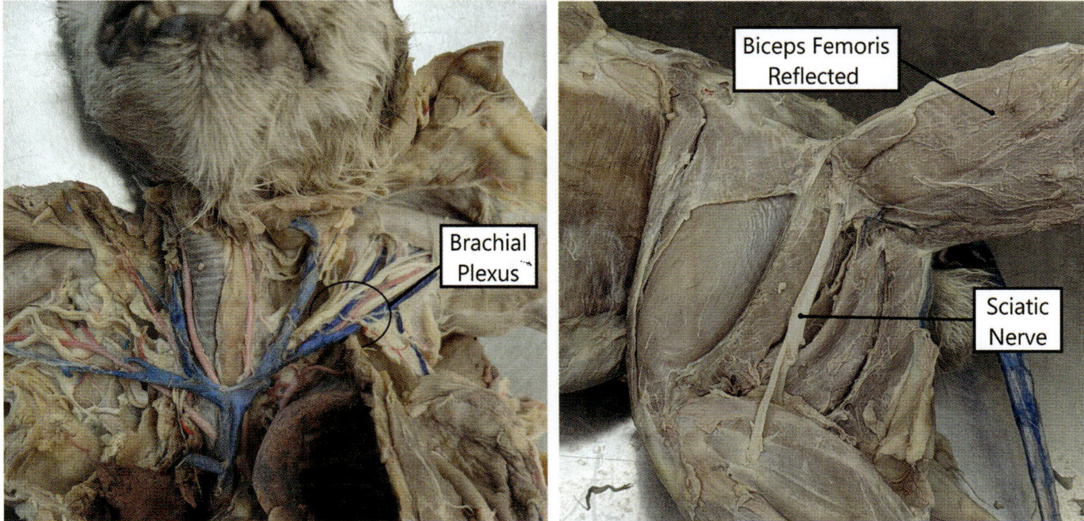

Figure 7.9 The brachial plexus and the sciatic or ischiatic nerve.

intramuscular injection. Some people avoid the problem entirely by using the cranial rather than the caudal thigh when giving an injection. Damage to this nerve can, at worst, cause complete loss of function of the limb.

The **pudendal nerve** arises from the area of the sacrum and has an impact on the pelvis, genitalia, rectum, and perineum. One of its branches is the **caudal rectal nerve**. This nerve supplies the external anal sphincter. Any surgery in the area of the rectum needs to be done avoiding this nerve. The consequence of damaging it can be incontinence for feces. Surgery done in this area might be removal of the anal sacs (sebaceous glands on either side of the anus) or repair of a perineal fistula (an opening into the body in the area of the anus, lateral to it).

Clinical Case Resolution: Petey

A physical exam is done on Petey, which is normal aside from his abnormal gait. Although he has a slightly thin body condition, he is well muscled and his coat appears improved from the owner's initial description. A neurologic exam is performed, which reveals a bright and alert disposition with intact reflexes. Upon attempting to play during the exam, Petey seems to have some head tremors. Bedside bloodwork is normal, and the remainder of his examinations are within normal limits.

*Based on the physical exam and blood results, it is presumed that Petey has cerebellar hypoplasia (CH). This congenital disease cannot be cured, but managed with safe indoor only areas, low entry litter boxes and flat no-spill food and water dishes. Most cats with CH have normal lives despite their poor coordination and the condition is non-painful. To confirm this diagnosis, imaging of the brain via CT scan or MRI can be performed but is often not necessary. CT scans get their abbreviation from **c**omputed **t**omography which uses radiation to produce an image of bones and soft tissue. MRI scans get their abbreviation from **m**agnetic **r**esonance **i**maging which uses magnetic fields and radio waves to produce an image of bones and soft tissue.*

Review Questions

1   What is an alternate name for the neuron cell body?
  A Dendrites
  B Soma
  C Nucleus
  D Axon

2   Which glial cells are found in the peripheral nervous system?

3   True or False: White matter has a myelin sheath and is always found in the deeper layers of the central nervous system.

4   Which part of the nervous system has vesicles filled with neurotransmitters?
  A The axon
  B The synaptic knobs
  C The postsynaptic tissue
  D The astrocytes

5   What is the name of the white matter tissue that allows the right and left cerebral hemispheres to communicate?

6   Mesencephalon is another term for:
  A The pons
  B The "in between" brain
  C The midbrain
  D The medulla oblongata

7   Explain the difference between the meninges in the brain and the spinal cord.

8 Which of the following cranial nerves arises from the cerebrum?
  A Cranial nerve III
  B Cranial nerve VII
  C Cranial nerve X
  D Cranial nerve II

9 In which area of the body can we find the brachial plexus?

10 What nerve is in a common location for intramuscular injections and should be avoided?
  A The ischiatic nerve
  B The femoral nerve
  C The radial nerve
  D The cauda equina

8

Anatomy of the Endocrine System

> **Clinical Case: Eloise, a 16-Year-Old Female Spayed Domestic Short Hair Cat**
>
> *Eloise has not been to the vet in a few years, but the owner is concerned about her. The owner notes that Eloise is losing weight despite eating more food and has become very vocal, particularly at night. She also notes that Eloise seems to be drinking and urinating more. Eloise is an only cat and only lives with her one owner.*

Introduction

The endocrine system is largely responsible for the metabolism of cats and dogs. Its malfunction is the cause of a wide variety of common chronic diseases. We will discuss the physiology of the system in detail in Chapter 21. Its systemic anatomy is somewhat unusual in that it is a single system which has components spread throughout the body. Remember that organ systems do not need to be in close anatomical proximity. The endocrine system works closely with the nervous system to orchestrate a unified response to any bodily changes. Sometimes the two systems are referred to together as the neuroendocrine system.

The constituents of the endocrine system are referred to as **glands**. Unlike other glands (e.g., those of the skin), they do not have ducts that conduct their products to other areas or organs. Their products, **hormones**, are carried through the body as a result of close contact between the endocrine gland and the bloodstream. Therefore in addition to rich neural innervations, they are well-vascularized.

The Hypothalamus

There are a number of sites throughout the central nervous system that play a role in the management of endocrine products or hormones. One of the primary sites for the endocrine system is in the brain, specifically the diencephalon, called the **hypothalamus**. The hypothalamus is made of grey and white matter, similar to other structures of the central nervous system. The hypothalamus produces **neurohormones**, which are chemical messengers that are able to be read and understood by the nervous system and the endocrine system. This is how the brain communicates to direct the endocrine system and maintain homeostasis. The hypothalamus transmits these neurohormones through the **portal system**, which is a series of blood vessels that take the message to the **anterior pituitary**. The hypothalamus can also communicate through the **pituitary stalk** which is a series of nerves and vessels that take the information or products to the **posterior pituitary gland**.

The Pituitary

The pituitary gland is a small but powerful bilobed gland on the ventral brain that sits in a small fossa on the ventral surface of the skull called the **sella turcica**. The pituitary is ellipsoid in shape and dark in color. Rostral and caudal to it is the cavernous sinus of the brain. The pituitary gland can also be referred to as the **hypophysis**. It is bilobed or divided into two lobes, and each side performs a different set of tasks. One side is called the **anterior pituitary**, which produces many hormones under the direction of the hypothalamus. The anterior pituitary can also be called the **adenohypophysis**, as microscopically it appears glandular in nature, and adeno is the root word for gland. The other side is called the posterior pituitary, which also communicates with, and stores products from, the hypothalamus. The alternate name for the posterior pituitary is the **neurohypophysis**, as it appears as nervous tissue under the microscope. Technically, there is a third portion of the pituitary called the **intermediate lobe**, which is a thin layer of cells in between the anterior and posterior pituitary. In humans, it is quite underdeveloped, it is absent in birds, but it may be significant in fish as it has an impact on the color change of scales. The large variety of hormones produced and released earned the pituitary the title of the "master endocrine gland."

Pineal Gland

Another gland in this area is the **pineal gland** or **pineal body**. Its name comes from the root word "pineapple," which it is said to resemble. It is in the area of the third ventricle of the brain. It is also known as the **epiphysis** and will not be readily identifiable on necropsy. The pineal gland is responsible for managing the circadian rhythm or sleep–wake cycles. In reptiles, some breeds have a pineal gland that resides on the dorsal brain and actually receives sunlight directly from the outside. This is useful for animals that govern their metabolism using hours of daylight to restrict or increase activity.

The Peripheral Endocrine System

Glands that function only in producing and/or managing the production of hormones are known as primary endocrine glands. There are several primary endocrine glands throughout the rest of the body including the thyroid, parathyroid, and adrenal gland. Secondary endocrine glands are areas manufacturing hormones that are within organs or tissues that have nonendocrine features. These include the pancreas, the gonads (either testes or ovaries), the kidney, the stomach, the small intestine, and the thymus.

The Thyroid

One of the major primary endocrine glands is the **thyroid gland**. It is a C-shaped gland that wraps around the trachea from the lateral to the dorsal surface and then to the other lateral surface. Depending on the species, the dorsal connection can be very thin or the same width as the rest of the gland. The thyroid is dark red in color and has a connective tissue covering. It is considered to consist of two lobes. Cytologically, the thyroid has a unique appearance, consisting of tens of thousands of **follicles**. They are rounded in appearance and full of **colloid**, which is the precursor to thyroid hormones.

Under normal conditions, it should not be easily palpable in dogs and cats. During the physical exam, running the fingers along either side of the trachea may yield the sensation of a swelling that interrupts the smooth flow of the palpation. This is known as "**thyroid slip**" and is associated with enlargement of the thyroid gland. This enlargement is associated with **hyperthyroidism**, a condition common in older cats that causes increased appetite and weight loss.

The Parathyroid

In viewing the thyroid gland on dissection, one may observe a small lump on the surface of the thyroid or partially embedded within it (Figure 8.1). There is one on each side, and they are referred to as the **parathyroid glands**. They are pale in color. As will be seen later, they have a great deal to do with calcium and phosphorus balance within the body. One reason that thyroidectomy, or removal of the thyroid, is rarely employed as a treatment for hyperthyroidism is that it is difficult to avoid disrupting the parathyroid glands in the process.

The Adrenals

Another primary endocrine gland is the **adrenal gland**. The adrenal glands are small, pinkish, smooth structures slightly cranial or craniomedial to the kidney (see Figure 8.2). There is one on each side of the body. The adrenals are firm and solid and have two sections: a **medulla** and a **cortex**. This gland will often be surrounded by fat, so careful displacement of the perirenal fat layer is important. Running on the ventral surface of the adrenal gland are the thoracolumbar vein and artery.

The adrenal gland has bands of tissue, each of which produces discrete hormones (Figure 8.3). The **adrenal cortex** produces glucocorticoids, mineralocorticoids, and reproductive hormones. The **adrenal medulla**, deep to the cortex and more or less in the center of the gland, produces important chemicals that can be considered both hormones and neurotransmitters.

The Pancreas

The best known of the secondary endocrine glands is the endocrine tissue within the pancreas. The endocrine areas of the pancreas are called the **islets of Langerhans**, where specialized cells called **alpha (α)**, **beta (β)**, and **delta (δ) cells** produce hormones. These areas are involved in the production of insulin, among other hormones. The function of the alpha, beta, and delta cells of the islets will be discussed in Chapter 21. Bear in mind that these structures are microscopic. Gross inspection of the pancreas on dissection will not yield an appreciable difference in structure between the endocrine and nonendocrine tissues within the pancreas.

Because the pancreas has a connection to the duodenum for the transfer of digestive enzymes, inflammatory bowel disease can be associated with pancreatitis. Pancreatitis, in turn, can be associated with inflammation of the endocrine sections as well, which is why diabetes mellitus (an insulin-based disorder) can be associated with chronic enteritis and/or pancreatitis.

The Gonads

Parts of the reproductive system have secondary endocrine tissue. These include the testes and ovaries. The **testes** in the male are located in the scrotum and are oval in shape. They comprise a series of interconnected tubules and channels that are related to the creation and movement of sperm. In between the tubules in the testes are **interstitial cells** which are responsible for producing male sex hormones, or **androgens**.

The **ovaries** are located in the caudal abdomen or in the pelvic canal, depending on the species. They are small and oval in shape

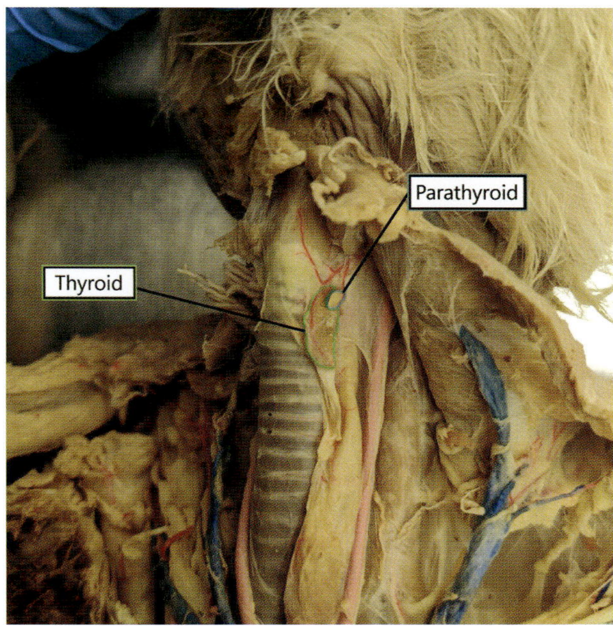

Figure 8.1 The thyroid and parathyroid glands viewed with the animal in dorsal recumbency. Note that they do not cover the ventral surface of the trachea. The cartilaginous rings that support the trachea are clearly visible as the white bands that wrap horizontally around the trachea.

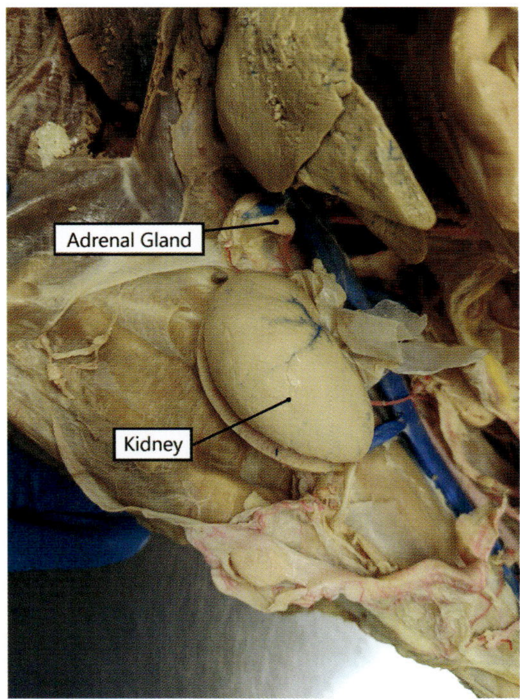

Figure 8.2 The adrenal glands just beyond the cranial pole of the kidney.

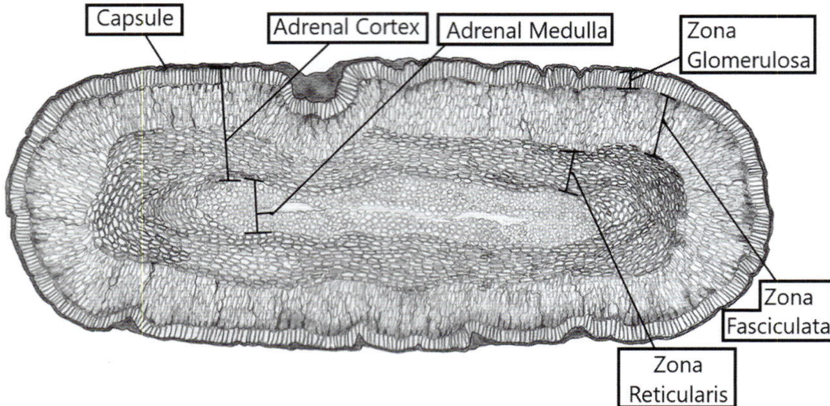

Figure 8.3 The bisected adrenal gland showing the cortex and medulla. The areas of the cortex are the zona glomerulosa, which produces mineralocorticoids; the zona fasciculata, which produces glucocorticoids; and the zona reticularis, which produces small amounts of sex hormones.

and are suspended by a thin tissue to secure them to the body wall and the remainder of the reproductive tract. The ovaries work to produce mature ova in a cyclical pattern, the timing of which is variable among the species. The ovaries work to produce hormones like **estrogens and progestins** in response to stimuli from the anterior pituitary. In pregnancy, **relaxin**, a hormone meant to help relax the muscle and ligaments of the pelvic girdle, may be produced by the ovaries or placenta.

The **placenta** is another reproductive organ formed during pregnancy that has endocrine function. It works to support the health of the fetus and maintain the pregnancy while also secreting small amounts of progesterone, estrogen, relaxin, and chorionic gonadotropin.

The Kidney

Another part of the secondary endocrine system is the **nephron**, the functioning unit of the kidney. A small number of endocrine cells within the nephron, particularly close to the glomerulus, produce a hormone called **erythropoietin**. This chemical messenger is vital in stimulating the bone marrow to produce red blood cells and is one of the reasons that we associate chronic kidney disease in its more severe states with anemia. Without those endocrine cells, bone marrow no longer produces sufficient red blood cells. There is another set of specialized cells in the kidney called **juxtaglomerular cells** which produce the hormone **renin**. Renin works in a multistep system to help regulate blood pressure.

The Gastrointestinal Tract

The gastrointestinal tract has a few areas that have some endocrine function. The stomach is a pouch in the abdominal cavity that receives food and water from the esophagus and moves it along to the intestines. The stomach has specialized cells, called **G cells**, in the stomach wall that produce **gastrin**. Gastrin helps to initiate and sustain the chemical digestion process.

The small intestine is the next part of the gastrointestinal tract after the stomach. This long narrow tube helps to move digesta forward and absorb nutrients. There are specialized cells in the small intestine that produce **secretin** and **cholecystokinin**. Both of these hormones work to help the effective digestion of food by a series of mechanisms which will be discussed in Chapter 25.

The Thymus

The **thymus** is a gland found in the mediastinum just ventral to the heart. This tissue can be seen if a dissection is performed by opening the thoracic cavity at the ventral midline. It will overlay the cranial heart or aortic arch and can easily be inadvertently removed as the tissue is delicate. The thymus produces **thymosin** and **thymopoietin** among other hormones that work to help the body produce and mature T cells, an important player in the immune system.

Small amounts of endocrine tissue are also found within other tissue like the liver. There are even small amounts of endocrine tissue in the heart. Again, none of these endocrine materials are macroscopic.

Clinical Case Resolution: Eloise

Eloise has a full physical exam which confirms the owners concerns of weight loss. It also shows some mild muscle loss and an unkempt haircoat. Upon palpation of the ventral neck, an approximately 2 cm unilateral mass is noted in the location of the thyroid on the right side. The patient history, presentation, and physical exam are all strongly suggestive of hyperthyroidism.

In order to substantiate these suspicions, blood work is performed to check a complete blood count, chemistry and electrolyte values, and thyroid levels. Blood work results confirm that Eloise has hyperthyroidism, and treatment options are discussed with the owner.

Please note—this case is continued in the Endocrine Physiology chapter, where a deeper look at the physiologic mechanisms of hyperthyroidism is explored.

Review Questions

1 Which endocrine organ is contained in the sella turcica?
  A The hypophysis
  B The hypothalamus
  C The thyroid
  D The G cells

2 Where can the parathyroid gland be found?
  A In the abdominal cavity, near the kidney
  B In the brain, near the hypothalamus
  C In the thoracic cavity, near the trachea
  D In the mediastinum, cranioventral to the heart

3 What function does the pineal gland serve?

4 Which organ has the islets of Langerhans?
  A The pancreas
  B The stomach
  C The kidneys
  D The brain

5 True or False: The hypothalamus directly communicated with the anterior and posterior pituitary.

6 Which endocrine gland is considered the "master endocrine gland"?
  A The hypothalamus
  B The hypophysis
  C The thyroid
  D The pineal gland

7 Which portion of the adrenal gland produces neurotransmitters?

8 Which organ would be responsible for communicating with the bone marrow that the body needs more red blood cells?
  A The stomach
  B The brain
  C The bones
  D The kidneys

9 Which endocrine organ directly helps in building and maturing cells of the immune system?

10 True or False: The testes have no exocrine function and only endocrine functions.

9

Anatomy of the Urinary Tract

> **Clinical Case: Bert, a 3-Year-Old Male Castrated Domestic Medium Hair Cat**
>
> *Bert is presented to the emergency room for lethargy and vomiting. The owner reports she has three other cats at home and Bert is the only one that appears ill. Upon brief triage examination, Bert's bladder is very firm and large.*

Introduction

The urinary system in cats and dogs shares many similarities to that of humans. The urinary system anatomy is contained in the retroperitoneal space and the peritoneum. The primary job of the urinary system is to filter blood and remove waste by creating urine. The urinary system consists of the kidneys, the ureters, the bladder, and the urethra and ends at the urethral opening (Figure 9.1).

The Kidneys

Physiologically complex, the urinary system can be said to begin with the kidneys. In dogs and cats, there are two, one on each side of the animal. They reside in the dorsal abdomen, approximately deep to the cranial lumbar vertebrae. The right kidney lies cranially in the abdomen relative to the left kidney. This spatial difference reflects the position of the heart toward the left of the midline, only leaving room for the left kidney more caudally. The cranial and caudal borders of the kidneys are called the **cranial** and **caudal poles**. The cranial pole of the right kidney is nestled against a hepatic fossa, which is a shallow depression, so named because it resembles the fossa of a bone. It is in a more fixed position as a result of this, compared with the left kidney.

In most species of mammals, the kidneys rest in the **retroperitoneal cavity**, which is to say dorsal to the peritoneal membrane that surrounds the abdominal cavity and most of its internal organs. They generally can be palpated with firm exploration of the cranial abdomen in smaller animals. The outer surface is often surrounded by a layer or partial layer of fat.

The superficial surface of the kidney is covered by the **renal capsule** composed of fibrous material (Figure 9.2). In life, the kidney has a dark red/brown color. Its shape is that of an oval with an indentation on the medial surface. This forms the derivation of the name of the kidney bean. This indentation is known as the **renal hilus** and is the point of entry and exit for the renal artery and vein, as well as the ureter. Note that not all mammals have kidneys in this shape. For example, the dolphin kidney resembles a cluster of grapes. The kidney of the horse has a Valentine heart shape and that of the bovine is lobed.

On the surface of the kidney, a large number of vessels are noted. In its role as the filter of all the blood in the body, its vascularization is complex. The interior layer of the kidney just deep to the capsule is referred to as the **renal cortex** (see Figure 9.3). It is a relatively narrow, brick-red area that has a granular appearance. This may appear beige in a preserved specimen. Its deeper border has a scalloped appearance. This border is referred to as the **corticomedullary boundary**. Deep to this boundary is the **renal medulla**. It is darker red than the cortex and has a striated appearance. It has a much larger surface area than the cortex.

Anatomy and Physiology for Veterinary Technicians and Nurses: A Clinical Approach, Second Edition. Lori Asprea.
© 2026 John Wiley & Sons, Inc. Published 2026 by John Wiley & Sons, Inc.
Companion website: www.wiley.com/go/asprea/anatomy_vettech2e

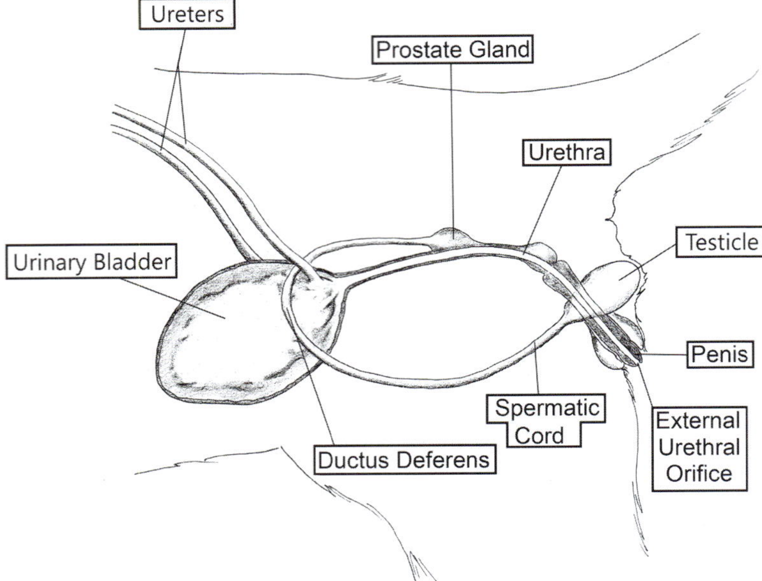

Figure 9.1 The general structure of the urinary system, which starts at the kidney and ends at the distal urethra. While this drawing is of a male (the prostate gland, testicles, and ductus defers/spermatic cord is only found in males), the female architecture is similar. Notice that the interior of the urinary bladder is wrinkled. This gives it extra surface area so that it can expand and contract.

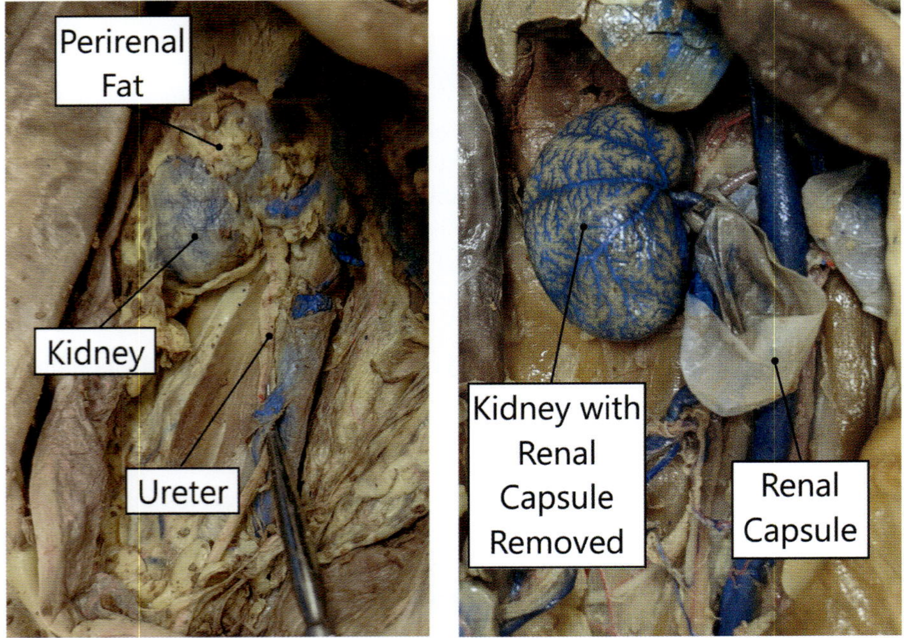

Figure 9.2 The kidney. In dogs and cats, the kidney is surrounded by the renal capsule.

The Nephron

The functional unit of the kidney is a microscopic structure called the **nephron** (Figure 9.4). The nephron travels between the cortex and the medulla. While there are many nephrons in all mammals, the exact number is species specific and relative to the size of the animal. For example, an elephant has more nephrons than a cat.

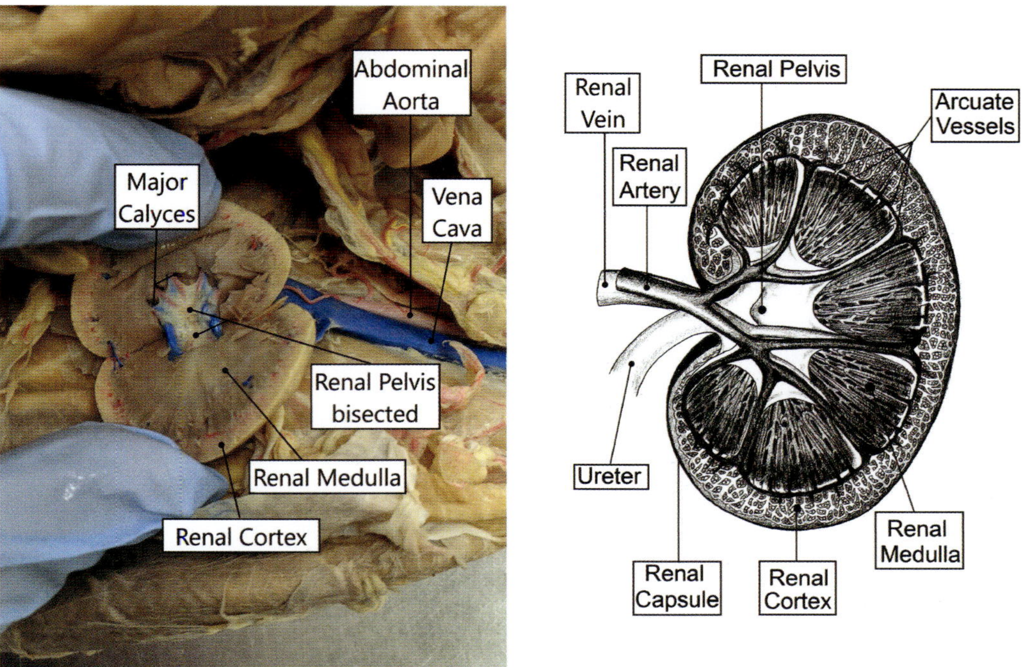

Figure 9.3 The bisected kidney. Note that the size of the animal will limit the visible detail within the bisected kidney.

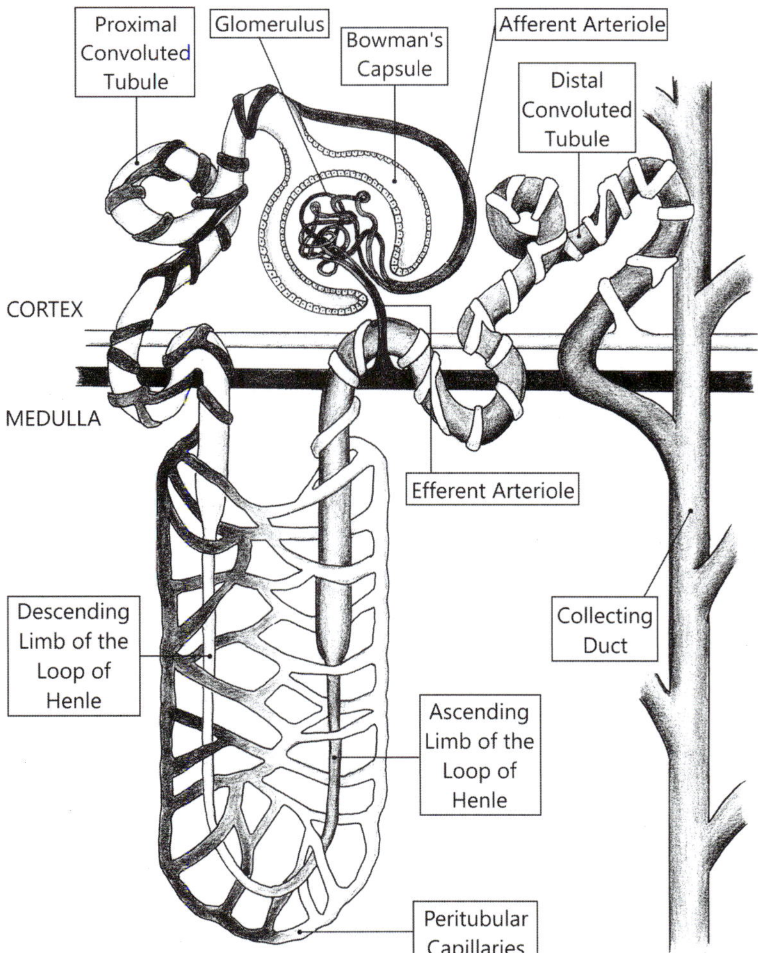

Figure 9.4 The nephron. This image also appears in Chapter 22.

The nephron has its own important anatomy, and the functions of the nephron will be discussed heavily in Chapter 22. The nephron begins with the **renal corpuscle**, a structure that has two distinct parts. The first part of the renal corpuscle is the **glomerulus**, which is a tuft of microscopic blood vessels that bring blood into the kidney from the renal artery. These vessels have small fenestrations, or holes, on the surface to allow for filtration. Surrounding the glomerulus is the second part of the renal corpuscle called **Bowman's capsule**. Bowman's capsule then funnels into a tube which is broken down into three parts. The first part of the tube is the **proximal convoluted tubule (PCT)** which is named as it is close to the renal corpuscle and is twisted on itself. The next portion of the nephron is the **loop of Henle**, which dips down through the medulla and then makes a U-turn and comes back up toward the cortex. Following the loop of Henle is the **distal convoluted tubule (DCT)**, named for being a twisted portion of the tube at the far end of the flow of the nephron. The distal convoluted tubule connects to a **collecting duct**. Multiple nephrons connect to each collecting duct. The collecting ducts come together as they progress deeper into the medulla of the kidney. They fan out into a series of **minor** and **major calyces** (singular calyx) which are funnels that take the liquid produced by the nephrons and help lead it out of the kidney. From the major calyces, a dilated area that is concave and whitish gray in color is formed called the **renal pelvis**. (Note again the importance of proper terminology. The *pelvis* is a bony structure; the *renal pelvis* is soft tissue.) Filtrate collects in the renal pelvis and is funneled into the **ureter**. As the liquid filtered by the kidney exits via the ureter, it is referred to as urine.

The Ureters

The ureter exits the kidney at the hilus and continues along the dorsal retroperitoneal cavity toward the urinary bladder. It curves medially, entering a connective tissue sheet called the **genital fold** in the male and the **broad ligament** in the female. The ureter enters the urinary bladder on its dorsal surface, near the neck of the urinary bladder. On rare occasions, the ureter enters the bladder in an abnormal place; this condition is known as **ectopic ureter**. Bear in mind that there will be a ureter entering the urinary bladder from each side. An important anatomical feature of the ureter is that it enters the bladder at an angle, which helps discourage the reflux of urine out of the urinary bladder when the bladder contracts.

In the intact female, the ureter runs alongside the **oviduct**, the connection between the ovary and the uterus. This is particularly important to keep in mind during ovariohysterectomy ("spay"). Severing the ureter instead of the oviduct will result in life-threatening injury. The surgeon will be careful to trace the structure carefully toward the ovary before incising it.

The ureter contains three layers of tissue. The outer layer is fibrous in nature, while the middle layer is made of smooth muscle. The inner layer is made of **transitional epithelial cells**. The middle layer of smooth muscle contracts in waves to help propel urine toward the bladder. This muscle can also go into painful spasm in certain conditions, such as when a calculus (stone) is present within it.

The Urinary Bladder

The **urinary bladder** is an oval, hollow organ that will have a gray appearance on dissection. Be cautious on incising the bladder; it may contain urine even after the death of the animal. Note the use of the phrase "urinary bladder." As there is another structure called a gallbladder in dogs and cats, the use of the single word "bladder" is imprecise.

In life, the urinary bladder is distensible and is found in the caudal abdomen. The cranial-most part of the urinary bladder is quite mobile; this allows it to fill with urine to a greater or lesser extent depending on the amount of liquid material involved. The fact that the position and size of the urinary bladder can vary means that it is very important to locate it exactly before performing **cystocentesis** (inserting a needle into the bladder to extract a sample of urine) during a physical exam. Blindly placing a needle into the abdomen in an attempt to extract urine may cause the examiner to perforate the intestine or a blood vessel. The **apex** of the bladder, the portion facing the abdominal wall, may have a short blind tunnel (a diverticulum). This is the remnant of a fetal vessel called the **urachus**. It is possible to have material, such as calculi (plural of calculus), trapped in this area. The entire urinary bladder is suspended from the dorsal abdomen by the **round ligament**, a fibrous tissue that is in part the remnant of the umbilical artery. The caudal section becomes quite narrow, and it is also referred to as the **neck of the urinary bladder**.

In the female, the urinary bladder is connected with the broad ligament, which also attaches to the uterus. In the male, the urinary bladder is within the genital fold of the membrane, which also contains the **ductus deferens**, a conduit for sperm, which will be discussed in the chapter on reproductive anatomy.

The urinary bladder has a number of layers on a gross and microscopic level. One of the important muscle layers is called the **detrusor muscle**. One of the layers of the interior epithelium is made up of **transitional cells**, similar to ureters. Seen more in dogs than in cats, **transitional cell carcinoma (TCC)** is the most common cancer of the urinary bladder.

Careful examination of the interior surface of the urinary bladder in the area of the neck may reveal three small openings. Two of these are the entrances of the right and left ureters. The other is the exit for urine as it enters the urethra. This area is the **trigone** (see Figure 9.5) and is the site of most transitional cell carcinomas.

The muscles that form the gateway between the urinary bladder and the urethra, a sphincter, have both skeletal and smooth muscle components. As such, there is both voluntary and involuntary control over the opening of the sphincter and thus of urination. Injury to the muscles or the nerves controlling them contributes to urinary incontinence, which is when the animal urinates when or where it ordinarily should not.

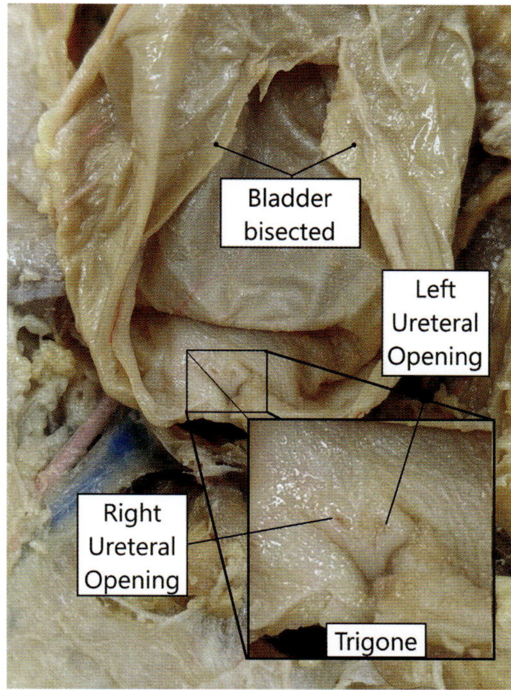

Figure 9.5 The trigone in the dissected bladder.

The Urethra

As urine exits the urinary bladder, it enters the **urethra**, which is a tube that leads to the outside of the body. This area will be difficult to uncover during dissection without fracturing or disassembling the pelvis; if observation *in situ* is desired, it is best to wait until all other dissection has been completed in order to view it.

In the female, the urethra runs along the ventral pelvis and is ventral to the reproductive tract. It passes into the vagina at the vestibular junction and becomes one passage toward the outside. As the urethra rises dorsally to make this entrance and because there can be a small turn in the vagina in that area, the placement of a urinary catheter in a female dog or cat is usually difficult. Substantial practice is required to do this effectively. The urethra is surrounded by the **urethralis muscle** and is innervated by the **pudendal nerve**. Its submucosal tissue has erectile tissue, which also contributes to continence. Otherwise, its structure is similar to that of the urinary bladder.

In the male, the urethra exits the urinary bladder and enters the penis. The pelvic part of the urethra is the section of it within the body. As the urethra exits the body, it is referred to as the **external urethra**. It is surrounded by spongy tissue as it travels the length of the penis. In the pelvic urethra, near the urinary bladder, it is joined by the reproductive ducts. This junction explains why the penis is able to discharge both urine and semen. The dorsal surface of the pelvic urethra is just deep to the rectum. For this reason, palpation of the rectum can cause muscular contraction of the urethra.

The course of the urethra in the male cat is a unique one. The cat is the only mammal whose penis faces caudally. Therefore, as the urethra extends away from the urinary bladder, it travels in a circuitous route, running caudally, then cranially, and then caudally again. This curve can cause material to become trapped if there is particulate matter (such as calculi) or mucus plugs. This results in obstruction of the urethra and causes urine to back up toward the urinary bladder, which is a critical emergency.

Avian

The avian system is quite different. From the kidney, waste material is transported to a central area in the caudal abdomen known as the **cloaca**. "Urine" is not actually liquid in the avian but is composed of urea-loaded crystals. The cloaca also accepts fecal material from the digestive tract. As a result, renal and digestive excreta exit from the same location in the animal. In fact, the egg also exits by way of the cloaca.

Clinical Case Resolution: Bert

*Upon feeling Bert's bladder, the owner is questioned on Bert's litter box habits. The owner notes they can't tell if Bert is uri-nating normally since they have multiple cats that share the litter box. Light pressure is put on the bladder, and it cannot be expressed. It is determined that Bert has a urinary obstruction, which is an emergency. It is likely that there is a stone or mucous plug lodged in the urethra, blocking the outflow of urine. Urinary obstruction causes **uremia**, or a build up of urine toxins in the blood. Refer to Chapter 22, Renal Physiology for more information.*

Bert is sedated and given pain medications, and a urinary catheter is placed into the urethra, clearing the obstruction. The urinary catheter is left in place, and Bert will stay in the hospital to be monitored for the next 2–3 days.

Review Questions

1 Which part of the urinary system resides in the retroperitoneal cavity?
  A The kidneys
  B The ureters
  C The bladder
  D The urethra

2 Which part of the kidney is deeper, the renal cortex or renal medulla?

3 What is the portion of the kidney contains the renal artery, renal vein, and ureter?
  A Renal pelvis
  B Renal capsule
  C Real poles
  D Renal hilus

4 What are the three points that make up the trigone?

5 Which is the correct order of flow?
  A Nephron → minor calyx → major calyx → collecting duct → renal pelvis
  B Major calyx → renal pelvis → minor calyx → nephron → collecting duct
  C Collecting duct → nephron → renal pelvis → minor calyx → major calyx
  D Nephron → collecting duct → minor calyx → major calyx → renal pelvis

6 Where can the detrusor muscle be found?
  A The kidney
  B The ureter
  C The bladder
  D The urethra

7 True or False: The urethra contains skeletal muscle.

8 Where can Bowman's capsule be found?
  A The renal capsule
  B The renal corpuscle
  C The renal pelvis
  D All of the above

9 Explain why the male cat has a higher likelihood of urinary obstruction.

10 Why is transitional cell carcinoma one of the most common cancers in the bladder?

10

Cardiovascular Anatomy

> **Clinical Case: Chiclet, a 3-Month-Old Female Intact Maltese**
>
> *Chiclet previously came in for a first appointment 2 days ago after being purchased from a family friend who had a litter. At the time of the first appointment, Chiclet was found to have a loud continuous heart murmur and a poor body condition. Chiclet is back today to be assessed by a cardiologist.*
>
> *A heart murmur is a sound heard in the heart that signifies blood turbulence. This means blood is not flowing in the exact right direction or is regurgitating backward around the valves or vessels. It is often described as a whooshing sound in between heartbeat sounds.*

Introduction

The circulatory system includes a number of structures and vessels. The heart, veins, arteries, and lymphatic vessels play a role in the passage of fluids throughout the body. They are aided by lymph nodes and (indirectly) by the spleen and the thymus. All of these organs and conduits have the same goal: to bring needed materials, oxygen, nutrients, inflammatory cells, and platelets, throughout the animal and to remove waste products, including carbon dioxide, cells, debris, and interstitial fluid. These processes will be discussed further in Chapter 23.

The Heart

The heart is a large organ within the thoracic cavity, situated near the midline, between the left and right lung lobes. It is covered by a connective tissue sac called the **pericardium** (Figure 10.1). The pericardium is composed of three layers. The superficial layer is called the **fibrous pericardium**. Deep to this is a two-layered membrane that forms the **serous pericardium**. The **parietal layer** of the serous pericardium is superficial to the **visceral layer**, which actually adheres to and combines with the outer surface of the heart, or the **epicardium**. Between the layers of the serous pericardium is a small amount of viscous fluid. In certain cardiac diseases or cardiac malfunction, excess fluid forms within the pericardium, and the increased pressure can then interfere with heart function. This condition is called **pericardial effusion** and makes the heart sound muffled on auscultation. The sac can be surgically fenestrated or even removed without significant consequences in order to decrease the pressure against the heart.

Deep to the epicardium is the myocardium, the actual heart muscle. It has a unique microscopic structure, partly like smooth muscle and partly like skeletal muscle. The myocardial layer is thicker in some areas than in others. In particular, the area around the left ventricle is much thicker. The endocardium is the lining of the interior chambers of the heart. It is contiguous with, and in fact becomes, the lining of some of the great vessels, such as the aorta.

When looking at a dog or a cat during a physical exam, the heart can be visualized as extending from the second or third intercostal space to the fifth or sixth intercostal space, about two-thirds of the way up from the sternum. In mammals, the heart has four chambers: a **right atrium, left atrium, right ventricle**, and **left ventricle**. Looking at the animal in

Anatomy and Physiology for Veterinary Technicians and Nurses: A Clinical Approach, Second Edition. Lori Asprea.
© 2026 John Wiley & Sons, Inc. Published 2026 by John Wiley & Sons, Inc.
Companion website: www.wiley.com/go/asprea/anatomy_vettech2e

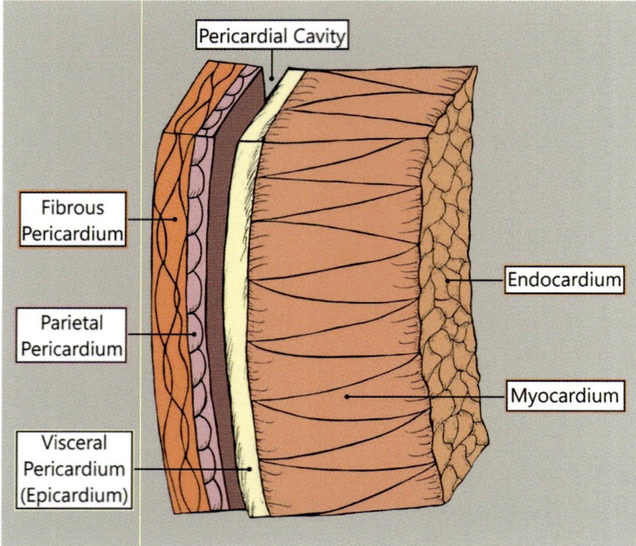

Figure 10.1 The layers of the heart and surrounding tissues.

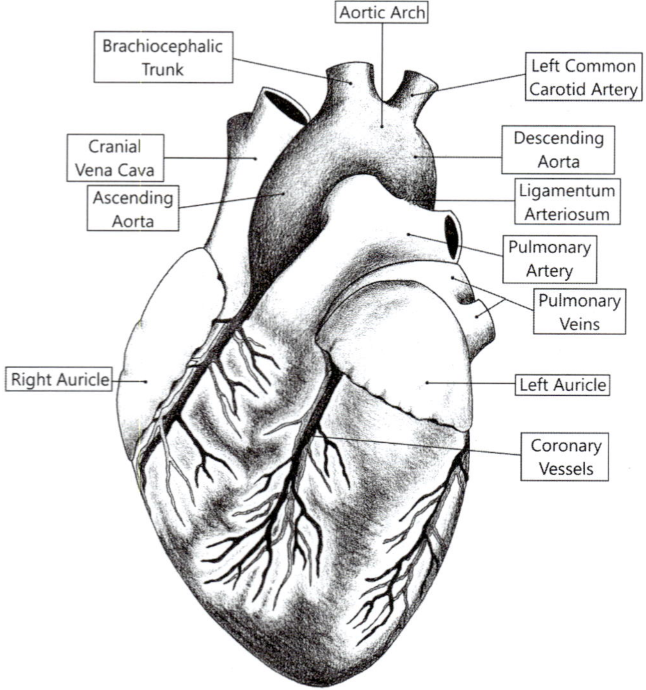

Figure 10.2 The great vessels of the heart.

dorsal recumbency, the atria are cranial to the ventricles. The wider part of the heart is cranial to the narrower part. The wider portion is the **base** of the heart, and the thinner caudomedial end is the **apex**. The great vessels are the **aorta, pulmonary arteries, pulmonary veins, cranial vena cava**, and **caudal vena cava** (Figure 10.2).

The basic circulation into and through the heart involves blood leaving the left ventricle via the aorta, passing through other arteries throughout the body and then returning to the heart by way of a number of veins that feed into the cranial and caudal vena cava (plural form: cavae). The vena cavae enter the right atrium of the heart. Blood flows into the right ventricle and is carried toward the lungs by the pulmonary trunk (pulmonary artery). Blood is thus transported to the lungs and oxygenated. It then is transported to the left atrium by way of the pulmonary veins. Blood travels from there to the left ventricle, and the cycle continues (Figure 10.3).

The heart itself has a circulatory system as well (see Figure 10.2). **Coronary arteries** and **coronary veins** supply the heart muscle and support structures and are visible on the heart once the pericardium has been removed. The coronary arteries branch directly off the aorta.

The heart is present in most vertebrate circulatory systems, but there is, as usual, a great deal of species differentiation. The heart of the dogfish has only two main chambers and two great vessels (one artery, one vein). Snakes and other reptiles have a three-chambered heart.

The Exterior of the Heart

Upon severing the ribs from the sternum on one side of the thorax, the heart will be revealed, nestled between the right and left lung lobes. The thickest vessel at the base of the heart, which travels a short distance cranially before turning and continuing caudally, is the **aorta**. It is the artery that gives rise to almost all the other arteries that course through the body. Note that arteries are vessels that travel away from the heart, and veins are those that travel to the heart. As a memory tip, think "artery begins with 'a,' 'a' for a̲way." On the exterior surface of the heart, two "leaves" can be seen near the base, in the area of the pulmonary trunk. These structures are known as **auricles**, from the root word for "ear." You may also see a small cord of fibrous tissue connecting the pulmonary trunk and the aorta. This is called the **ligamentum arteriosum** (Figure 10.2). It is the remnant of a fetal vessel, the **ductus arteriosus**, that circulates blood from the aorta to the pulmonary artery, diverting it from the lungs. This is because the fetus does not rely on its lungs to obtain oxygen, instead receiving it from the mother. Immediately after birth, this vessel closes, stopping communication between the two great vessels and redirecting the blood to now travel through the lungs to pick up oxygen. If the duct does not close properly once the puppy or kitten is born, blood flow is not normal, and blood

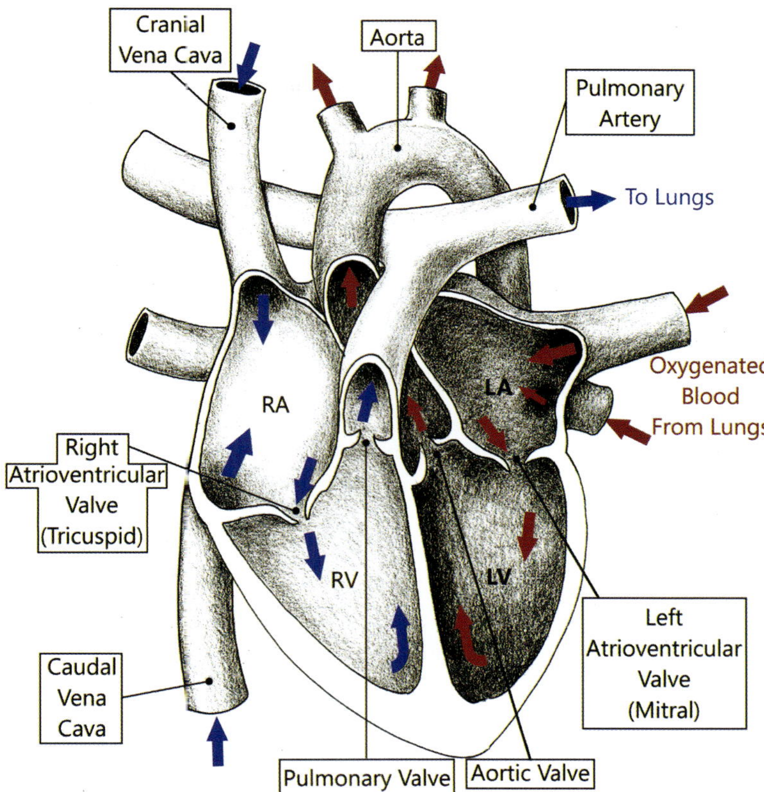

Figure 10.3 The great vessels of the heart and the major valves with normal blood flow. The aortic and pulmonary valves are referred to as semilunar valves because of their reported resemblance to the shape of the crescent moon.

cannot be oxygenated properly. This birth defect is found most often in certain dog breeds and is known as **patent ductus arteriosus (PDA)**.

The Interior of the Heart

Within the heart there is a sort of "skeleton" made of dense fibrous rings made of connective tissue. Each portion encircles the valves to act as a support and anchor system for the valves. It also helps to provide some electrical insulation between the chambers. Embedded within the heart is a small electrical system that controls cardiac muscle contractions. The electrical function of the heart will be discussed in a later chapter.

Dissect the heart along the long axis, along its midline. Four chambers are revealed (Figure 10.4). The ventricles are longer than the atria and sit caudal to the atria. Separating the atrium from the ventricle on each side is a fibrous structure known as an **atrioventricular valve (AV valve)**. On the right side of the heart, the AV valve is known as the **tricuspid valve**. It actually only has two cusps (leaves) in the dog. The left AV valve is known as the **mitral valve**, as it supposedly resembles a bishop's hat called a miter. An alternate name for the mitral valve is the **bicuspid valve**. It is also correct to call these the right or left AV valves. Supporting these valves are two structures: **papillary muscles** and **chordae tendineae** (Figure 10.2). The papillary muscles are anchored in the endocardium. The chordae tendineae are fibrous strands that have tremendous tensile strength. In ruminants and older horses, there is actually a bony attachment to the valves called the **os cordis**.

The entrances to the aorta and the pulmonary trunk are also covered by valves. The leaflets are considered to resemble a half-moon and are referred to as **semilunar valves**. The **aortic valve** separates the aorta from the left ventricle and has three cusps, while the **pulmonary valve** separates the pulmonary artery from the right ventricle and only has only two cusps.

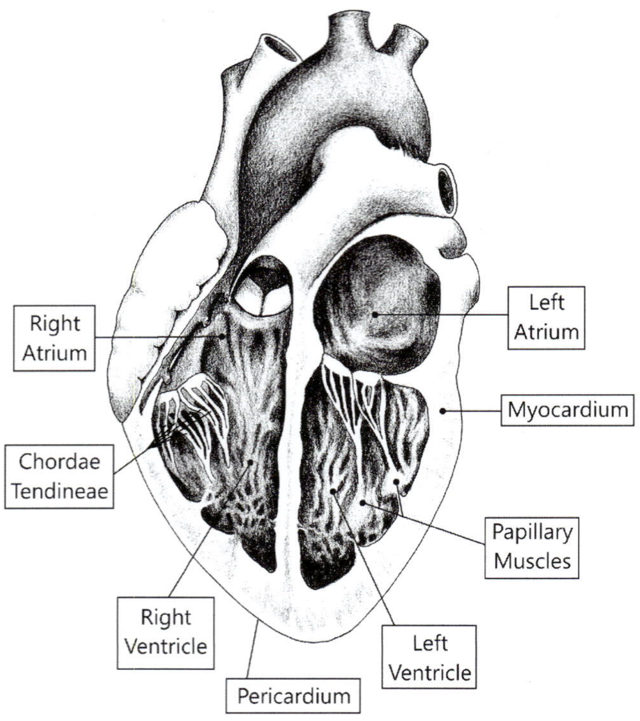

Figure 10.4 The chambers of the heart and internal features.

When auscultating the heart on the left side of the body, sounds associated with the mitral valve can be best heard at the fifth intercostal space, at the level of the olecranon. The pulmonary valve can be heard at the third intercostal space, at the same level. The aortic valve is best heard at the fourth intercostal space, near the shoulder. In order to remember this architecture, some use the device PAM left, T right (pulmonary, aortic, mitral on the left side and then tricuspid on the right side of the animal).

Dividing the left and right sides of the heart is a thickened wall called the **atrioventricular septum**. The cranial part of the wall between the atria is referred to as the **interatrial septum** and is relatively thin. In the fetus, there is an opening in the septum between the atria called the **foramen ovale**, allowing for blood to flow from one side of the heart to the other freely, as it does not need to travel to the lungs. This serves a similar purpose to the ductus arteriosus. Also similarly, the foramen ovale closes abruptly when the infant is born. If it does not close properly, the condition is called **atrial septal defect**. It, too, is somewhat common in certain dog breeds. The caudal portion of the atrioventricular septum that separates the ventricles is called the **ventricular septum** and is thicker than the interatrial septum.

The heart moves blood toward the lungs from the right ventricle. This is the beginning of what is called the **pulmonary circuit**. The left ventricle launches blood toward the rest of the body, referred to as the **systemic circuit**. As can be imagined, a great deal more force is needed to propel blood throughout the body. Therefore, it is not surprising that the left ventricular wall is thicker than the right wall and the aortic valve is thicker than the pulmonary valve.

Peripheral Circulation

The rest of the circulatory system consists of vessels that carry blood or other fluids throughout the body. Most often, the smallest of the arteries and veins are connected via very narrow vessels called **capillaries**. There are occasions where arteries connect to each other directly. These are called **anastomoses** and allow multiple arteries to serve a given area. The open space at the center of a hollow vessel or organ is called a **lumen**. Thus, the luminal surface is the one that is innermost, lining the "hole" through the center of the vessel (or organ, such as the interior of the intestine, gallbladder, or urinary bladder).

Arteries

Arteries tend to course in protected areas, deep within the trunk or on the medial surface of the limbs. Their route is often circuitous. Small arteries are referred to as **arterioles**. The largest of the arteries is the aorta, which arises directly from the left ventricle of the heart. Most of the larger branches of the aorta divide off at an angle to it in order to decrease some of the force of the blood flow; the strong pulse is a direct reflection of the fact that the aorta exits the heart itself, rather than branching from another vessel. Arteries tend to have a smaller lumen, or inner diameter, and a thicker smooth muscle layer in their walls.

The layers of arteries are called **tunics** (from the Latin word for covering). The outermost layer is a fibrous coat of connective tissue, which protects against excessive expansion and possible rupture. The middle layer is the thickest and consists of elastic tissues and occasional stretches of smooth muscle. The innermost layer is the **endothelium**, which consists of elastic connective tissue as well as epithelial cells. The connective tissue in the arteries of domestic animals does not generally become very stiff; in humans, however, this is common with age and is informally called "hardening" of the arteries **(atherosclerosis)**.

The arteries arising directly from the heart, and some of their major branches, are mostly elastic tissue, with little or no muscle in the middle tunic. Note that the pulmonary trunk, which arises from the right ventricle of the heart and heads toward the lungs, is an artery. The term artery refers not to oxygen content but to whether blood is flowing away from the heart or not.

Some named arteries have more muscle tissue. Contraction of these muscles can decrease the diameter of the vessel and helps control the pressure of the blood flow. This is called **vasoconstriction**.

The arteries branch and become progressively smaller turning into **capillaries**, which are small, narrow vessels that are extensions of the endothelial tissue, with a delicate connective tissue covering. Some fluid passes from the capillaries into the interstitial space, and some transfers directly to the veins. Some capillaries, particularly in the intestines and part of the kidney, are **fenestrated** (have small window-like pores allowing the exit or entrance of larger molecules). **Sinusoids**, which are wider and often fenestrated groups of capillaries, can actually take in very large particles. Sinusoids are found in the liver, the spleen, and the bone marrow. A group of arterioles can form anastomoses, as noted above. These structures, in turn, can form a network (cluster) called a **rete**. The best-known rete is the renal glomerulus, a part of the nephron (Figure 9.4).

Veins

Compared to arteries, veins have thinner walls and are not situated deeply in the body. They generally have a greater diameter and/or capacity to carry blood, with the exception of the aorta. The smallest veins are called **venules**. Unlike arteries, most veins of the trunk and limbs have **valves** within their lumen, composed of two or three semilunar cusps. These help to keep blood flow unidirectional since veins return blood from the far reaches of the body back toward the heart.

In contrast to most arteries, the outer tunic of veins is mostly elastic connective tissue, with the middle layer mostly muscle. The endothelium is thin, with no elastic tissue. Folds that descend into the lumen of the vessel form the valves. Given that the vessels are composed of living tissue, they themselves need a blood supply. Small vessels called the **vasa vasorum** supply the blood vessels with a blood supply of their own.

The blood vessels have extensive innervation. Among other functions, these nerves help control blood pressure, which is discussed in Chapter 23.

Many animals presented for classroom necropsy have been injected with a silicone-based material to make the vessels stand out. By convention, the arteries are colored red, the veins blue, and possibly include a third yellow dye for lymphatics. Occasionally, excessive force is used in injecting the dye, leading to large clumps of plasticine material appearing within the vasculature or to a lack of coloring in the distal vessels. This is a postmortem phenomenon and does not represent pathology.

Lymphatics

The other major type of vessel is the **lymphatic vessel**. These mostly arise from a group of capillaries called a **venous plexus** (in order to distinguish it from a nerve plexus). The lymphatic vessels have the capacity to pick up larger molecules, such as proteins and other particulate matter, which have ended up in the **interstitial fluid**. The interstitial area is the material between the cells and cavities. The lymphatic vessels have closely spaced valves and sometimes will have a beaded appearance. Unlike arteries and veins, lymphatic vessels start off very small and become larger as they travel. Eventually, they form major vessels, or trunks, which eventually empty into veins.

Many lymphatic vessels pass through a **lymph node** as they travel. These are firm, smooth structures covered by a capsule (thin "overcoat"). In the carnivore, there are relatively few lymph nodes, but they are large and tend to be found in clusters. In contrast, equines have small lymph nodes that spread all over the body. In dogs and cats, a number of lymphatic vessels will enter the node at once, but material exits the node in one vessel. The function of these nodes will be discussed later. For now, note that in an animal that has active inflammatory disease, these nodes may appear quite large; this is referred to as a **reactive lymph node**. The nodes can also be enlarged in other disease states, such as the cancer known as **lymphoma**.

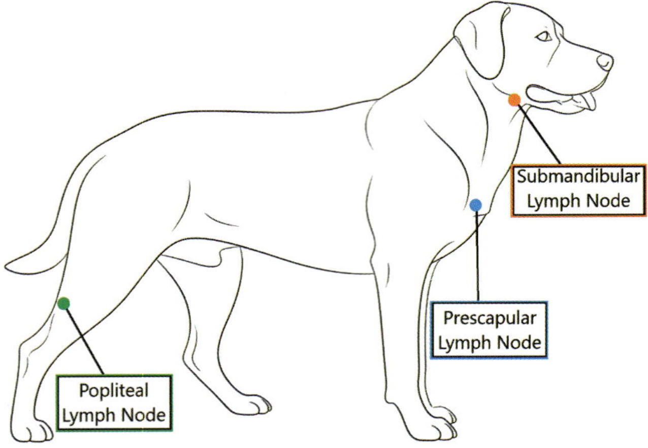

Figure 10.5 The palpable, or easily felt, lymph nodes: the submandibular, the prescapular, and the popliteal.

A **tonsil** is a special type of lymph node. Tonsils do not have a capsule and are generally not associated with lymphatic vessels. They occur in the **pharynx, genitals**, and **intestines** and are available to filter contaminated material away from the area.

Certain lymph nodes can be palpated during a physical exam. In dogs, we can check the **submandibular, prescapular, axillary, inguinal**, and **popliteal lymph nodes** (Figure 10.5). The submandibular lymph nodes are ventral to the caudal mandible. The prescapular lymph nodes are in the cranial thorax, close to where the trunk meets the leg. The axillary lymph nodes are in the axillary or "armpit" area, and inguinal lymph nodes are in the inguinal or groin area where the hind limb meets the body. The popliteal lymph nodes are found just caudal to the stifle. These nodes are so close to the surface that they are readily palpable. In cats, the popliteal lymph node is not generally palpable unless it is responding to disease. In bovines, you may be able to palpate the prescapular nodes.

The Named Arteries

As the aorta exits the heart itself, it has a widened appearance, referred to as the **aortic bulb**. It can be identified nestled between the atria, approximately above the area of the mitral valve. The **coronary arteries** arise from the aortic bulb, supplying the heart itself with oxygen. As the aorta exits the pericardium, it travels cranially and is called **the ascending aorta**. The part that starts to bend around is called the **aortic arch**. Arteries leading from the aortic arch include major vessels such as the **brachiocephalic trunk, the left subclavian artery**, and **the common carotid artery** (see Figure 10.2).

The common carotid artery splits into **left and right carotids**, which travel all the way to the brain. In cats, the left and right common carotid arteries branch from the brachiocephalic trunk. There is **an external carotid** and **an internal carotid** on each side, which diverge approximately at the level of the larynx. The internal carotid, protected by being deep within the body, goes directly to the brain. The external carotid has a number of branches that supply other areas of the neck and head. These include the **facial artery**, which runs along the mandible. Other branches include the **maxillary artery**, supplying the teeth and eye, and the **superficial maxillary artery**, supplying the masseter muscle and the eyelids.

The carotids, if occluded, will choke off the supply of oxygen, glucose, and other materials the brain needs to stay alive. As is true for all major arteries, they have a pulsing movement that reflects the heart pumping the blood along. In dogs and cats, the carotid artery is one vessel we use to check the pulse. In the horse, where this vessel is not accessible, we use the facial artery instead, easily felt ventral and slightly medial to the lateral mandible.

The **subclavian artery** diverges into a number of branches. The **vertebral artery** moves cranially to supply the spinal cord and brain. Another branch is the **internal thoracic artery**, which courses caudally and becomes the **cranial epigastric artery**.

The internal thoracic artery may be hard to locate on dissection. The epigastric artery assumes importance in large-scale skin grafts, such as after a burn injury; the artery is often diverted to provide blood to the grafted skin

The subclavian artery also courses along to the axilla (essentially, the armpit), where it is called the **axillary artery**. It continues distally along the medial brachium to the cranial elbow, where it becomes the **median artery**. It gives off a number of branches, including one called the **superficial brachial artery**. This artery is important in that it runs along the **cephalic vein** and **radial nerve**. The cephalic vein is one of the most commonly used vessels for routine phlebotomy in the dog. It is important to avoid the nearby artery during this procedure. Other branches continue toward the paw (Figure 10.6).

In dissecting into the axilla, a tangle of vessels and nerves will be noted. The nerves are off-white in color and resist breaking even when tugged firmly. This nest is called the brachial plexus. Again, since there are so many important vessels and nerves, it is no surprise that it is in such a protected area.

After giving off the major vessels, the aorta executes a turn and begins to course caudally. Once this happens, it is referred to as the **descending aorta**. The thoracic section runs next to the **azygous vein** and the **thoracic duct** (a major lymphatic vessel) and enters the abdomen through a hole in the diaphragm called the **aortic hiatus**. The abdominal section of the aorta continues caudally and has many arteries that branch off it.

The first visceral branch of the abdominal aorta is the **celiac artery**. The celiac is easily visible on necropsy. It continues to become **hepatic, splenic**, and **left gastric arteries**. The latter supplies the duodenum, the liver and spleen, and the stomach. The hepatic artery branches to the gallbladder, stomach, duodenum, and pancreas.

The next major artery branching from the abdominal aorta moving caudally is the **cranial mesenteric artery**. It branches in such a way as to eventually supply the jejunum,

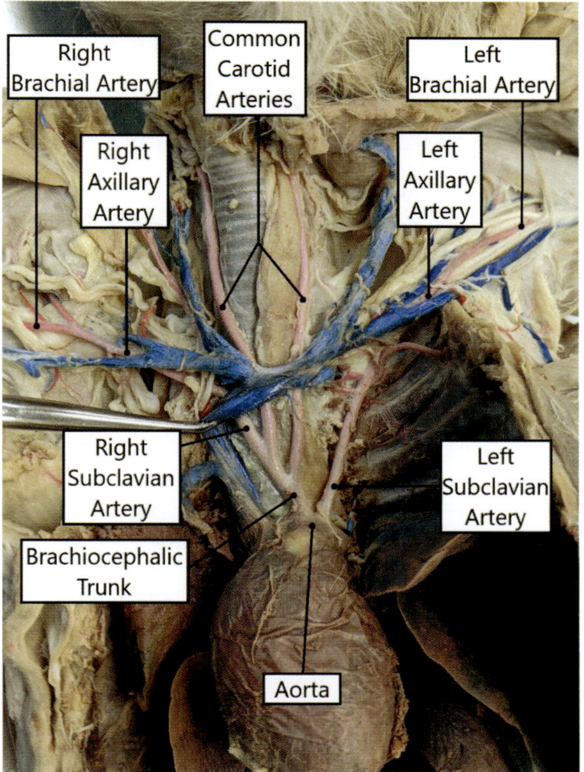

Figure 10.6   The thoracic arteries.

ileum, and colon. In this manner, it contributes to the collateral circulation of the intestines. Viewing the mesentery will reveal a network of numerous small arteries. Each section of the small intestine has several arteries supplying oxygen and nutrients. Interruption of any of these arteries thus does not completely deprive any one section of a blood supply. The term "**collateral circulation**" means that there are many vessels contributing to one area.

Caudal to the cranial mesenteric is the **renal artery**. This travels directly from the aorta to the kidney. The direct supply from the major artery underscores the importance of the kidney as a filter for the entire bloodstream. Continuing caudally to a point near the termination of the abdominal aorta is the **caudal mesenteric artery**, which supplies the colon and the rectum.

As the abdominal aorta continues to move caudally, it splits into a series of main arteries. The first split is a pair of **external iliac arteries** and the second is a pair of **internal iliac arteries**. The aorta does continue past this point, but here it is a very thin vessel called the **coccygeal artery**, which supplies the tail. The fork at the distal aorta, where the iliac arteries branch off, is an important landmark. In cats, where a blood clot forms in the heart or in the arterial system, the clot will travel along the aorta and come to rest at this fork. This condition is referred to as a **saddle thrombus**. The clot is unable to move further because of the abrupt change of direction and narrowing of the vessel. Blood supply to the pelvic limbs and tail is cut off. In addition to being extremely painful, this condition is difficult to treat. A cat coming into the clinic showing signs of extreme pain, and whose rear paws are cold, may be suffering from this condition. This is a medical emergency and demands immediate attention (Figure 10.7).

As mentioned above, the two caudal-most major branches of the aorta are the external iliac and internal iliac arteries (each one on each side). The external iliac artery is the primary supplier of blood to the hind limb. The **femoral artery** branches from the external iliac artery. Checking for a pulse is often done using this vessel. In fact, timing the pulse of the femoral artery in contrast to the heartbeat can reveal something called **pulse deficit**, an important indicator of circulatory system pathology. Pulse deficit is when the heartbeat and femoral arterial pulse are not synchronized.

The internal iliac artery brings blood to the pelvic viscera and walls of the caudal abdomen. By way of its branches, it helps supply the urinary bladder via the **umbilical artery**, caudal muscles of the proximal pelvic limb, and gluteal

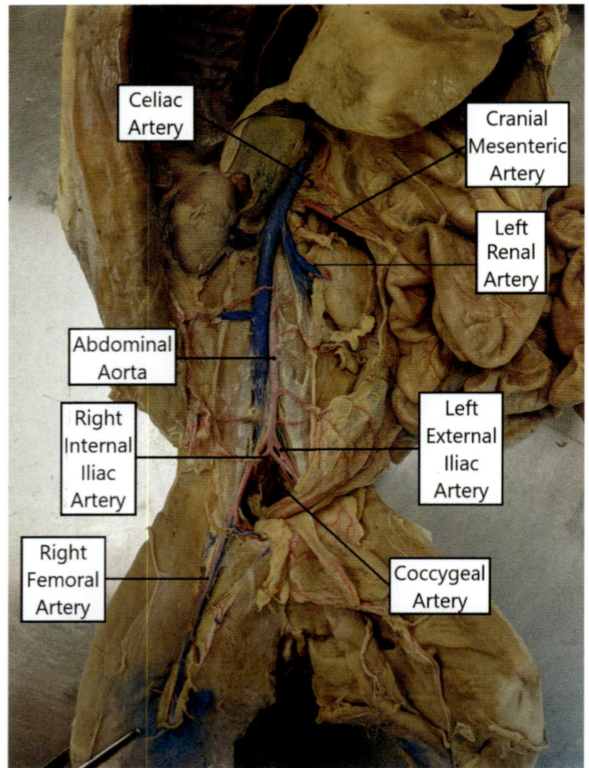

Figure 10.7 The abdominal arteries.

muscles via the **caudal gluteal artery**. The **internal pudendal artery** branches from the internal iliac artery. Its first branch is the **prostatic artery** in the male or the **vaginal artery** in the female. They supply the rectum, urinary bladder and urethra, and the reproductive areas. There are also branches that bring oxygen rich blood to the ovaries called the **ovarian arteries**.

The **external pudendal** artery supplies the groin and prepuce, which is the tissue surrounding the penis. The femoral artery courses along the medial part of the proximal pelvic limb and then crosses to the caudal part of the limb. It passes the caudal to the stifle, where it is called the **popliteal artery**. This artery, in turn, divides into the **cranial and caudal tibial arteries**. The cranial tibial artery will be easily found on dissection, but the caudal tibial artery may be more difficult to uncover. The popliteal lymph node will be easily visualized in the fat caudal to the stifle, appearing as a dark, smooth, firm, approximately pea-sized structure.

The medial femoral artery gives way to the **saphenous artery** branches and continues distally by way of various branches all the way to the paw. The vein that runs alongside it called the **saphenous vein**, is the point where we generally obtain blood samples in cats.

The Named Veins

The major veins entering the heart are the cranial and caudal vena cavae. The cranial vena cava brings deoxygenated blood from the head and cranial body and the caudal vena cava the rest of the body. They return the blood to the right atrium of the heart. Blood is carried away from the right ventricle via the pulmonary artery to the lungs. Returning from the lungs with their load of oxygen are the **pulmonary veins**. The number of these veins varies among species. In dogs, there are two of them; large animals generally have three. The pulmonary veins have no valves. They enter the left atrium. Eventually, the blood enters the left ventricle before being pumped out of the heart.

It is notable that most arteries have a vein paired with them and have essentially the same name. For example, there is a **brachiocephalic vein** and a brachiocephalic artery. They usually travel next to each other. There are, however, some exceptions.

The aorta does not have a paired vein. Analogous to the aorta is the vena cava; there is no "aortic vein." The same is true for the celiac artery in that there is no celiac vein.

By the time blood starts to return to the heart, it no longer is receiving the strong "push" from the pumping of the heart. Therefore, veins do not pulse as blood moves through them. This plays a role in phlebotomy; if it is pulsing, it is not a vein. We usually sample venous blood for laboratory testing purposes (Box 10.1). We can sample arterial blood in very specific circumstances, but different steps must be taken.

Blood returning from the head is carried in the **jugular veins** on each side. The jugular vein is often used to obtain a blood sample in dogs and cats. It is the blood vessel we use in almost all cases to obtain blood in equines and bovines as it is readily accessed and big enough to obtain a good sample easily.

The **subclavian vein** brings blood from the thoracic limbs toward the trunk. One of the distal vessels that feed into the subclavian vein is the **cephalic vein**. As we mentioned, this is the vein that we use most often to obtain blood from dogs. Both the jugulars and the brachiocephalic veins feed directly into the cranial vena cava (Figure 10.8).

Coming from the caudal part of the animal, the **internal and external iliac veins** drain the hind limb and wall of the pelvic area. The external iliac vein is supplied by a vein coming from the crus and femoral part of the limb. This

> **Box 10.1   Phlebotomy**
>
> Phlebotomy is the procedure of using a needle to take blood from a vein.
> In order of preference, vessels from which we take blood are:
>
> - Dog: cephalic vein, lateral saphenous vein, jugular vein
> - Cat: medial saphenous vein, cephalic vein, jugular vein
> - Equine: jugular vein
>
> It is important to note that blood draw locations are selected based on patient temperament and tolerance as well as patient illness or pain levels.

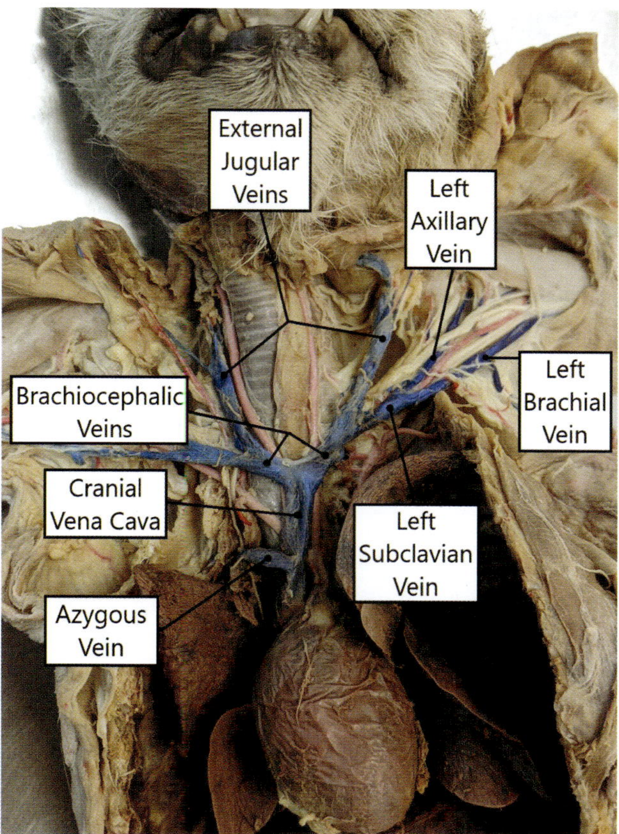

Figure 10.8   The thoracic veins.

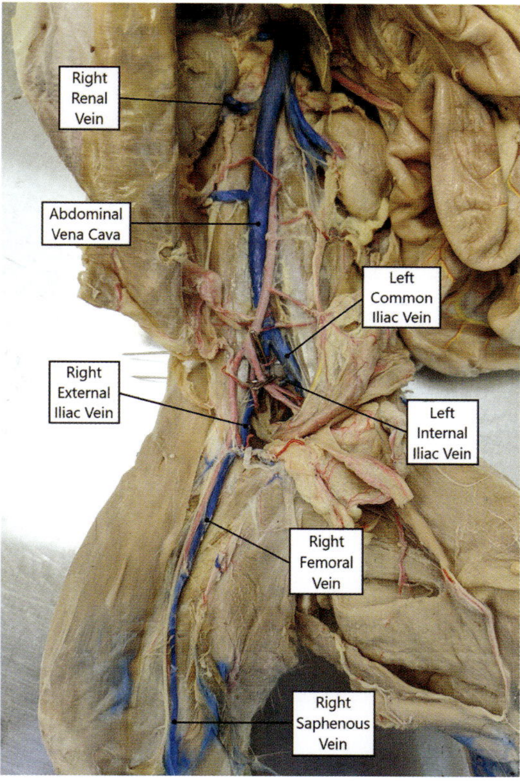

Figure 10.9   The abdominal veins. Note duplicity of the left renal vein, which can be a variant of normal.

vein is called **the medial saphenous vein** and a **lateral saphenous vein**. The saphenous vein can be used in dogs to obtain a blood sample but is used most frequently in cats. The iliac veins all feed into the caudal vena cava (Figures 10.9 and 10.10).

The **portal vein** eventually receives input from the spleen, digestive organs, rectum, and even the caudal esophagus. This vein plays a major role in the filtering roles of the liver and digestive tract. The **renal vein** as well as the portal vein eventually feed into the caudal vena cava. As the caudal vena cava tunnels through the liver, it is fed by the **hepatic veins**.

The **azygous vein** travels a long course and runs alongside the aorta as it travels into the thorax. It continues cranially and enters the cranial vena cava or the coronary sinus of the right atrium (a shallow bowl where the vena cavae enter the right atrium).

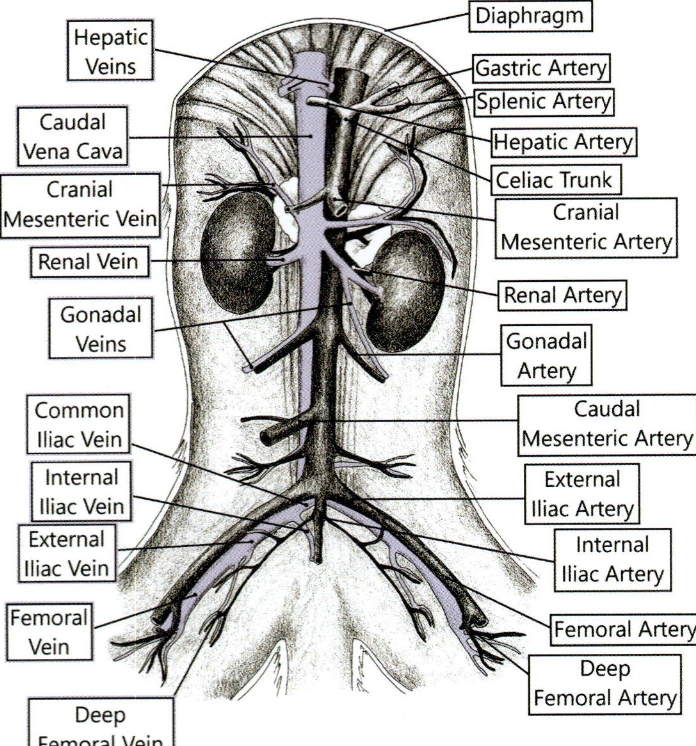

Figure 10.10 The abdominal vessels.

Clinical Case Resolution: Chiclet

Chiclet was assessed today by a cardiologist. The loud murmur is still present, and a thrill can be felt on Chiclet's body wall. A thrill is a palpable vibration felt over the heart that indicates turbulence. This is only felt in patients with severe murmurs.

After an exam, thoracic radiographs, an EKG, and an echocardiogram, it is determined that Chiclet has a PDA. Once this diagnosis is made the next steps are repair of the PDA. There is no way to manage the condition with medication alone, as the issue is a result a physical defect. Surgical intervention includes cardiac surgery or a less invasive method of blocking the ductus arteriosus through a cardiac catheter, depending on what it best for each specific case.

Review Questions

1 What is synonymous with the epicardium?
   A The myocardium
   B The serous pericardium
   C The parietal pericardium
   D The visceral pericardium

2 What chamber of the heart does the aorta come from?
   A The left atrium
   B The left ventricle
   C The right ventricle
   D The right atrium

3 What is the name of the vessel that brings blood to the lungs to be oxygenated

4 Which valve separates the left atrium from the left ventricle?
A The pulmonary valve
B The tricuspid valve
C The mitral valve
D The aortic valve

5 What are the smallest arteries called?

6 Which vessel supplies the tail with oxygen-rich blood?
A Coccygeal artery
B Coccygeal vein
C Renal artery
D Azygous vein

7 Which vessel brings deoxygenated blood away from the kidney?
A Renal artery
B Renal vein
C Cranial mesenteric artery
D Celiac vein

8 Which of the following vessels is most likely to be used for venipuncture (phlebotomy) in a feline patient?
A Subclavian vein
B Axillary vein
C Brachial artery
D Medial saphenous vein

9 True or False: The vena cavae has a thoracic and abdominal component.

10 Which of the following lymph nodes is palpable in the pelvic limb of the dog?
A The prescapular lymph nodes
B The popliteal lymph nodes
C The submandibular lymph nodes
D The inguinal lymph nodes

11

Respiratory Anatomy

Clinical Case: Perdue, a 3-Year-Old Male Intact German Shorthaired Pointer

Perdue is brought in by his handlers with a 2-day acute history of sneezing and nasal discharge. Perdue is a hunting dog that has been in the field multiple times in the previous months. His handler reports that his energy and appetite remain normal, but they have pulled Perdue from work for now. He has had no other signs aside from sneezing and nasal discharge, which seem to be progressive. He is fully vaccinated but does stay in kennels frequently with other hunting dogs.

Introduction

The respiratory system begins at the nose in most terrestrial animals. In dogs and cats, the nose is merged into the muzzle. Its **mucocutaneous border**, where skin transitions into the mucous membrane, is often the site of skin diseases associated with autoimmune disorders, so its superficial surface always requires close inspection on physical examination. The nose provides not only a conduit for the passage of air but is also involved in olfaction. It also warms and humidifies air, reducing irritation to the tissues of the upper respiratory system. It is also noteworthy that the **tear ducts** empty into the nostrils; one way that we can assess the patency of the tear duct is to introduce saline into the duct and see if it runs out of the nose. The role of the respiratory system is to bring fresh air into the body through inhalation, allowing oxygen (O_2) to bind to red blood cells and be dispersed to all tissues. This is simultaneously done while carbon dioxide (CO_2) is carried out of the body through exhalation, ridding the body of acidic waste. The role and importance of these gasses will be further discussed in Chapter 24.

Entry into the Respiratory System

The external opening into the nasal passage is known as the **nostril**. The nostrils are also referred to as **nares**, and the terms are essentially interchangeable. The outer walls of the nostrils are made of cartilage. The lateral surfaces of these walls are referred to as **nasal alae** (from the Latin root meaning "wings"). The exterior central groove visible between the nares is referred to as the **nasal philtrum** (see Figure 11.1). The flat area between the nostrils, including the philtrum, is the **nasal planum**. The nasal philtrum is a known acupressure point that can sometimes be used to stimulate breathing in neonatal patients. In this procedure, a small-gauge needle is inserted into the nasal philtrum at the base of the nares until it contacts the bone, and then the needle is rotated. Stimulation of this acupressure point can help initiate breathing.

The short tunnel at the entrance to the nasal passage is called the **nasal vestibule**. It narrows slightly as it runs caudally on each side; each passage is separated by a cartilaginous wall called the **nasal septum**, which runs medially and caudally. The wall becomes bone by the time it reaches the level of the **ethmoid bone**.

The lining of the interior surface of the nasal passages is a mucous membrane, with many ciliated cells. Some of these tissues are erectile; this function is particularly triggered in cases of inflammation.

Anatomy and Physiology for Veterinary Technicians and Nurses: A Clinical Approach, Second Edition. Lori Asprea.
© 2026 John Wiley & Sons, Inc. Published 2026 by John Wiley & Sons, Inc.
Companion website: www.wiley.com/go/asprea/anatomy_vettech2e

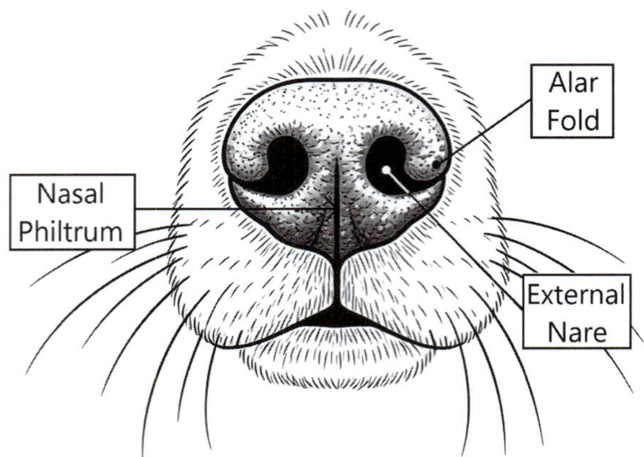

Figure 11.1   The nares and nasal philtrum.

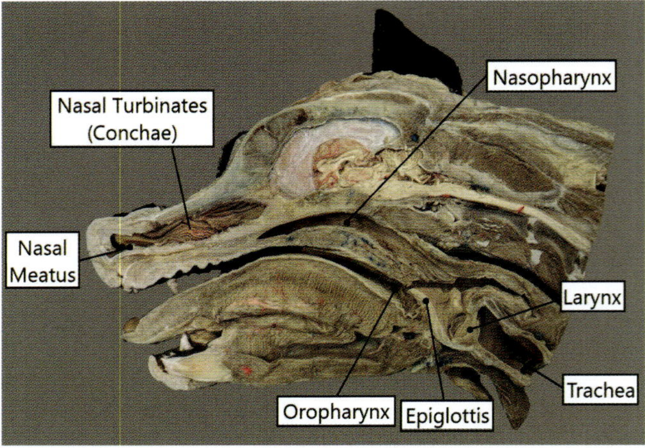

Figure 11.2   A bisected canine head. Note the complex folding of the nasal conchae and the pharyngeal and laryngeal components.

As the cartilaginous section ends, there is a bony wall composed of shell-like scrollwork called the **conchae**, or **nasal turbinates** (Figure 11.2). The concha is divided into three major openings, called the **dorsal, middle**, and **ventral meatus**, respectively. As air passes through the dorsal meatus, it flows over the olfactory mucosa. Air that continues via the middle meatus directs air to the **pharynx**.

The **frontal sinus** is dorsal to the ethmoid area; the **maxillary sinus** is deep and ventral to the eye. Both are lined by a mucous membrane that is continuous with that of the nasal mucosa. This is how inflammation travels into the sinuses. Note that the respiratory mucosa is involved in the pathway to the olfactory system as well; it is for this reason that a diminished sense of smell often accompanies upper respiratory inflammation. This factor is a particular issue in cats, who depend to a great extent on their sense of smell as a stimulus to appetite.

As air continues ventrally from the nasal passage, it passes through the **oropharynx**, which includes the caudal section of the oral cavity and the dorsal section of the throat, or more appropriately, **the pharynx**. As the air continues caudally, it arrives at the **larynx**, which is the boundary between the pharynx and the **trachea**.

The Larynx

The larynx itself is composed of a series of cartilages. The largest is the cranial-most and is called the **thyroid cartilage**. It forms the palpable sides and the ventral surface of the larynx. The rostral part of it comes to a point that, in humans, is referred to as the "Adam's apple."

The cranial part of the larynx has connections to the **hyoid apparatus** (the chain of small bones running from the skull and connecting with the larynx and the base of the tongue), which is why the larynx moves when the animal swallows. A stalk of cartilage, in the shape of a leaf, is attached to the cranial larynx and is referred to as the **epiglottis**. The epiglottis closes over the laryngeal opening when the animal swallows so that liquid and solid materials go into the esophagus instead of the trachea and then the lungs.

The name of the next cartilage in the series, the **cricoid cartilage**, comes from the Latin root for a signet ring, which it resembles. It is caudodorsal to and articulated with the thyroid cartilage. The third structure is a pair of somewhat triangular cartilages that sit inside the cricoid cartilage and rock back and forth. They provide the attachment for the **vocal folds**, and the mobility of the cartilage allows for the vibration of the folds. These are called **arytenoid cartilages**.

The opening between the vocal folds is known as the **glottis**. It is lined by epithelium and a thick layer of mucous membrane. When the glottis is open, then air passes through into or out of the trachea. Air passing on its way out causes the vocal folds to vibrate, which is part of how the animal makes sound. Again, this has tremendous import from a clinical standpoint; when placing an endotracheal tube, it must be placed between the vocal folds, through the glottis, in order to secure an airway for the patient.

The Trachea and Lungs

The continuation of the airway past the larynx is the **trachea** (Figure 11.3). It is a fibrous tube marked by a series of **cartilaginous rings** (Figure 11.4). These rings are incomplete in the dog and cat in that the dorsal surface is composed of fibrous tissue rather than cartilage. The inner lining of the trachea consists of ciliated cells, with the middle and outer linings made of fibrous material. When performing a tracheotomy, the goal is to surgically form an opening in between the rings. The trachea and remaining branches of the bronchial tree have a smooth muscular component that can constrict or dilate the airways.

The trachea enters the thorax at the **mediastinum**, the medial space between the lung lobes. Dorsal to the heart, the trachea branches into the two **main bronchi**. This spot is considered to be the division between the upper and lower respiratory tracts. Each main bronchus maintains the rings as it enters each side of the lung, after which the rings disappear.

These main bronchi carry air toward the lobes of the lungs. The number of **lobes** (sections) the lung has varies greatly by species, as does their outside appearance. In dogs and cats, there are three lobes on the left and four on the right (see Figure 11.5). On the left, there are the **cranial, middle,** and **caudal lobes**. Note that some people refer to these lobes as **the cranial part of the cranial lobe and the caudal part of the cranial lobe**. They are followed by the left caudal lobe. On the right, there are **cranial, middle,** and **caudal lobes**, as well as a smaller section called the **accessory lobe**. The accessory lobe is in a caudodorsal position and fits into a fold in the parietal pleura. In dogs and cats, the connective tissue that makes up the lungs has small, thickened fibers that give the lungs their "cobblestone" appearance.

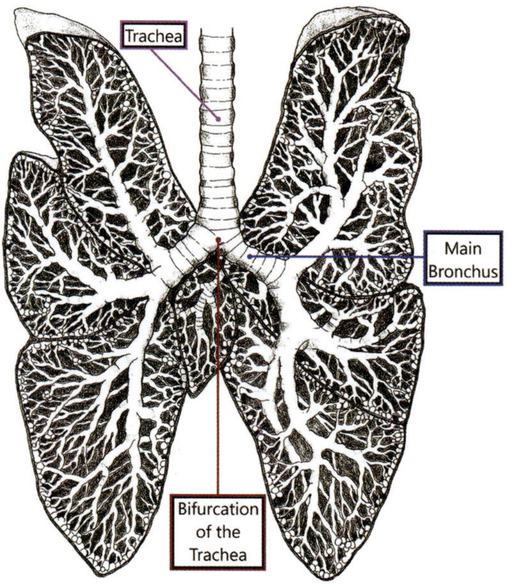

Figure 11.3 The lungs with the trachea splitting into the main bronchi and the remainder of the bronchial tree.

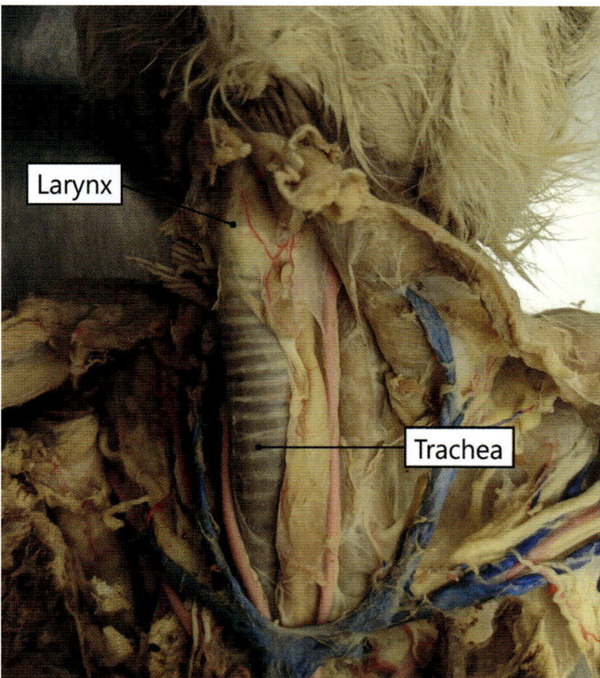

Figure 11.4 The trachea with cartilaginous rings.

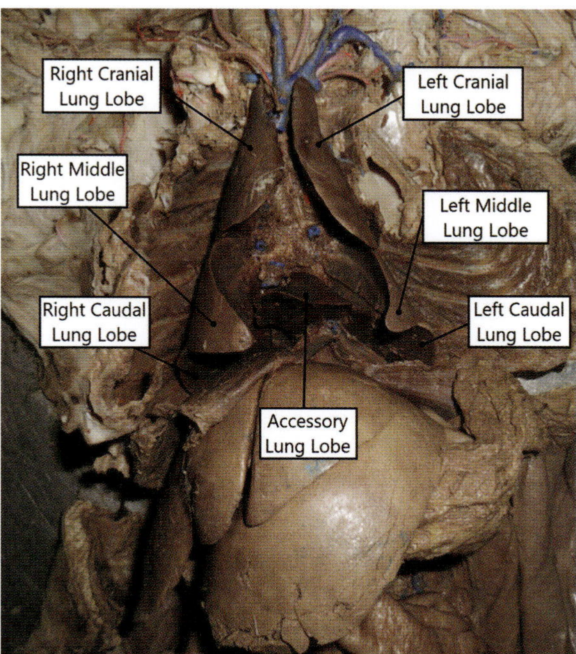

Figure 11.5 The lobes of the lungs. Note that the heart has been removed.

Within each lung lobe, the branch of the main bronchi divides into a series of smaller and smaller branches of tubes. The smallest are known as **bronchioles**. The bronchioles branch into smaller pathways called **alveolar ducts**. At their terminus, they become a series of small sacs known as **alveolar sacs**. The alveolar sacs are clusters of **alveoli**, similar in appearance to a cluster of grapes. These clusters have a highly vascular network of capillaries covering them. Each individual alveolus is a small sac that is one cell layer thick, comprised of the thinnest epithelium in the body. Their function is crucial to respiration, which will be discussed in Chapter 24.

Pulmonary tissue itself is composed of elastic, spongy material. In the moments after birth, the lungs fill with air. One way to determine if a dead neonate has passed away before or after birth is to take a sample of lung tissue and see if it floats. Before birth, it will not have any air in it yet, so the tissue will sink in water. If the newborn died after birth, when the lungs had filled with air, the tissue will float.

The Pleura

The **pleura** is a thin layer of protective tissues in the thoracic cavity. It consists of two layers of **serosal material**: the **parietal pleura** lines the interior of the thoracic cavity, and the **visceral pleura** covers the lungs themselves. There is a small amount of viscous material in between the layers, which lubricates the tissues and helps maintain negative pressure within the chest cavity. The concepts of **pleural effusion** (fluid buildup in between the lungs and the thoracic wall) and **pleuritis** (inflammation of the pleura), then, refer not to the lung tissues themselves but to the surrounding layers.

The visceral pleura folds around the cranial part of the lungs, near the branching of the main bronchi. While the main bronchi cannot be seen on radiography, the borders of the mediastinal space are visible on radiography. The ability to see it is important in diagnosing many disease conditions. The area where the main bronchi diverge is the only place at which the lungs are anchored to the body; the rest of the lungs are free-floating within the thoracic cavity.

The Anatomy of Breathing

At the caudal portion of the thoracic cavity is the **diaphragm**. The diaphragm is a sheet of skeletal muscle that spans the width of the thorax and plays a major role in respiration. There are openings for the aorta and the veins, called the **aortic hiatus**, and the esophagus, called the **esophageal hiatus**. A hiatal hernia is an abnormal opening or tear in the diaphragm; diaphragmatic hernia can be congenital or caused by trauma and can actually allow parts of the abdominal organs to be pulled up into the thorax.

The diaphragm is not the only muscle used for inhalation and exhalation. The **intercostal muscles** are a series of skeletal muscles in between the ribs. They are comprised of the **internal** and **external intercostal muscles**. During inhalation, the diaphragm and internal intercostal muscles contract, while during expiration, the diaphragm relaxes and the external intercostal muscles contract. It is important to remember that the lungs don't take air in by an active forcing motion but rather use a pressure gradient. The pressure within the thoracic cavity is negative compared to the normal atmospheric pressure on earth. As a result, when the diaphragm contracts, it increases the amount of space in the thoracic cavity, which gets filled by the air from the environment.

Because the muscles involved with breathing are skeletal muscles, technically breathing can be controlled to a certain point. Deep breathing or shallow breathing techniques can be used, and we know humans can decide to hold their breath. Although breathing utilizes muscles under conscious control, the medulla oblongata in the brain subconsciously keeps breathing going on an autopilot-like setting.

Species Differentiation

The nasal passage in the nose of the horse has a small diverticulum, or blind alley. Caution needs to be exercised when placing a feeding tube into the nose. The tube could inadvertently be guided into the diverticulum, which would not be helpful.

The pig has a bony plate in the area of the canine/feline philtrum. This is known as the rostral plate.

The horse has a third main bronchus on the right side of the mediastinum.

The pig has a highly lobulated appearance to the lungs, the surface of which appears as pebbles. The lungs of the horse are smooth.

The lungs of the avian are rather small and do not expand in the process of inhalation and exhalation. The gas exchange of respiration takes place in the lungs. On the other hand, there are air sacs, which look like bubble wrap, which are spread throughout the thorax and abdomen and perform the actual expansion and contraction (Figure 11.6). This will be discussed further in Chapter 23.

Clinical Considerations

The function of the system is dependent on each of its parts, from the opening of the nostrils to the air exchange at the surface of the alveoli. The distinction between the upper and lower respiratory systems is particularly important from a clinical standpoint. When using a stethoscope to auscultate the sounds of the airway, we must distinguish between upper and lower respiratory noise when present.

If a patient has narrowed, or **stenotic**, nares like in most brachycephalic animals, it can cause **stertor**. Stertor is the snorting-like sound from having anatomically narrowed nares, an elongated soft palate, or the presence of laryngeal saccules. It is the sound of turbulent airflow. This sound can be heard without a stethoscope but can make lung auscultation difficult, as the sound can permeate all listening fields. When we hear upper respiratory noise in the lower airways, we call it **referred upper airway sounds**. Alternatively, there is **stridor**, another upper airway sound that is much more melodic and higher pitched and is accompanied by wheezing. Stridor is also an anatomical anomaly sound. It generally represents laryngeal or tracheal disease and should be further investigated to determine the cause. Both stertor and stridor can represent underlying issues that can lead to an airway crisis.

Many sounds can be appreciated in the lower airways. In a normal patient, we expect to hear a very quiet passing of air in and out that matches respiration. Over the trachea, we expect to hear **bronchial breath sounds**, which have a prominent inspiratory and expiratory sound. **Bronchovesicular sounds** are heard in the chest and consist of soft inspiratory sound and soft short expiratory sound. **Vesicular sounds** can be heard in the periphery of the lung fields and are very soft. Abnormal sounds can be **crackles or wheezes**, which represent a variety of airway issues, including pulmonary edema or asthma, respectively. Absent lung sounds are also abnormal and can represent lung collapse or fluid interference.

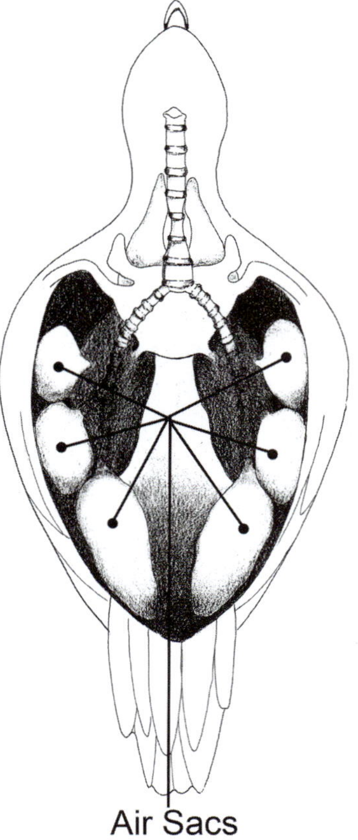

Figure 11.6 The avian air sacs.

Clinical Case Resolution: Perdue

Perdue has a physical examination performed which reveals a good body condition score, healthy coat, and normal hydration. Thoracic auscultation confirms normal heart and lung sounds, along with mild referred upper airway noise. Perdue has unilateral yellow and blood-tinged mucoid discharge (R Nare) and sneezes multiple times throughout the appointment. The owner reports that he has not been coughing, which is supported by normal lung sounds and respiratory rate.

The remainder of Perdue's physical examination is within normal limits. He is normothermic and energetic with a great interest in treats with normal mentation. Based on his history, the veterinary staff are concerned about infectious etiology versus foreign body. Thoracic radiographs are taken and are normal. Additional diagnostics offered include a CT scan and rhinoscopy. This will require general anesthesia and is planned 3 days from the appointment time.

Perdue is sent home with a course of antibiotics and instructions to carefully observe and chart symptoms at home.

Two days later, the handlers report that although Perdue's nasal discharge has less yellow color, it is still persistent along with the sneezing. The plan for advanced diagnostic imaging and rhinoscopy remains in place.

> *The following day, Perdue is placed under general anesthesia and has a CT scan of the head and neck performed, followed by a rhinoscopy. CT shows normal anatomy with no signs of neoplasia or bony destruction of the nasal passages. It shows the right dorsal meatus, right middle meatus, and right side of the conchae are fluid-filled, likely with mucous. In rhinoscopy of the right nasal passage, a grass awn foreign body is visualized 3.7 cm past the nasal entrance. The foreign body is removed, and Perdue will finish his course of antibiotics.*
>
> *The handlers are notified of what was found and the risks associated with grass awn foreign bodies. It is recommended that the hunting area be assessed for this risk moving forward. Perdue will be monitored for any further signs, including developing chronic rhinitis secondary to the foreign body.*

Review Questions

1 What is the goal of the respiratory system?
   A Retrieving nutrients
   B Performing gas exchange
   C Ridding the body of urea
   D Providing the tissues with a rich supply of CO_2

2 What area can be stimulated to induce respiration in neonates?
   A The nares
   B The nasal planum
   C The nasal philtrum
   D The nasal conchae

3 What are the scroll-like plates in the nasal passages?
   A The bronchi
   B The alveoli
   C The alveolar ducts
   D The conchae

4 True or False: The larynx contains a series of three sets of cartilage that includes an anchor point for the vocal cords.

5 What is primarily responsible for protecting the trachea when an animal swallows food or water?
   A The epiglottis
   B The cricoid cartilage
   C The arytenoid cartilage
   D The nasal philtrum

6 True or False: Cats and dogs have complete cartilaginous rings that line the entire bronchial tree.

7 How many lung lobes exist in the cat?
   A Three
   B Four
   C Six
   D Seven

8 True or False: The parietal serosa creates a layer directly on top of the lung tissue.

9 What is the large muscle that separates the thoracic cavity from the abdominal cavity and helps control breathing?

10 Which species has a rostral plate?
   A Feline
   B Equine
   C Swine
   D Canine

12

Gastrointestinal Anatomy

> **Clinical Case: Tucker, a 1.5-Year-Old Male Intact Labrador Retriever**
>
> *Tucker is brought into the clinic because the owner says he is reluctant to eat or drink. The owner reports that for the last 2 days, Tucker has been drooling a lot and not really interested in eating. Initially, he was drinking, but he kept "spitting up" the water he drank. She noticed him swallowing and gulping frequently and making some sounds like he was trying to cough or clear his throat.*
>
> *According to the owner, there is no history of trauma or diet change. She does give braided rawhide chew bones once per week, but Tucker has always had them without issue.*

Introduction

The anatomy of the digestive tract is amazingly variable among species. The importance of the metabolic processing of foodstuffs dictates examination of the significant differences among them. Dogs and cats will be discussed first. The digestive tract in mammals also includes the liver and pancreas, organs that have digestive and nondigestive functions.

Canines and Felines

The **alimentary tract** is a tube within the body, stretching from the mouth to the anus. There are certain structures that connect to the tract by ducts, such as the **salivary glands**, the **gallbladder**, and the **pancreas**.

In order, from cranial to caudal, the parts include the **lips, the teeth and oral cavity, the pharynx, the esophagus, the stomach, the small intestine, the large intestine, the rectum**, and **the anus**. Ancillary structures will be discussed along with each major organ.

The Oral Cavity

The mouth is used for prehension or gathering of food and includes the lips, teeth, tongue, and salivary glands. Note that some of these structures have functions beyond ingestion. These include aggression, defense through biting, grooming, conduction of gases to the airway when breathing, and amplification of sound when vocalizing.

The **outer vestibule** of the mouth includes the lips and cheeks, as well as the oral cavity up to the **palatoglossal arch**, which is the soft tissue border of the caudal oral cavity, approximately at the level of the ramus of the mandible. Depending on the species, the lips can be thick and mobile or thin and less mobile. They consist of skin, mucosa, nerve endings (supplied mostly by the seventh cranial nerve), and salivary glands. The border between the epidermal and mucosal tissues is referred to as a **mucocutaneous border**. Some of these borders are associated with certain diseases (e.g., lupus erythematosus).

Movement of the ingesta within the oral cavity is assisted by the **buccinator muscles** within the cheeks. Recall that the temporal and masseter muscles also control this function. The dorsal oral cavity consists of the **hard and soft**

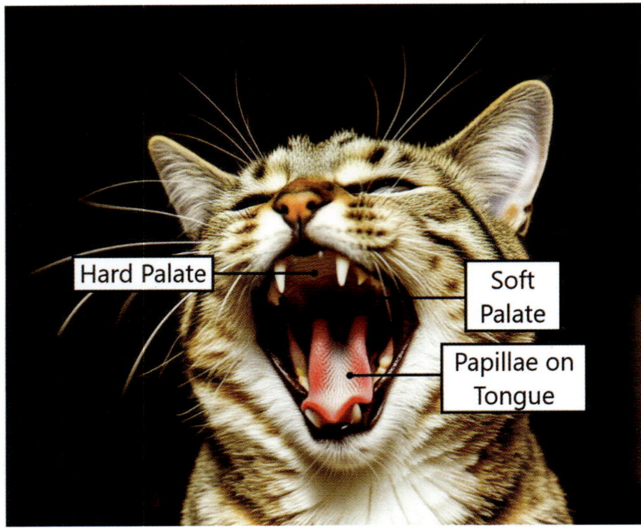

Figure 12.1 The hard palate overlies the palatine bone. Its rugae (ridges) are clearly visible. The soft palate helps guide food down the digestive tract as the food is chewed and swallowed. The papillae are an important part of the sense of taste. *Source: Generated with Gemini AI.*

palates. The hard palate covers the ventral palatine bone, while the soft palate does not have a bony backing (see Figure 12.1). The hard palate has ridges, called **rugae**, which are caudally facing and help direct food further into the digestive tract. The roof of the oral cavity also contains a duct that connects to the nasal cavity. As air passes through this duct, it is conveyed along the nasal cavity to the olfactory mucosa of the vomeronasal organ. This enhances the strength of food odors, which play a large role in the stimulation of appetite. A cat will often, upon encountering an interesting smell, hold his/her mouth open for several seconds to stimulate this organ; this adds to the intensity of the olfactory experience. This is discussed further in Chapters 3 and 16.

The **tongue** is a mostly muscular feature. The **root of the tongue** is anchored to the caudal area of the oral cavity and is connected in part to the mandible. The **apex of the tongue** is the freely mobile, rostral part. Its dorsal surface is covered by thin hairs, composed of connective tissue. It is also the home of small "mounds" of tissue called **papillae**, which are involved in the sense of taste. Of clinical note: It is important to deflect the root of the tongue ventrally in order to visualize the vocal folds when placing an endotracheal tube.

The salivary glands can either enter from outside the oral cavity or are completely contained within it. Some of the key salivary glands are the **parotid, mandibular**, and **sublingual** salivary glands. A parotid gland is located on each side of the head. It sits within a nest of fascia, ventral to the pinna. It opens into the oral cavity from the area of the maxilla, around the teeth called premolars. The mandibular glands open onto the ventral mouth. The sublingual glands are rostral to the mandibular glands and have numerous small ducts. Certain disease states can cause the salivary glands to become inflamed. If indicated, removal of some of these glands can be accomplished. However, this is done with great difficulty due to their size and location within other important areas of the oral cavity.

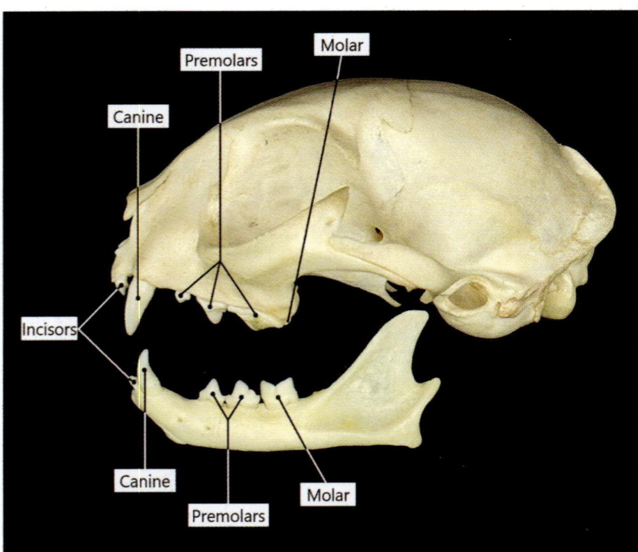

Figure 12.2 Position of the teeth: the upper teeth are rooted in the incisive and maxillary bones, and the lower ones in the mandible. There are no teeth on the ramus of the mandible.

The mucosal tissue that contains the teeth is referred to as the **gingiva**. Their color can be a major indicator of disease states. A pale pink or white color is often associated with anemia. A blue tinge may indicate **cyanosis**, a lack of sufficient oxygen within the bloodstream. Yellow can be an indication of hepatic disease. A brown, muddy color may reflect **methemoglobinemia**, associated with carbon monoxide poisoning or acetaminophen ingestion in cats. In addition, a tacky (sticky), dry condition of the gingiva reflects dehydration. Palpation of the gingiva should be a part of any physical examination.

Dentition

The teeth are variable in number among species (see Figure 12.2). The upper set of teeth is referred to as the **maxillary arcade**, and the lower teeth as the **mandibular arcade**. The names of the teeth are characterized by their location and shape. The rostral-most rectangular teeth are referred to as **incisors**. Caudal to them are longer,

Table 12.1 Canine and feline dental formula.

Canine Maxilla (3142)	Canine Mandible (3143)	Feline Maxilla (3131)	Feline Mandible (3121)
3 – Incisors	3 – Incisors	3 – Incisors	3 – Incisors
1 – Canine	1 – Canine	1 – Canine	1 – Canine
4 – Premolars	4 – Premolars	3 – Premolars	2 – Premolars
2 – Molars	3 – Molars	1 – Molars	1 – Molars

cone-shaped teeth referred to as the **canine teeth**. Caudal to them are the **premolar teeth**, which often have a sharp or irregular dorsal surface. The caudal-most teeth are the **molars**.

In order to identify teeth, a formula is utilized. The number of each type of tooth is listed from rostral to caudal, with the maxillary teeth above the mandibular teeth, separated by a line. The formula represents half of the arcade. An adult dog's formula is 3142/3143. This indicates that on each side of the maxilla, there are three incisors, one canine, four premolars, and two molars. Note that each mandibular section includes one additional molar. The formula for the adult cat is 3131/3121. The teeth are identified by a letter and a number, or just a number. For example, I2 refers to the second incisor (counting from the midline). The other abbreviations are C, PM, and M. See Table 12.1. Additionally, a method of assigning numbers to each tooth is the Triadan system, used in dental settings (Figure 12.3).

Please note that each of the above dental formulas only represents one half of the arcade. For example, in the canine maxilla, the left half of the arcade is comprised of 3142, and this repeats on the right half.

As in primates, there are **deciduous** ("baby") teeth, which are ejected as the permanent ("adult") teeth grow in. It is useful to reassure a client that the deciduous teeth are rarely found once they come out and that there should not be any concern if these teeth are "missing." Generally, many cats and dogs swallow these deciduous teeth without notice. In some animals, we can see a condition known as **retained deciduous teeth**. This is when the deciduous teeth do not fall out, and the adult teeth grow in alongside them. This results in sets of baby teeth and adult teeth together. This is overrepresented in smaller dog breeds and brachycephalic breeds. These retained deciduous teeth must be extracted to prevent future concerns.

The tooth itself is called the **dens** (see Figure 12.4). It is composed of a number of parts. The **crown** is the visible part and is covered by a hard material called **enamel**. The **root** of the tooth, which should be completely embedded within the gingiva, is covered by a different material called **cementum**. Cementum and enamel cover a substance called **dentin**, which makes up the bulk of the tooth. Between the crown and the root, there is a slight indentation called the **neck of the tooth**.

The socket in which each tooth sits is called the **alveolus**, and the joint where the tooth and the socket come together is called the **gomphosis** (refer to Figure 5.3). The gingiva should extend up to the neck of the tooth. Exposure of the neck and root of the tooth is an indication of dental disease. At the very center of the tooth is a connective tissue called **pulp**. The nerve supplying each tooth runs through this area. The roots of the teeth are eventually embedded in the jaw.

The different shapes of each tooth facilitate their function. The incisors have a single root as do the canines. The root of the canine is particularly long, anchoring this large tooth securely. Premolars have two roots, as do molars. In cats, the third maxillary premolar and first mandibular molar are known as the **carnassial teeth**; in dogs, it is the fourth maxillary premolar and the first mandibular molar that are the carnassial teeth. These teeth have three roots and are particularly difficult to extract.

Beyond labeling and numbering the teeth, it is also important to note that the teeth have their own direction terms so that specific anatomical areas can be described. The **buccal surface** of the teeth is the outer surface that faces the cheek as the side of the mouth. The **labial surface** is the outer surface of the teeth that faces the lips at the front of the mouth. On the mandible, the inner surface of the teeth is called the **lingual surface**, as it faces the tongue, whereas on the maxilla the inner surface of the teeth is referred to as the **palatal surface** since it faces the palate. The **occlusal surface** of the tooth is the area where the teeth meet when the mouth is closed. The **mesial surface** of the tooth is the outer surface of the tooth facing the midline and the **distal surface** of the tooth is facing away from the midline. The term **coronal** refers to toward the crown of the tooth, whereas **apical** refers to toward the root of the tooth.

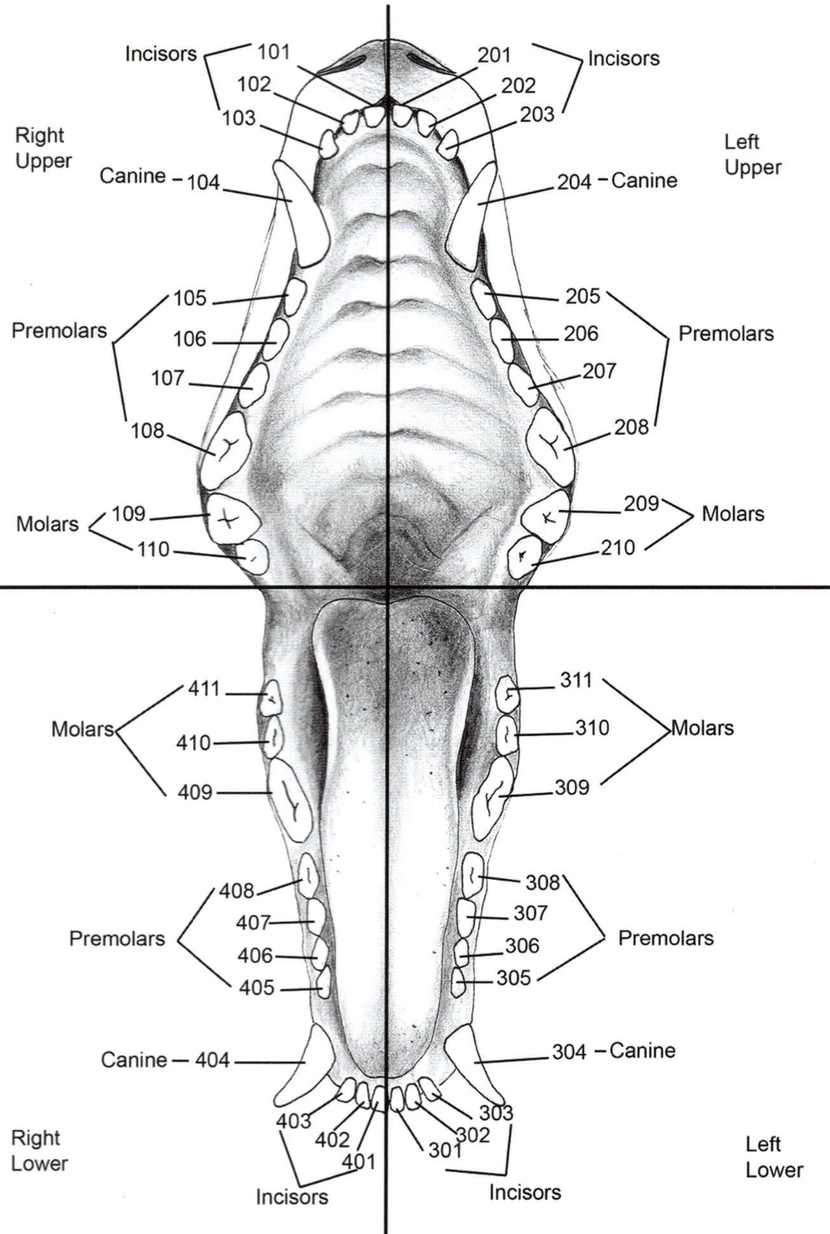

Figure 12.3 The modified Triadan chart is a way of identifying each tooth by a separate number, such that it is clear which teeth are on the left or right, and which are maxillary or mandibular. For numbering purposes, the mouth is divided into four quadrants: upper left, upper right, lower left, and lower right. This image also appears in Chapter 25.

The Pharynx and Esophagus

The vestibule of the oral cavity opens into a large space called the **pharynx** (essentially, the throat). The area immediately caudal to the vestibule is referred to as the **oropharynx**. It merges with the **nasopharynx**, which is caudal to the nasal passages. Thus, the pharynx carries both air and food (and whatever else the animal has eaten). The pharynx narrows as it approaches the **larynx**, where it is referred to as the **laryngopharynx**. Ingesta are conducted through the pharynx into the **esophagus**, a tube which connects with the **stomach**.

Passing the pharynx into the esophagus, ingesta must go through the **upper esophageal sphincter**, which allows food and water to enter. Next, the **cervical esophagus** courses through the neck of the animal. It is crucial to remember that the esophagus runs to the left of the trachea (the animal's left) in this area. When placing an esophageal feeding tube, the animal should be in right lateral recumbency so that the left side, and thus the esophagus, is available.

The section of the esophagus from the thoracic inlet to the diaphragm is known as the **thoracic esophagus**. The esophagus passes through an opening in the diaphragm called the **esophageal hiatus** as it travels toward the stomach. The short

Figure 12.4 Parts of the tooth. The crown is covered by enamel. The bulk of the tooth consists of dentine. The pulp cavity contains vessels and nerves. The neck of the tooth intersects with gingiva. Each of the two roots is seated in the alveolus, which is the socket in the bone the tooth sits in.

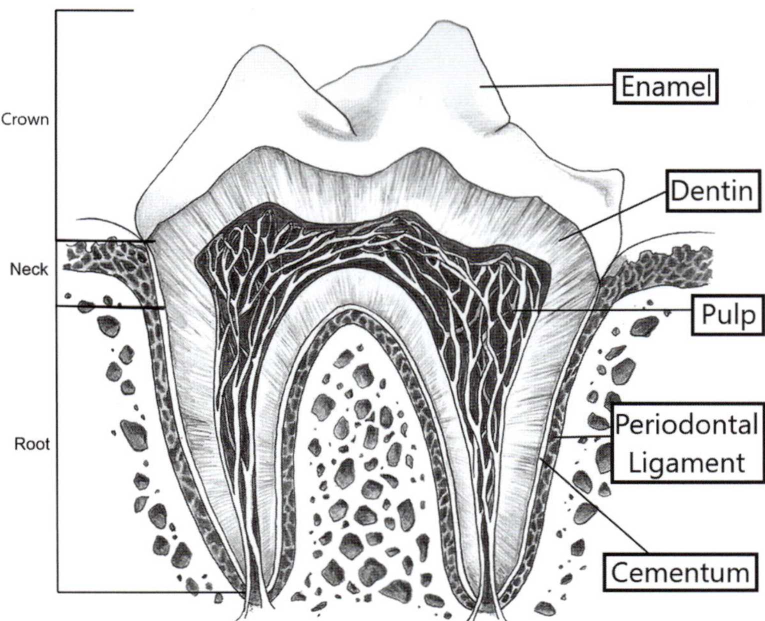

section from the diaphragm to the stomach is referred to as the **abdominal esophagus**. Note that these divisions represent sections of the same long tube and are used for convenience in description rather than for reasons of microanatomy.

The esophagus is composed of several layers. The outer layer, **the serosa**, is composed of connective tissue. There is a **muscular layer** deep to the serosa and the **luminal layer** which is mucosal tissue. There are two layers of muscle tissue, one longitudinal and one circular. Even within small animal species, there are structural differences. In dogs, the esophagus is lined by striated muscle throughout its length. In cats, the distal (caudal) section of the esophagus is smooth muscle. The lower esophageal sphincter is called the **cardiac sphincter**.

Once the esophagus passes the diaphragm, it has entered the abdominal cavity. The esophagus itself enters the stomach. Further discussion of the abdomen is warranted here. The **abdominal cavity** is the space caudal to the diaphragm, extending to the **pubic brim** (pelvic cavity). It is the largest of the body cavities. It is further divided into two sections: the **peritoneal space** and the **retroperitoneum**. The peritoneum is a membranous sac, within which are most of the visceral organs. The sac itself, composed of connective tissue, also covers the serosal surface of many of the organs. The accumulation of fluid within the peritoneal space is referred to as **ascites** and is an indication of severe disease states such as cardiac or hepatic dysfunction, or the viral disease feline infectious peritonitis (FIP). The retroperitoneum, an area in the caudal abdominal cavity, is the space between the peritoneum and the body wall. It contains lymph nodes, the kidneys, the ureters, and parts of the reproductive tract.

Within the peritoneum are folds of connective tissue that suspend the small and large intestines from the body wall. This is referred to as **mesentery** and carries blood vessels and lymphatic vessels to and from the digestive tract. They arise from a thick base, called the **root of the mesentery**, present in the dorsal part of the cavity.

For the purpose of description, the abdomen is divided into parts. The divisions are right cranial, right middle, right caudal, left cranial, left middle, and left caudal. The area of the caudal abdomen just medial to the pelvic limbs is referred to as the inguinal area. When noting in a medical record, using specific descriptive terms helps the medical team better understand what, if anything, was found.

The Stomach

The structure of the **stomach** is particularly species specific. In dogs and cats, which are omnivores and carnivores, respectively, the high level of concentration of nutrients in their food allows stomach structure to be relatively simple. The superficial layer, **the serosa**, is connective tissue. Deep to this is a layer of **smooth muscle**. Next is a layer including elastic fibers, nerves, and blood and lymphatic vessels. The **luminal surface** is composed of epithelium and mucosa, as well as a large number of glands. The elastic fibers corrugate to form **rugae (ridges)**. Rugae are folds that increase the surface area of the digestive tissue. The fuller the stomach is, the less prominent they are.

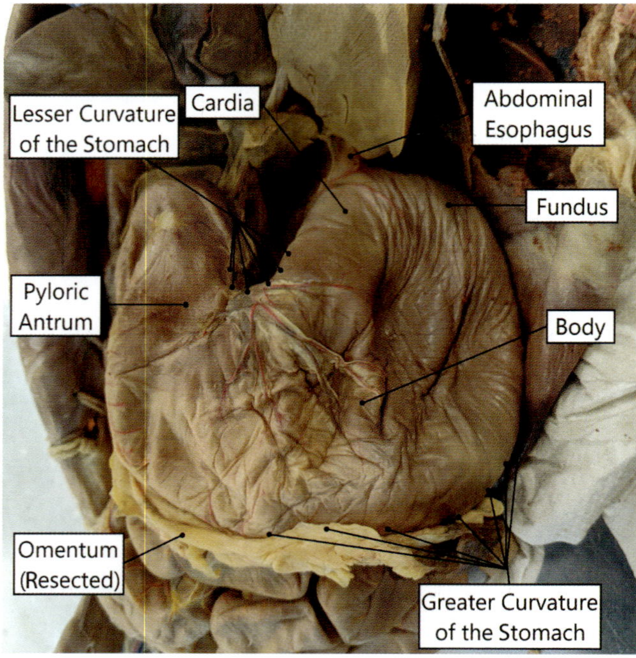

Figure 12.5 Sections of the stomach. The animal's head is toward the top of the picture. The greater curvature anchors the omentum, which is a fatty "blanket" that covers the viscera along their ventral surfaces.

The stomach has named areas. The **cardia** is a short section where the esophagus enters. The tubelike section caudolateral to it is the **fundus**, which can expand to accommodate food. This opens into a large cavity running on a transverse axis across the cranial abdomen, called the **body of the stomach**. The body of the stomach is the primary churning area. Continuing on is a short, narrower section called the **pyloric antrum**, which moves food forward. Medioventral to this is the **pylorus**, a short canal that contains the **pyloric sphincter**. This smooth muscle sphincter opens when food is ready to travel through it (Figure 12.5).

The craniomedial curve of the body of the stomach is known as the **lesser curvature**. It is linked by connective tissue to the liver. The longer, bowl-shaped, caudolateral border is known as the **greater curvature of the stomach**. Attached to the greater curvature of the stomach is a large sheet of fat and connective tissue called the **omentum**. It has a lacy appearance and covers the ventral surface of the peritoneal cavity like a curtain. Within the omentum is the **gastrosplenic ligament**, providing the spleen with an anchor to the stomach. The majority of the omentum is superfluous and is often used as graft tissue; that is, a section of omentum can be excised and placed into a gap to form a soft-tissue bridge when tissue is damaged.

The major blood supply of the stomach is the **celiac artery**. Most of the veins of the stomach join the **portal vein**. There are many lymphatic glands and vessels. Innervation of the stomach is both sympathetic and parasympathetic.

The Liver

The liver is a multilobed organ which is situated around the **gallbladder**. The gallbladder is a hollow organ that stores and releases bile under control of hormones, which will be discussed in Chapter 25. The liver lobes, beginning from the left and moving to the right, are as follows: **left lateral lobe, left medial lobe, quadrate lobe of the liver, right medial lobe, right lateral lobe**, and **caudate lobe** (Figure 12.6). The gallbladder is normally situated in between the quadrate lobe and the right and medial lobe. It is important to note that these liver lobes can appear markedly different from one animal to the other during dissection, with some lobes occasionally not as clearly demarcated. The patterns of the lobes also vary between species: for example, the equine liver is less lobated and there is no gallbladder present, while the ruminant liver has fused lobes that sit mostly to the right side, and in avians, the liver has two lobes.

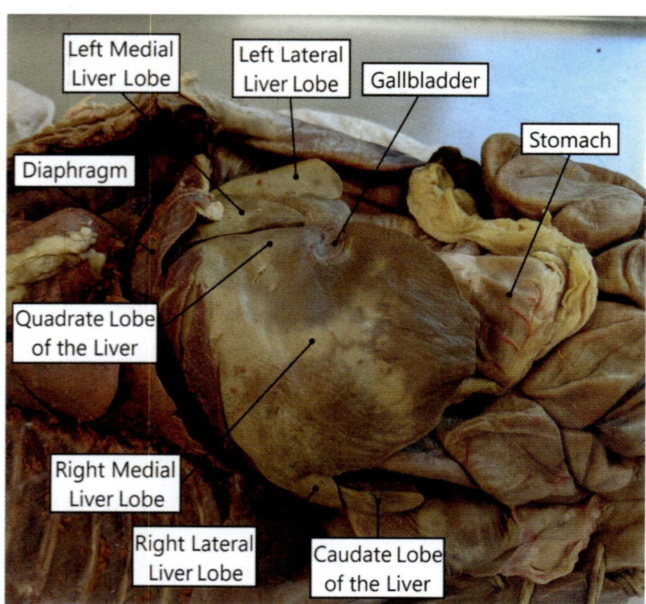

Figure 12.6 The lobes of the liver.

The Intestines

The intestines are often referred to as the gut. In the carnivore, it is relatively short – approximately three to four times the length of the trunk. In comparison, the gut is 25 times the length of the trunk in sheep.

The pyloric sphincter is the gateway to the **small intestine**. In order of the passage of nutrients, the sections are the **duodenum**, **jejunum**, and **ileum**.

The duodenum is a relatively short section forming a "J" shape (see Figure 12.7). The descending limb heads toward the right kidney, with the ascending limb curving around to point toward the stomach. The curve itself is the medial section between them. Contained in the descending limb are the **major and minor papillae** (in the dog; there is only one in the cat). These openings accommodate the **bile duct** and the **pancreatic duct**. In some animals, there are actually two pancreatic ducts. On careful examination of the luminal surface of the duodenum, you may see the papillae.

The **pancreas**, an organ with both endocrine and exocrine functions, runs along the medial surface of the duodenum. Its exocrine functions, those that relate to sending out enzymes or other chemical messengers, include releasing digestive enzymes into the intestinal tract. Its larger amount of tissue is devoted to the production of digestive enzymes. In life, it has a pink, cobblestone appearance. It is supplied by the **celiac and mesenteric arteries** and drains to the **portal vein**. As is true for most of the gastrointestinal (GI) tract, there is sympathetic and parasympathetic innervation. Note that the pancreas has endocrine tissue as well; one of the crucial hormones it produces is insulin. When we discuss endocrine physiology, we will describe the function of this hormone; abnormalities of its production or function are involved in a common metabolic disease, diabetes mellitus.

From the duodenum, the small intestine coils numerous times into the jejunum and then the ileum. The small intestines are suspended from the mesentery and are not anchored to any other part of the abdomen. When serial radiographs are taken, the small intestine will change its position as it contracts and expands these coils. A lack of change over a number of hours can help verify intestinal stasis, known as **ileus**; this is a potentially fatal condition wherein the intestines no longer contract and expand as they usually do and must be managed medically.

The border between the **jejunum** and the **ileum** is merely a functional one. On gross visual inspection, it is hard to point to the spot where the change occurs. This can only be determined on a microscopic level. When performing a dissection, you can be sure to identify the ileum if it is immediately proximal to the colon, as we know that a portion of small intestine must be ileum (see Figure 12.8).

The tissue of the small intestine has several layers, also called **tunics**. They include a serosal layer, a layer of muscle and elastic tissue, and a layer of epithelial tissue. The ileum turns toward the right as it runs toward the **cecum**. The **ileocolic junction** denotes this connection. A condition called **intussusception** occurs when part of the intestine telescopes into another. **Ileocecal intussusception** is a common type of intussusception in dogs and is readily surgically cured if it is treated quickly.

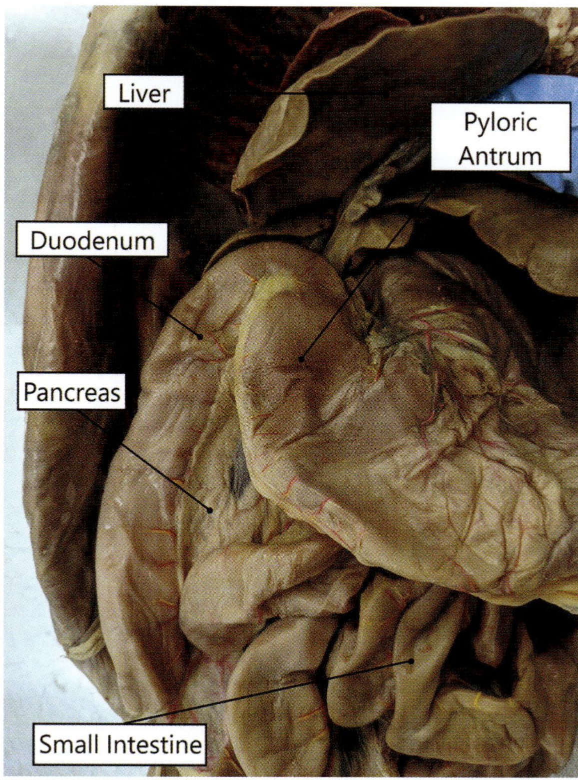

Figure 12.7 The duodenum is the next portion of the gastrointestinal tract after the stomach. A portion of the pancreas runs alongside the duodenum.

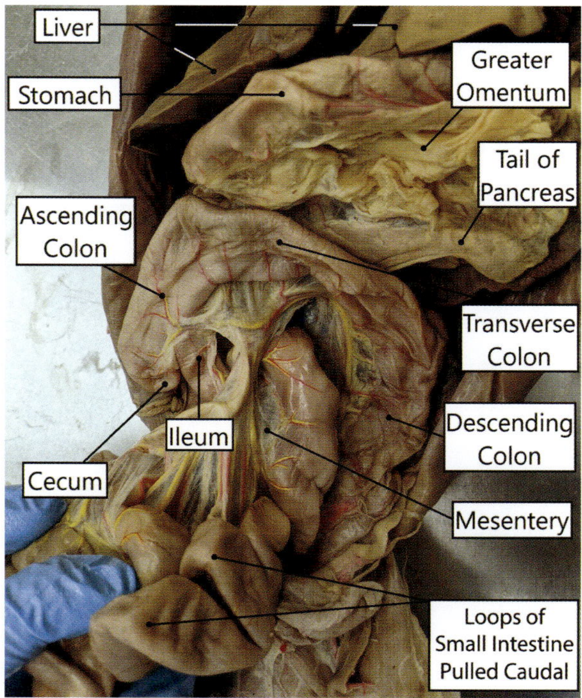

Figure 12.8 The ileum enters the cecum, which in dogs and cats is vestigial, as the ingesta continue toward the colon.

In dogs, the cecum connects to the **ascending colon**. The cecum is a blind alley that forms a slight spiral. In dogs and cats, the cecum is vestigial, or no longer physiologically necessary. In contrast, the cecum is well developed and crucial to digestion in species such as rodents, rabbits, and equines. Exiting the ileum and passing the cecum, the small intestine becomes the large intestine, or the **colon**. At the caudal end of the colon, the lumen widens into a chamber called the **rectum**. Material exits the body at the **anus**, a sphincter with smooth and striated muscle components.

The colon is divided into three parts. The **ascending colon** emerges after the ileum and is relatively short in the carnivore. The **transverse colon** travels from the right toward the stomach, in an area between the stomach and the small intestine. Again, note that the intestine is mobile, so the exact positioning of the transverse colon will vary. The longest part of the colon is the **descending colon**. It runs along the left flank, turns slightly medially at the pelvic cavity, and widens to become the rectum. The distal descending colon exits the peritoneum to course in the retroperitoneum. The rectum is dorsal to the reproductive organs. It has a connective tissue attachment to the vagina in the female and to the urethra in the male.

In a ventrolateral position between the internal and external anal sphincters are the **anal sacs**. There is one on each side of the anus, and their opening can be seen from the outside of the animal. These glands are compressed and emptied during defecation. They are sebaceous glands whose viscous fluid has a strong odor. This fluid can be discharged under stress. Skunks can voluntarily expel this fluid, which is an effective defense mechanism. The anal glands of dogs and cats can become clogged and may need to be manually expressed during physical examinations in the clinic. Animals that "scoot" (rub their perineum along the floor while moving forward) often have impacted or blocked anal glands.

The blood supply of the intestines originates mostly from the **cranial and caudal mesenteric arteries**; the proximal duodenum is supplied by the **celiac artery** and the caudal rectum by the **internal pudendal artery**. Many of the veins eventually empty into the **portal vein**. There is a tremendous amount of lymphatic drainage, most of which goes to the thoracic duct. There are many lymph nodes within the mesentery. Notice that the vessels are present in very large numbers within the mesentery and that each section of the intestine gets blood from a variety of arteries. This is the basis of collateral circulation, which refers to redundancy in the blood supply. If one or even a few of these vessels are damaged or surgically interrupted, the intestine still has a sufficient number of circulatory vessels to compensate. Sympathetic and parasympathetic innervation is present.

Species Variation

The lips of ruminants, and equines to an even larger extent, are much thicker and more mobile than in dogs and cats. This assists in the prehension of food. These areas are well innervated. This innervation can cause the release of endorphins, which is useful in some forms of large animal restraint. When a twitch is wound around the lips of a horse, the large number of nerve endings that are present cause sufficient distraction and a surge of endorphins that allow for handling and restraint.

The dentition of the ruminant is unique (see Figure 12.9). There are no maxillary incisors. In their place, there is a thick mass of tissue called a **dental pad**. This allows the tough, fibrous material they eat to be ground against the pad's flat surface.

Equines and lagomorphs (rabbits) have a great deal in common from a physiological standpoint. Unlike mammals, the majority of their food is digested in the cecum as opposed to the stomach. Thus, the cecum is relatively much larger, and the stomach much smaller, than in dogs and cats. As their diet has almost no fat, equines do not require bile for digestion. Rats, equines, and lamoids do not have a gallbladder.

One of the most striking adaptations to diet is present in ruminants (see Figure 12.10). Ruminants have a four-chambered stomach, which receives the crushed food

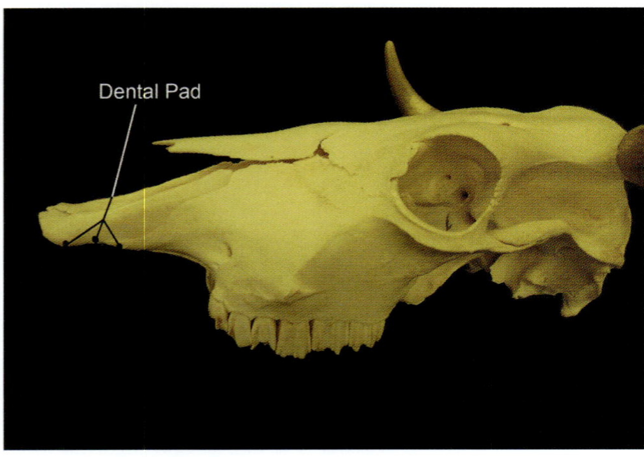

Figure 12.9 The dental pad is not actually pictured here; the lines point to where it would be. Note the absence of teeth. In the living animal, it forms the area where the maxillary incisor teeth would be and allows the crushing movement necessary to process grasses and fibers.

materials from the oral cavity. The cranial-most part of the stomach is the **reticulum**, where food undergoes fermentation. Its lining contains many small compartments and may be familiar as the food item tripe. This cavity lies directly caudal to the heart. In foraging for food, ruminants will occasionally take in nails, fence wire, and other sharp items. They can actually penetrate the reticulum and perforate the heart. The condition, formally known as **traumatic reticulopericarditis** and informally known as "**hardware disease**," is fairly common. The treatment for this is to have the animal swallow a magnet, which prevents any future metal from migrating outside the reticulum.

Caudal to the reticulum is the largest chamber, the **rumen**, which comes from the root word of the species designation, ruminant. The next chamber is the **omasum**, and the last is the **abomasum**. The abomasum is closest to the mammalian stomach in structure and function. In young ruminants that are dependent upon milk, there is a temporary muscular structure called the **esophageal groove**. This allows milk to bypass the rumen, reticulum, and omasum and travel directly to the abomasum to avoid fermentation of the milk or colostrum.

In some ruminants, there is a short section of the intestine that ends in a descending colon. In goats, the colon has a spiral shape.

The equine colon is particularly long and consists of a tube that folds over on itself, then travels to the other side of the animal and folds over on itself again. There are smaller folds called **haustra** along some of the length of the colon. They can be palpated on a rectal exam and help the examiner pinpoint his/her location within the cavity.

Avians have a quite different system. They have a beak rather than lips and do not have teeth. As food enters the oral cavity, it is often stored in a space called the **crop**, in the ventral neck. Food travels along the esophagus to the stomach, which has two chambers, the **ventriculus** and the **proventriculus**. Material is then discharged via the **cloaca**, a chamber that is shared with the reproductive tract (Figure 12.11).

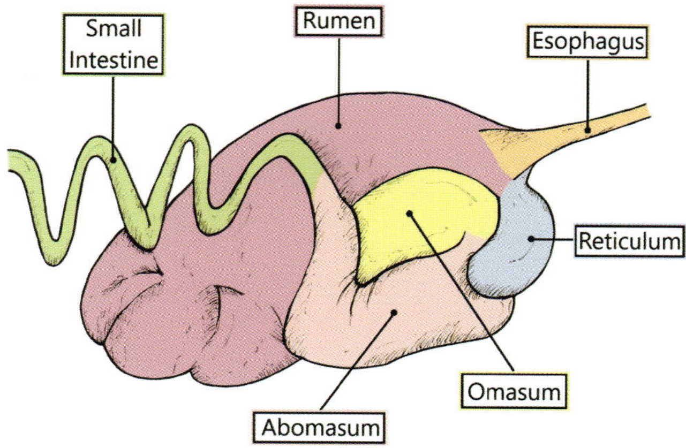

Figure 12.10 Features of the bovine gastrointestinal tract. Note the bovine does not have four separate stomachs but one stomach with four chambers.

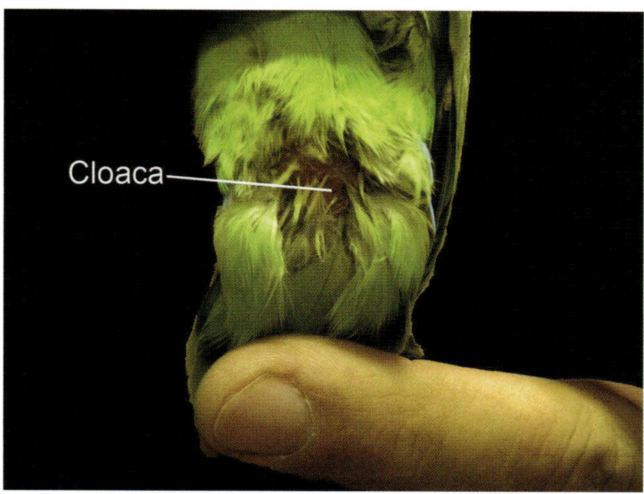

Figure 12.11 The cloaca is the common exit from the avian body for the digestive, urinary, and reproductive tracts.

Clinical Case Resolution: Tucker

Tucker has a thorough oral exam, which appears normal aside from ptyalism (hypersalivation). After an otherwise unremarkable physical exam, Tucker has radiographs of his cervical and thoracic area, as well as his abdomen. Radiographs reveal an esophageal foreign body. This means there is something stuck in the esophagus that must be removed.

Tuckers owners agree to a procedure for removal using endoscopy as a minimally invasive option. Tucker is placed under anesthesia the endoscope is carefully introduced into the mouth and the proximal esophagus. It is revealed that a piece of rawhide was stuck in Tucker's thoracic esophagus. Once carefully removed, there is some ulceration of the esophagus in areas that the rawhide was rubbing against. Tucker is woken up and sent home on a soft diet, medications to help heal the esophagus and reduce acid production, and strict instructions to no longer offer rawhides or chews that may be swallowed. They are also advised to watch out for any signs of nausea, regurgitation, drooling, changes in breathing pattern, or decreased appetite. It is recommended they return in 2 weeks for a recheck appointment.

Review Questions

1 What are the ridges on the palate called?
  A The mandible
  B The buccinator
  C The rugae
  D The ileum

2 The apex of the tongue is closest to:
  A The incisors
  B The molars
  C The throat
  D The soft palate

3 According to the dental formulas, how many premolars are in the canine mandible?
  A 4
  B 6
  C 7
  D 8

4 Deciduous teeth are the same as permanent teeth.
  A True
  B False

5 Which portion of the esophagus is immediately caudal to the diaphragm?
  A The cervical esophagus
  B The upper esophageal sphincter
  C The thoracic esophagus
  D The abdominal esophagus

6 Which cavity contains the kidneys?
  A The thoracic cavity
  B The retroperitoneal cavity
  C The peritoneal cavity
  D The mediastinal cavity

7 Which portion of the stomach is the primary mixing and churning area?
  A The body
  B The cardia
  C The greater curvature
  D The fundus

8 The pancreas runs alongside which portion of the digestive tract?
  A The ileum
  B The cecum
  C The duodenum
  D The mesentery

9 Which portion of the large intestine runs from the right cranial abdomen to the left cranial abdomen?

   A The cecum

   B The ascending colon

   C The descending colon

   D The transverse colon

10 Which species uses the cecum as a primary digestion site?

   A The skunk

   B The rabbit

   C The canine

   D The equine

13

Reproductive Anatomy

> ### Clinical Case: Boots, a 2-Year-Old Male Intact Mixed-Breed Dog
>
> *Boots was recently adopted and is believed to be approximately 2 years old. He is presenting today for his first appointment with his new owners and to get preanesthetic blood work and an exam for his orchiectomy (neuter). The records from the adoption indicate that upon palpation, only one testicle was identified.*

Introduction

The anatomy of the reproductive system varies remarkably in structure across mammalian species. In addition, the system in reptiles and fish is quite different from that in mammals. The reproductive system changes shape and size during adulthood as well as in youth, under certain neural and endocrine influences. It is particularly affected by age-related factors, both at the beginning and the end of life. Each species and sex has its own terms to identify them. A sample of these terms can be seen in Table 13.1.

The offspring of breeding animals also have their own terms for young. A sample of these can be viewed in Table 13.2.

The basic functioning units of the reproductive system are the **gonads**, with their associated ducts and glands. Here we will review the anatomy of the female and male gonads and related organs, while in Chapter 26, the functions and physiology of each sex will be described.

The Female

At the cranial most portion of the female reproductive system is the **ovary**. It is solid and ellipsoid, and within a given species, it is of a constant size regardless of body weight. There is significant species variation, however. For example, the ovary of the mare is a very large, kidney-shaped organ. The ovary in dogs and cats is comparatively smaller and located in the dorsal abdomen. It will be found just caudal to the kidneys (see Figure 13.1).

The entire reproductive tract is suspended from the body wall by a thin, semitransparent membrane called the **broad ligament**. Although continuous throughout its length, the part suspending the ovary is known as the **mesovarium**.

The **estrous** (reproductive) cycle is dominated by hormonal control and will be elucidated later. On dissection, some small protrusions may be noted on the surface of the ovary. These are called **follicles** and contain the **ova**. They change in size throughout the estrous cycle and regress completely at some points.

In horses and cows, the follicles are easily rectally palpated during the examination of the pelvis as part of a routine physical exam. This has great economic significance. For example, the presence and size of follicles in cows can indicate their stage of pregnancy. As one might imagine, the early stages of pregnancy in cows can be difficult to observe on gross examination of the animal. Particularly in dairy cattle, the discovery of pregnancy and its relation to lactation is crucial to the commercial value of the animal.

Anatomy and Physiology for Veterinary Technicians and Nurses: A Clinical Approach, Second Edition. Lori Asprea.
© 2026 John Wiley & Sons, Inc. Published 2026 by John Wiley & Sons, Inc.
Companion website: www.wiley.com/go/asprea/anatomy_vettech2e

Table 13.1 This table outlines the terms used for each sex within each species. It also includes notes where certain health or reproductive factors alter the name.

Species	Male	Female	Notes
Canine	Dog	Bitch	—
Feline	Tom	Queen	—
Horse	Stallion	Mare	Neutered male: Gelding
Donkey	Jack	Jenny	—
Bovine	Bull	Cow	Neutered male: Steer Female who has never had a calf: Heifer
Sheep	Ram	Ewe	Neutered male: Wether
Pig	Boar	Sow	Neutered male: Barrow Female who has never had a piglet: Gilt
Goat	Billy	Doe	Neutered male: Wether
Ferret	Hob	Jill	Neutered male: Gib Spayed female: Sprite
Rabbit	Buck	Doe	—
Deer	Buck	Doe	—
Llama	Sire	Dam	Neutered male: Gelding

Table 13.2 The term for the young of each animal.

Species	Young
Dog	Puppy
Cat	Kitten
Horse	Foal
Donkey	Foal
Bovine	Calf
Sheep	Lamb
Pig	Piglet
Goat	Kid
Ferret	Kit
Rabbit	Kit
Deer	Fawn
Llama	Cria

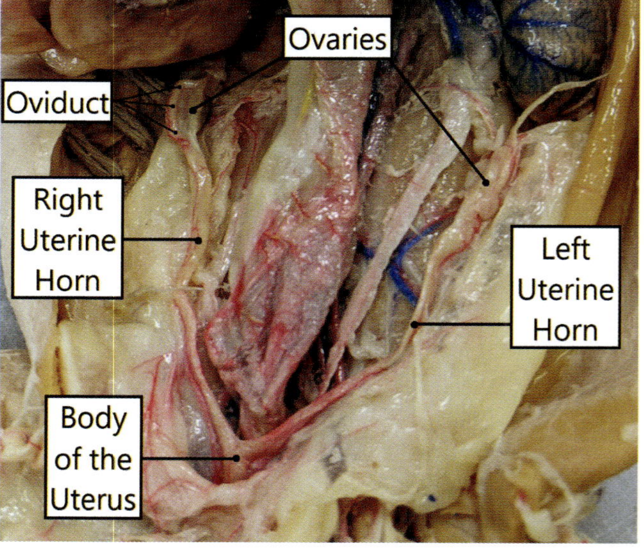

Figure 13.1 The female reproductive system. The animal's head is toward the top. The white pouch that appears to be caudal to the body of the uterus is actually the urinary bladder, which has been reflected back from its normal position ventral to the reproductive tract.

Surrounding the ovaries are the **oviducts**. The ovum, or mature egg, is funneled from the cranial end of the oviduct by the **infundibulum**, a hollow tunnel. It has a fringed end with fingerlike projections that help guide the ovum into the oviduct. These fringes are called **fimbriae**. In dogs, there is actually a small amount of space between the infundibulum and the oviduct. As a result of this, some ova can escape into the abdominal space (Figure 13.2).

The section of the broad ligament that suspends the oviduct is called the **mesosalpinx**. In most domestic animals, fertilization actually occurs within the oviduct, which is quite different from the process occurring in primates.

The oviduct on each side leads into a larger tunnel that proceeds caudally and medially. This section of the system is called the **uterine horn**. Dogs and cats, unlike primates, have a bicornate uterus, where the uterus is a V shape (refer to Figure 13.1). The section of the broad ligament suspending the uterine horns is the **mesometrium**, which continues to become the outer lining of the body of the uterus.

After fertilization in the oviduct, the embryo comes to rest in the horns, where it implants in the uterine tissue to develop. The fetal puppy or kitten develops within the horns of the uterus, which are highly distensible. While the horns of the uterus are relatively straight in dogs and cats, they loop extensively in sows.

The uterine horns meet at a common chamber called the **body of the uterus**. In dogs and cats, this area is very short. It is situated in a relatively more caudal position in cats than in dogs. This necessitates a different incision for ovariohysterectomy in each species. The head of the uterus is connected to the body wall by the suspensory ligament. In dogs, this is a thick connection that requires some force to sever in surgery; in cats, the ligament is thin and can easily be broken with the finger.

The uterus is a hollow muscular organ that has multiple layers. The outermost layer is the **perimetrium**, which is covered by a layer of **peritoneum**, the tissue that lines all the organs within the abdominal cavity. The middle layer is the **myometrium**, which is the muscle layer responsible for uterine contractions. The inner layer of the uterus is called the endometrium. It is a thick, layered, highly vascularized tissue. In cows, the embryo attaches to the endometrium via a structure called a **caruncle**.

The ovaries and uterus have strong vascularization and neural input, as well as a great deal of lymphatic drainage. The **ovarian artery** brings oxygenated blood to the ovaries and comes directly off the aorta, following a torturous path.

The body of the uterus narrows as it travels caudally. A sphincter muscle called the **cervix** is positioned between the uterus and the vagina, controlling access to the uterus. The cervix stays closed except during some parts of the estrous cycle and during **parturition** or giving birth. It has mucus-producing glands that assist in sealing the opening (Figure 13.3).

The area from the cervix to the **urethral orifice** is known as the **vagina**. It is relatively thin and distensible and courses through the retroperitoneal area. It has a smooth outer lining, with muscle and mucous glands within. The vagina serves to receive the penis during breeding and act as the birth canal during parturition. It runs dorsal to the urinary bladder and urethra and ventral to the rectum. There is a large venous plexus extending ventrally from the body of the uterus along much of the vagina, necessitating caution during abdominal surgery. Note that the possum actually has two vaginas, designed to accept the "double" penis of the male.

The **urethra** is the tube that carries urine from the bladder to the urethral orifice during urination. It opens into the vagina at an area called the **vestibule** of the vagina. This resides caudal to the ischial arch and slopes toward the **vulva**, where the vagina/urethra exits the body (Figure 13.4).

The vulva contains the only external portions of the female reproductive system. It is categorized into three parts: the vestibule, as mentioned above, the **clitoris**, and the **labia**. The clitoris is homologous to the penis and contains **erectile tissue** and is extensively supplied with

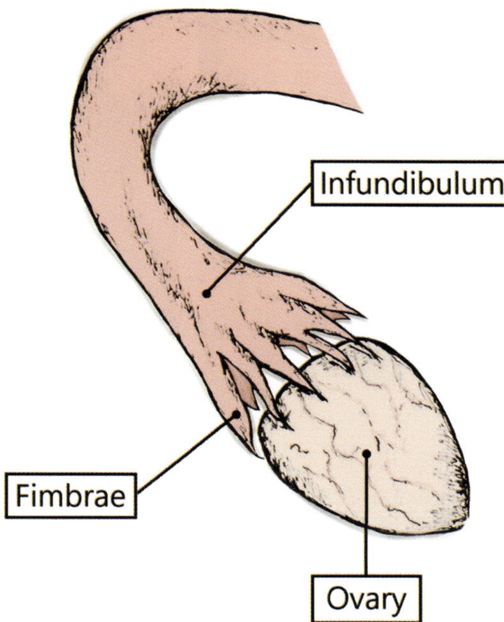

Figure 13.2 The infundibulum with fimbriae which will gently guide and accept the ovum into the oviduct.

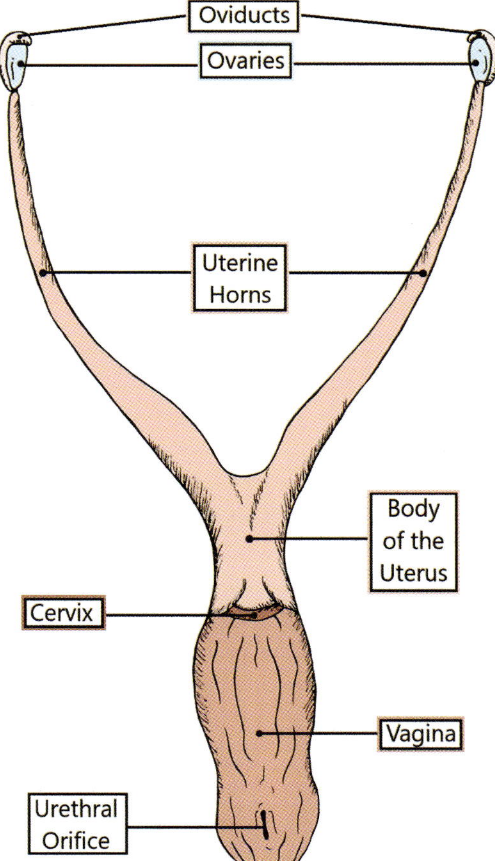

Figure 13.3 The female reproductive system with the ventral vagina canal removed to view the cervix and urethral orifice.

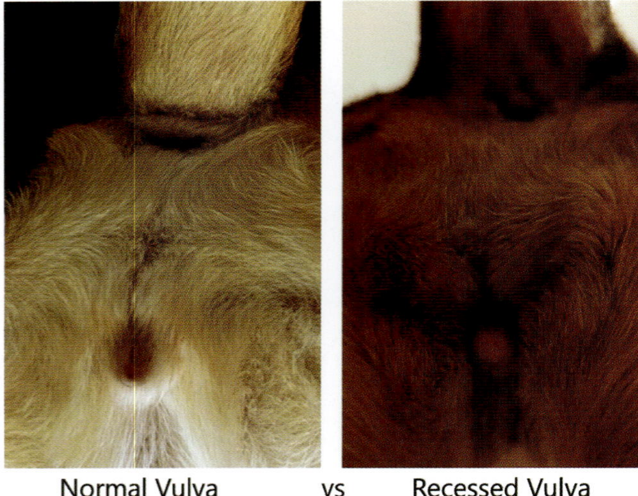

Figure 13.4   The canine vulva. A normal, partially haired vulva compared to the animal on the right with a recessed vulva.

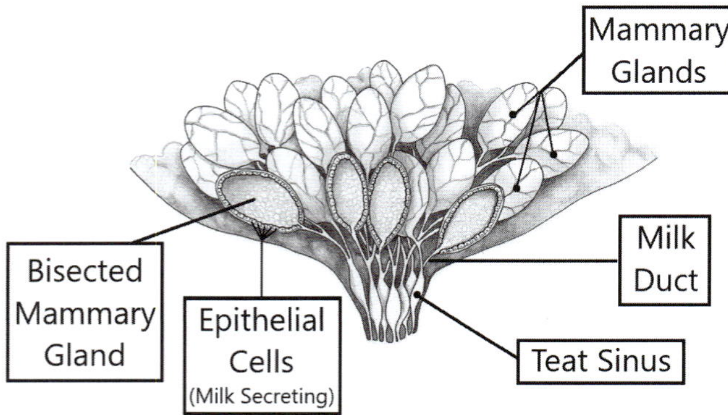

Figure 13.5   The mammary gland and alveoli.

Table 13.3   Each animal has a differing normal number of mammary glands and associated teats. this table lists some of the more common animals encountered in veterinary medicine. You can see that the number of teats is relative to the number of offspring in a singe litter.

Species	Total number of mammary glands/teats
Dog	8–10
Cat	8
Horse	2
Donkey	2
Cow	4
Sheep	2
Pig	14, but can go up to approximately 30
Goat	2
Ferret	8
Rabbit	8–10
Deer	4
Llama	4

nerve endings. The vulva ends in two soft-tissue flaps called the labia, from the root word for lips. An anatomical issue called **recessed** or **hypoplastic vulva** results in the vulva being completely or partially hidden by the surrounding skin. This can predispose animals to recurrent peri-vulvar dermatitis, vaginitis, or urinary tract infections, as the folding of skin around the area traps moisture and heat and makes an ideal environment for bacteria to grow. This can be rectified with medications to treat the infections as well as proper hygiene tips to help keep the area clean. Weight loss can help overweight animals to reduce the size of the tissue surrounding the vulva. Alternatively, a surgical intervention, called a **vulvoplasty** or **epesioplasty**, may be considered to correct the anatomical defect.

Another important part of the female reproductive anatomy is the **mammary glands**. The mammary glands are specialized glands of the skin that produce **colostrum** and milk. Colostrum is the first liquid produced by the mammary glands for the neonate after parturition and is rich with antibodies to help protect the newborn. In most mammals, there are two chains of mammary glands, one on the right and one on the left, although the number varies widely in different species (see Table 13.3).

Note that many animals have **supernumerary**, or extra, nipples.

Each mammary gland is comprised of **alveoli**, which are hollow cavities clustered like grapes within the mammary tissue (see Figure 13.5). Lining the alveoli are specialized cells that produce milk and then secrete that milk into a series of ducts that lead to the teat. The act of suckling causes the release of **oxytocin**, a hormone that causes the cells around the alveoli to contract. This process is called **milk let-down** and allows the milk to come from the alveoli, through the ducts to the exit of pores or openings on the teat (Figure 13.6).

The Male

The purpose of the male reproductive system is to produce male sex hormones, develop spermatozoa, and deliver those spermatozoa to the female to create offspring. In order to achieve this, there is a system of tissues, organs, glands, and ducts.

The **testicles** (or testes) are the analogues of the ovaries. They are smooth, solid, and ellipsoid in shape. Embryologically, the testes form in the cranial abdomen and descend to their location, generally within the **scrotum**. This is performed by a connective tissue called the **gubernaculum**. The gubernaculum is attached to the testicle and in the scrotum. As the animal develops, the gubernaculum pulls the testicles down toward and into the scrotum. If the testicle fails to descend at the proper time, it may remain in an ectopic (abnormal) position. This condition is known as **cryptorchidism**. The problem is usually hereditary, so it is important that cryptorchid animals are not used as breeders. Unilateral cryptorchidism is most common, although bilateral abnormality is seen on occasion. The problem is solved surgically. Most often, the testicle travels as far as the area of the inguinal canal, close to the scrotum. It can, however, remain in the cranial abdomen. Therefore, removing it requires some searching to identify its location. Undescended testicles should always be removed, not only to prevent breeding of the animal but because the retained testicle(s) have a higher incidence of becoming cancerous. Further, the undescended testicle continues to produce hormones, which in some specific cases may contribute to unwanted behaviors such as urine marking.

In dogs and cats, the testicles reside in the scrotum, a sack of skin. The scrotum has a median groove distinguishing one side from another. This division can result in asymmetrical sections. The skin is relatively thin and has many sweat and sebaceous glands. The testicles sit directly on the ventral scrotum.

In species such as most domestic animals, sperm must be produced at a lower temperature, so the testicles are located outside of the abdominal cavity within the scrotum. The scrotum can be alopecic, as in ruminants, sparsely haired, as in dogs, or heavily haired, as in cats. There is a muscle within the scrotum called the **cremaster**. The contraction of this muscle can pull the testes closer to the body in colder temperatures to maintain the appropriate environment for spermatozoa production.

In some animals, the testicles remain within the abdominal cavity to achieve the proper temperature for the production of sperm. Pachyderms (elephants, hyrax) are an example of this type of system. In some animals, for example, the bat, the testes descend at breeding season and then retract. Rabbits can retract their testicles at any time, which can make neutering a challenge.

Another species difference has to do with the relative size and position of the testicles. In the bull, the long axis of the testicle is vertical, and the size of the testicle and scrotum relative to the size of the rest of the body is quite large. In contrast, the long axis of the canine testicle is horizontal, and its relative size is smaller. The testicles of the cat actually slant slightly toward the anus. The testes are suspended within the scrotum at the end of the **spermatic cord**. The spermatic cord contains a large number of blood vessels, nerves, lymphatics, and a tube called the **vas deferens or ductus deferens**. The arteries contained in the spermatic cord are responsible for bringing oxygen-rich blood to the testicles and surrounding tissues, while the veins are organized into the **pampiniform plexus**. The testicular artery, like the ovarian artery, branches directly off the abdominal aorta. It too follows a contorted path to allow greater surface area. The pampiniform plexus is a fishnet-style web of small veins that help to thermoregulate the testicles. This plexus of veins drains back into the caudal vena cava.

The testicles are covered by a connective tissue called the **vaginal tunics**. The **visceral vaginal tunic** surrounds the testes, while the **parietal vaginal tunic** is the thicker outer layer. Immediately deep to the tunics is the **capsule**. The capsule is made of dense connective tissue and works to protect and support the testes.

Within the testes are a series of tightly coiled tubes called the **seminiferous tubules**. These seminiferous tubules are where spermatogenesis, or the creation of sperm, occurs with the support of **Sertoli cells**. Sertoli cells act as nurse cells to the forming sperm cells to provide nutrition as well as protection from the body's own immune system. Once the sperm cells are almost fully mature, they move into storage through the **efferent ducts** to the **epididymis** to complete maturation.

The epididymis is a flat ribbon-like structure that lies along the surface of the testis that contains a long-coiled tubule. The epididymis runs along the dorsal surface of the testicle in dogs, following a rather convoluted course. The epididymis

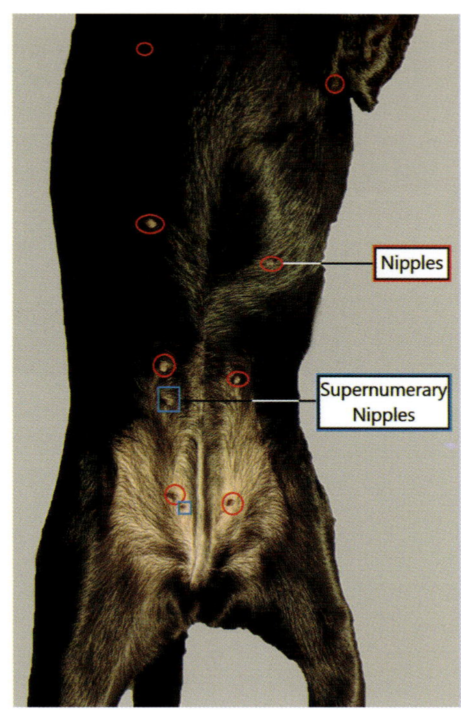

Figure 13.6 The nipples of a canine. Note that the normal paired nipples are outlined in red, while the supernumerary, or extra, nipples are outlined in blue.

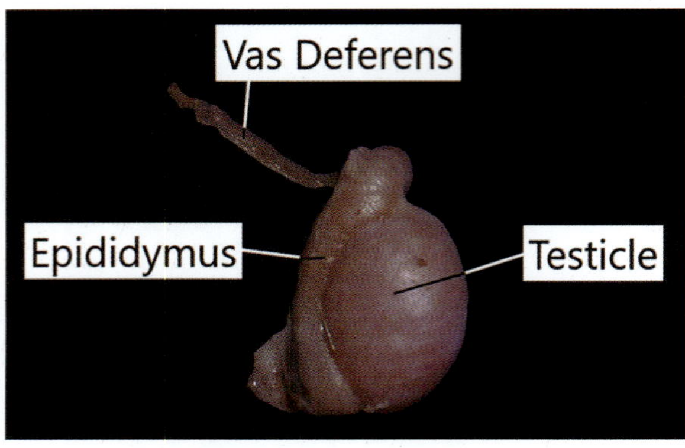

Figure 13.7   The testicle.

has three parts: the head, the body, and the tail. The head is where spermatozoa enter from the efferent ducts, the body is the main portion lying against the testis, and the tail is the distal portion that continues on to the **vas deferens**. The vas deferens, or ductus deferens, emerges at the distal end of the epididymis and proceeds dorsally over the urinary bladder, through the **prostate gland**, and enters the urethra. The vas deferens is supported within the abdomen by a peritoneal fold called the **mesoductus**. It is over the dorsal surface of the urinary bladder that the duct from each side joins to form one passage. The vas deferens carries sperm away from the testicle and toward the urethra for ejaculation (Figure 13.7).

Many mammals have what are known as **accessory reproductive glands**, which play an important physiological role. The **prostate gland** is present in dogs and cats. The **bulbourethral gland** is present in dogs but is vestigial in cats. The **vesicular gland**, which can be found where the deferent duct enters the urethra, is not present in dogs or cats. Of all of these, the one most likely to be seen on dissection is the **prostate**, which surrounds the urethra shortly after the urethra exits the urinary bladder. As in humans, enlargement of the prostate can either be benign or malignant. Prostate cancer in animals is much rarer than in humans but does occur.

The pelvic urethra (the part within the abdomen) is joined by the deferent and prostatic ducts and courses toward the outside of the body. It is highly vascular. It has a substantial layer of the **urethralis muscle**. The urethra runs ventrally to the rectum and can be palpated on rectal exam. In bovine practice, an instrument called an **electro-ejaculator** is inserted in the rectum to cause contraction of the urethra and to stimulate the discharge of semen; evaluation of sperm is critical in reproductive studies.

As the urethra exits the body via the **penis**, it is surrounded by an even more complex environment of vascular and **erectile tissue**. It courses all the way to the distal opening of the penis. The penis is broken down into three main parts: **the root, the body**, and the **glans**. The root is where the penis is connected to the pelvis with muscles and connective tissue. The body is the largest portion of the penis and contains bundles of erectile tissue. Erectile tissue is spongy like in nature and has open spaces called sinuses that fill with blood when an erection occurs, allowing the penis to become firm for vaginal insertion. The glans is the distal, free end of the penis, which is richly supplied with nerves.

The penis is suspended from an area ventral to the trunk in most species, in the area of the caudal abdomen. A notable exception is the cat. The feline has the only rearward facing penis among mammals. It travels a relatively short distance once it emerges from the body.

The **prepuce** is the external protective layer of tissue around the penis. It is a fold of abdominal skin that sheaths the body and glans of the penis. The outer layer of the prepuce is skin that can be somewhat haired, depending on the species. The inner layer of the prepuce is a moist mucous membrane.

Species differentiations are notable. In dogs, there is a small bone within the exterior penis, called the **os penis**. It is generally visible on radiography. In pigs and some small ruminants, the penis has a prominent **sigmoid flexure** (S-shaped curve). Some species have a small protrusion of soft tissue at the distal end of the penis called the **urethral process**. The dorsal penis in the bull has an **apical ligament** holding it to the prepuce. If this ligament is too short, the penis deviates to one side on erection, making copulation unsuccessful. The cat penis has spines on it that help tie the male and female together.

Clinical Case Resolution: Boots

A physical exam of Boots determines that the original records appear correct, as only one testicle is palpable within the scrotum. Boots is believed to be unilaterally cryptorchid. An abdominal ultrasound is performed to attempt to locate the abdominal testicle.

After explaining these findings to the owners, they elect to move forward with a neuter and laparotomy (abdominal exploratory) to remove the retained testicle. Due to the more invasive nature of this surgery, the recovery time will be slightly prolonged in comparison to a routine neuter.

Review Questions

1 True or False: Many domesticated animals have an os penis
   A True
   B False

2 What does the spermatic cord contain?
   A Nerves
   B Vessels
   C Ductus deferens
   D All of the above

3 What is the role of the cremaster muscle?
   A To move ejaculate out of the penis
   B To provide lubrication
   C To withdraw the testicles closer to the body
   D To provide blood flow necessary for an erection

4 Where is the site of fertilization in most female mammals?
   A The oviduct
   B The ovary
   C The uterus
   D The infundibulum

5 Which portion of connective tissue is responsible for suspending the oviducts to the body wall?
   A The mesometrium
   B The mesovarium
   C The mesosalpinx

6 True or False: Most domestic animals have one uterine horn.
   A True
   B False

7 Which portion of the epididymis receives spermatozoa from efferent ducts?
   A The head
   B The tail
   C The body
   D None of the above

8 True or False: The vagina is an external reproductive organ
   A True
   B False

9 What portion of the female reproductive tract is responsible for guiding the mature oocyte into the oviduct?
   A The infundibulum
   B The mesosalpinx
   C The mesometrium
   D The os penis

10 What are the specialized hollow cavities that create milk in the mammary glands?
   A The teats
   B The infundibulum
   C The alveoli
   D The prostate gland

Section 2

Physiology

14

The Cell and Hematology

Clinical Case: Noodle, a 10-Week-Old Female Intact Yorkshire Terrier

Noodle is presented to the emergency room for extreme lethargy and possible seizures. The owner has one other puppy from the litter at home with the whelping bitch. The other puppy is reportedly fine at this time.

Introduction

While it is possible to consider the matter at a subatomic level, and it can be argued that, in its own way, even this level of analysis relates to the function of all living (and other) structures, it is not germane to our discussion. Therefore, to investigate the basis of physiology, it is best to begin at the level of the cell.

The cell is recognized as a microscopic entity having a border, a nucleus, and an internal power mechanism. This is not true of pathogens. for example, while they are microscopic, and many have a border, they may not have a membrane-bound nucleus (bacteria), or they may obtain the energy to exist by living inside another cell (viruses).

The cells that make up plants have a cell wall, which is to say that their border is less permeable and has materials not found in the borders of most mammalian cells. The matter of walls becomes particularly important in considering bacteria; whether their borders are walled or not plays a role in how easy it is for antibiotics to penetrate them and disrupt their activities. This is one of the reasons that certain antibiotics are more effective against a given bacterium than others.

Here, we will review basic cell functions and roles, then explore the cells of the blood and their respective roles within the body.

Mammalian Cell Anatomy

The borders of mammalian cells are circumscribed by the **cell membrane**. This is a flexible barrier that has many folds which help to increase surface area. The membrane is mainly composed of **phospholipids**. This has significant implications. Disease states that cause a phosphorus imbalance can disrupt the cell membranes themselves and lead to cell death. Drugs that are **lipid soluble**, or fat soluble, will penetrate the cells more easily than those that are not. All along the cell membrane are a variety of receptor sites and channels that interact with anything that needs to enter, exit, or communicate with the cell.

The remainder of the mammalian cell is comprised of **the cytoplasm** and **the nucleus**. Each of these pieces plays an integral role in the cell's function. The cytoplasm is the inner substance of the cell and contained within it is **cytosol, the cytoskeleton, the organelles**, and **inclusions**. The cytosol is the liquid portion of the cell that contains dissolved electrolytes (like potassium), simple sugars, and amino acids. The cytoskeleton is a flexible structure just under the cell membrane to provide shape and structure as well as aid in metabolic activity. Organelles are like tiny organs that carry out the metabolic functions of the cells, while inclusions are small packages of engulfed or metabolic products. Inclusions can be used to store or transport these products.

The nucleus is the largest organelle and is essentially the brain of the cell. It contains the genetic material of the cell along with the blueprints for thousands of proteins that the cell might make. Cells can be **mononuclear, multinuclear,**

Anatomy and Physiology for Veterinary Technicians and Nurses: A Clinical Approach, Second Edition. Lori Asprea.
© 2026 John Wiley & Sons, Inc. Published 2026 by John Wiley & Sons, Inc.
Companion website: www.wiley.com/go/asprea/anatomy_vettech2e

or **anucleate**. Mononuclear cells contain one single nucleus, while multinuclear cells have more than one nucleus per cell. Anucleate cells are cells with no nucleus, and this is usually before the nucleus has formed in the developing cell, or by design after the cell has matured. For example, the red blood cells of mammals are anucleate, but before the red blood cell is fully mature, a nucleus is present.

The Production of Energy

Living tissue, including bones, organs, and connective materials like skin, is composed of cells. Within each cell is a collection of structures that perform operations such as replicating genetic material and maintaining electrolyte balance. The cell requires energy in order to carry out these activities.

The mammalian cell performs both **catabolism** and **anabolism**. Catabolism involves breaking materials such as nutrients down into other materials that can be used by the cell at the moment. Anabolism occurs when the cell takes materials and combines them to make a new molecule. An example of the latter would be the cell using **amino acids** to build a protein, as amino acids are the building blocks of proteins.

The breakdown of glucose, a simple sugar used by the body for energy, is accomplished by **oxidation**. In breaking down the glucose molecule, oxygen and carbon dioxide are produced. The complex series of chemical interactions that accompany this activity results in the production of **adenosine triphosphate (ATP)**. The breaking of the ATP molecule by removing one phosphorus liberates a large amount of energy, and thus ATP is utilized frequently. This series of steps occurs in the **cytosol** and in the **mitochondria** themselves, making mitochondria the main producer of ATP. Cytosol is the liquid portion of the cell in which structures like the **nucleus** and mitochondria are embedded. Since oxygen is used, the process is called **aerobic metabolism**.

The reaction was first described by a scientist named Krebs, so the set of reactions is known as the **Krebs cycle**. The crucial element is that oxygen is required and that nutrients are converted into energy. The end result of the process is the incidental production of water and carbon dioxide, which are excreted.

Along with the conversion of nutrients into energy by chemical means, there are also changes in **electrical charge**. Ion exchange is a part of the process of producing energy across the cell wall. At rest the cell wall is said to be **polarized**, or carrying a charge, in which the inside of the cell is more negatively charged than the outside of the cell.

Homeostasis is the maintenance of a steady and balanced state to allow normal function. The homeostasis of any cell, or for that matter any body system, is what makes for normal function. In other words, the healthy state of the individual depends on maintaining a balance in many things, including energy production and ion exchange. When discussing the balance of charged molecules that involves oxygen, such as occurs in the production of ATP, the homeostatic balance is referred to as **oxidation-reduction**.

At its most basic, **oxidation** refers to the addition of oxygen, and **reduction** refers to its removal. The addition and removal are accomplished by way of chemical reactions using other molecules in the cell. When the reactions are carried out properly, the animal is said to be in **redox balance** (reduction/oxidation).

A consequence of oxygen deprivation is a disruption of normal energy production and, ultimately, cell death. One way we attempt to address this problem is to provide oxygen directly to the animal as a gas to supplement his/her own respiratory system. Note that if oxygen is replaced too quickly or at too high a level, it can actually result in a flurry of activity that leaves an extra electron in the cell. This unbalanced negative charge can damage the cell significantly. If the blood supply to a previously poorly supplied area is restored too rapidly, or an animal in respiratory distress receives too much oxygen too quickly, more harm may be done than good. This is called **reperfusion injury**. It is important to be aware of this when working in an emergency or critical care area.

It is important that the animal has another way to make energy at times when oxygen levels are decreased. This decrease can be temporary from high levels of exercise or significant changes in altitude or long term, as in disease states and/or injury. Energy production can occur without oxygen, to some extent, in a process called **anaerobic metabolism**.

Aerobic catabolism uses materials such as glucose and its derivatives to make energy. The brain cannot use any other pathway to make energy than aerobic metabolism. It is for this reason that hypoglycemic puppies and kittens often show neurological symptoms; the brain cannot function without the oxygen and glucose it needs to make energy. Aerobic catabolism produces a large amount of energy.

However, there is a way to make low levels of energy, at a relatively fast rate, in some cells of the body. The anaerobic route of energy production also uses glucose; in fact, it can only use the sugars provided in food, as opposed to sugars produced as byproducts of other metabolic activity. Muscle cells in particular are capable of anaerobic metabolism.

The drawback to anaerobic energy production is that a byproduct called **lactic acid** is produced. Lactic acid is capable of damaging local tissue. During anaerobic metabolism, it can be converted to a less damaging molecule. However, if there is an overwhelming amount, it will be difficult or impossible to extract energy and allow the process to continue. Muscle cramping can occur due to lactic acid buildup.

Muscle cells also use an anaerobic pathway that produces **creatine phosphate**. Creatine phosphate can be used to make ATP in the absence of oxygen. In addition, muscle tissue can store oxygen in the form of myoglobin.

Aerobic metabolism can continue uninterrupted if oxygen is available and the animal is eating. Anaerobic metabolism only occurs under specific circumstances. In either case, the organism can sustain energy production.

Mammalian Cell Boundaries

The metabolism of the entire body is dependent on the ability of materials such as gases, particularly oxygen, and nutrients to enter or exit the cell membrane. This occurs by way of a variety of transportation mechanisms. Materials can move in or out of the cell using **passive transport** (movement without requiring energy) or **active transport** (movement requiring energy).

Passive transport, or transport in and out of the cell without the use of energy in the form of ATP, can be done in a variety of ways. **Diffusion** is the passive movement of particles across the semipermeable cell membrane from areas of low concentration to areas of high concentration. This is similar to a person riding a train. If you were to board a train that had some very crowded cars and some empty cars, you would move to the train cars with more space. The process of diffusion is the same as particles move from a crowded or concentrated area to a less crowded or concentrated area.

Another passive process is **facilitated diffusion**, in which particles can move through the cell membrane but require a carrier protein to do so. This is usually reserved for larger molecules or molecules that are not lipid soluble. **Filtration** is also a passive cell membrane process in which the forces of liquid on the cell wall force small particles through. Think of this concept as coffee and a coffee filter. Coffee grounds are placed in a filter and water is poured over. The pressure of the water causes small particles (caffeine, tannins, vitamins, and antioxidants) to pass through, while the coffee grounds stay behind.

Another important concept when discussing transport into and out of a cell is that of **osmosis**. At its simplest, osmosis refers to the tendency of water to be attracted to areas where the solution is concentrated. In a mammalian cell, the membrane is semipermeable. It does not let all molecules move in and out freely; if it did, it would soon be empty. If there is more material inside the cell than outside, water will be drawn in. On the other hand, if there is a great deal of material in the fluid around the cell, water will be drawn out. There is no energy required to make this occur. Osmosis is a type of passive transport, then, in that it does not need energy to work.

It is important to consider the number of particles both inside and outside of the cell, as these conditions can impact cell function and survival. In an **isotonic** setting, there is the same concentration of particles in the fluid outside the cell, as there are inside the cell. This means an even exchange of water in and out of the cell, leaving the cell unharmed. In a **hypotonic** setting, there are fewer particles outside the cell than inside the cell, resulting in the movement of water into the cell, where the particle concentration is higher. Remember that water wants to move from areas of low concentration to areas of high concentration. This can result in cell injury or death as the cell will bloat with water. Opposite this is the **hypertonic** setting, in which there is a higher concentration of particles outside the cell compared to inside the cell. This can lead water to exit the cell in high quantities, dehydrating or shrinking the cell which can also lead to cell death. These must be considered when administering fluids to a patient. As a general rule, we use isotonic fluid as intravenous supplementation, as it should not harm the cells as described above; however, there are instances or disease processes where hypertonic or hypotonic solutions may be selected.

There are also mechanisms that require the use of energy to transport things through the cell membrane. These **active membrane processes** can be done using ATP or by changing the electrical charges on the cell wall. This is generally used to move molecules or products against the concentration gradient. Where in diffusion, particles can passively move from an area of high concentration to an area of low concentration, active transport can move more particles into the areas of high concentration. This can be used for both **exocytosis**, pushing something out of the cell, and **endocytosis**, or taking something into the cell.

Hematology

Now that we have a basic understanding of mammalian cells and their functions, we can explore the cells of the blood. Blood is a fluid connective tissue, in that the liquid and cellular portions of blood serve to connect all the functioning systems of the body. The liquid portion of blood is **plasma** which is mainly water and dissolved solutes. Floating in plasma are the blood cells, which include **erythrocytes, thrombocytes**, and **leukocytes**. Also contained in plasma are proteins like **albumin**, factors for clotting, nutrients, waste products, gases, hormones, and more. All the blood cells are formed from stem cells. Each of these stem cells is called a **multipotent cell**. This cell then gets direction from the body to follow certain paths, leading to all types of mature blood cells.

Red Blood Cells

The formation of red blood cells or erythrocytes is called **erythropoiesis**, and it occurs in the bone marrow. The timeline from a stem cell to a mature red blood cell varies widely by species and can also be influenced by hormones and the availability of building material like iron. The main job of the mature red blood cell is to take care of gas exchange, by taking oxygen to tissues and carrying away the waste material, carbon dioxide.

The red blood cell in mammals contains no nucleus, as it is dissolved in the maturation process. This allows it to be more efficient in gas exchange for the mammal. In some other animals like reptiles and birds, the red blood cells maintain their nucleus (Figure 14.1). The red blood cell contains **hemoglobin** and iron, which provide the binding site for oxygen (Figure 14.2).

Platelets

Thrombocytes, or **platelets**, are created by a process called **thrombopoiesis**. Thrombocytes are unique as they are not actually complete cells, but rather fragments of another, larger cell called the **megakaryocyte** (Figure 14.3). The megakaryocyte is formed in the bone marrow, and it does not leave the bone marrow. Fragments of the megakaryocyte cytoplasm break off and enter circulation as platelets. These small pieces of cytoplasm contain clotting factors that help to stop or slow bleeding.

White Blood Cells

Leukocytes or **white blood cells** come in a variety of cell lines. The formation of white blood cells is called **leukopoiesis**. The white blood cells are **neutrophils, lymphocytes, monocytes, eosinophils**, and **basophils**, listed in the order of which they occur most frequently.

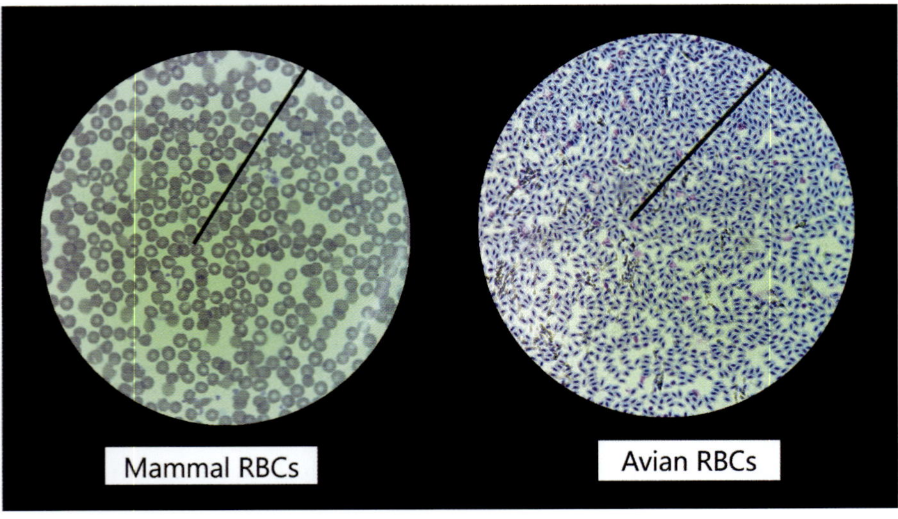

Figure 14.1 Red blood cell smears that have been prepared using a Romanowsky stain variant. Note that mammal red blood cells are non-nucleated as compared to the nucleated avian red blood cells.

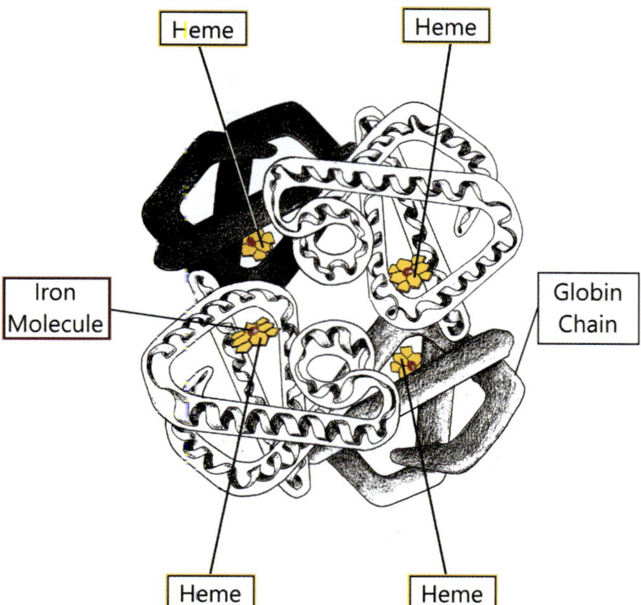

Figure 14.2 A hemoglobin molecule. Hemoglobin is comprised of four globin chains, each one containing a heme unit and an iron molecule.

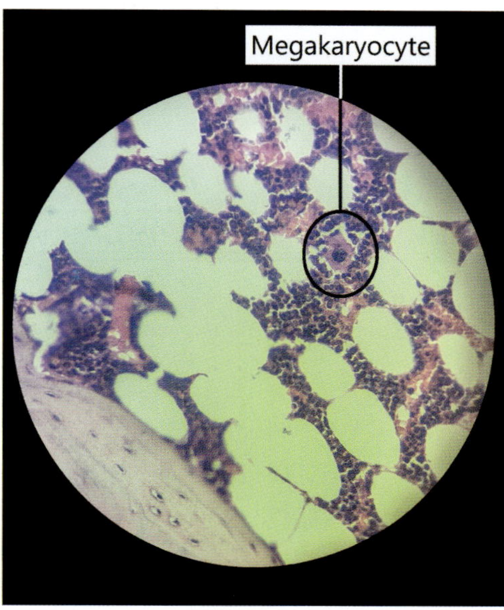

Figure 14.3 A microscopic view of the bone marrow to focus on the large Megakaryocyte. It is surrounded by open white areas which are adipose cells and red bone marrow producing other cell lines.

Neutrophils are the highest number of circulating white blood cells. They have a multilobed two to five-segment nucleus, and as such are sometimes referred to as **polymorphonuclear cells**. They are the first white blood cells on the scene in response to any insult like inflammation, bacteria, or viruses. Neutrophils are **granulocytes**, or cells containing granules that secrete products. In neutrophils, the granules secrete digestive enzymes that help to destroy foreign invaders. They also help recruit other immune cells to the area to help fight infections.

Lymphocytes are the second most commonly occurring white blood cells in circulation. They come in different types including **T-lymphocytes, B-lymphocytes**, and **natural killer cells** or NK cells. T-lymphocytes are the type of lymphocyte most frequently seen in circulation. They are **agranulocytes**, or cells with no granules, that are produced in the bone marrow and mature in the **thymus**, a small gland in the mediastinum. They have many different roles and subtypes but help to assist the immune system by killing infected cells and help the immune system to recognize and remember pathogens that have been encountered in the past by forming memory cells. Perhaps one of the most important things T-lymphocytes do is engage B-lymphocytes to join in the immune response.

B-lymphocytes are agranulocytes rarely seen circulating in blood. They are recruited by specific T-lymphocytes to participate in immune responses to foreign invaders. B-lymphocytes gain information about the pathogen from the T-lymphocytes and begin multiplying to help fight the infection. Once activated and multiplying, many B-lymphocytes turn into plasma cells which begin producing **antibodies**. Antibodies are proteins that destroy harmful invaders and are specific to each pathogen. For example, the antibodies to the common cold will not be useful against strep throat infections.

Natural killer cells or NK cells are another type of lymphocyte, but they differ in that they are a granulocyte. They also have a type of enzyme in their granules that kill cells. Natural killer cells are not specific like B-lymphocytes or antibodies.

Monocytes are the largest-sized white blood cells in circulation. They are agranulocytes that participate in inflammatory responses and help to clean up cellular debris. When monocytes leave circulation and enter tissue, they are called **macrophages**.

Eosinophils and basophils are rarely seen in circulation in dogs and cats, but this can vary in different species. Eosinophils are a type of granulocyte with a bi-lobed nucleus. When prepared on a microscope slide, the granules in the cytoplasm stain a red/pink color, making them easier to distinguish when looking at blood under the microscope. Eosinophils help to fight parasitic diseases and allergens. Basophils are another granulocyte rarely seen. They are mononuclear. The granules in basophils appear dark purple in color when prepared for microscopic examination, making them stand out among other cells in the blood. Basophils also play a role in fighting parasitic infections and allergens similar to eosinophils. The granules in basophils contain **histamines**, which are released during allergic reactions. In chronic or acute allergies, **antihistamine medications** can help combat the side effects of histamine release (Figure 14.4).

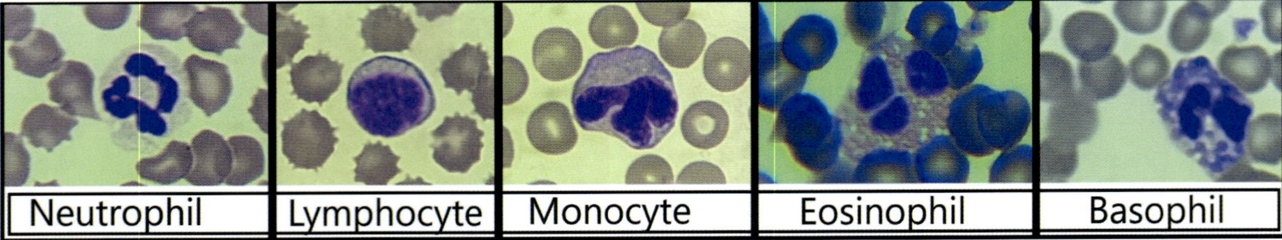

Figure 14.4 A comparison of each type of white blood cell organized from most commonly seen in normal canine and feline blood to least commonly seen in normal canine and feline blood.

Clinical Case Resolution: Noodle

Noodle is examined and point-of-care bloodwork reveals a very low blood sugar or hypoglycemia. Examination reveals a postictal (postseizure) state in which Noodle is weak and lethargic and seemingly disoriented.

There is a direct correlation between blood glucose levels and brain function. Glucose is a powerful source of energy for the survival of body cells. The brain itself cannot undergo anaerobic metabolism at all. If a low level of glucose in the blood persists, one of the most dangerous consequences is that neurological functioning will be adversely affected.

Noodle is hospitalized and given supplemental intravenous sugar and put on a frequent feeding schedule. With strict monitoring and treatment, her blood sugar normalizes, and she is sent home for monitoring. No permanent neurological effects are noted.

Review Questions

1 What is the mammalian cell wall mostly comprised of?
   A Phospholipids
   B Cytosol
   C Organelles
   D Mitochondria

2 Which organelle is responsible for creating the majority of adenosine triphosphate?
   A The nucleus
   B The mitochondria
   C The phospholipid bilayer
   D Oxygen

3 When discussing diffusion, we expect the following:
   A Particles will move from areas of low concentration to areas of high concentration
   B Water will move from areas of high concentration to areas of low concentration
   C Particles will move from areas of high concentration to areas of low concentration
   D None of the above

4 Which of the following fluid types fits the description "The extracellular fluid contains MORE particles than intracellular fluid"?
   A Hypertonic
   B Hypotonic
   C Isotonic

5 True or False: A megakaryocyte circulates around the body dropping off platelets as it goes.
   A True
   B False

6 Which of the following is not a granulocyte?
  A Eosinophil
  B Neutrophil
  C T-Lymphocyte
  D Basophil

7 If a patient is experiencing an allergic reaction, which cell line would be activated as a direct result of the allergy?
  A T-Lymphocytes
  B Monocytes
  C Macrophages
  D Basophils

8 True or False: The mature erythrocyte in domestic mammals contains no nucleus.
  A True
  B False

9 What does a monocyte become once it enters tissue?
  A Monocyte
  B Macrocyte
  C Monophage
  D Macrophage

10 Which of the following is responsible for production, storage, and release of antibodies?
  A T-lymphocytes
  B Eosinophils
  C Plasma cells
  D Natural Killer Cells

15

Functions of the Common Integument

<table>
<tr><td>Clinical Case: Sam, An 8-Year-Old Male Neutered German Shepherd</td></tr>
<tr><td>Sam is presented to the clinic for an appointment due to hair loss around his nose and muzzle. The owners report that they noticed a lightening of the nasal planum and hair loss over the last 2–3 months.</td></tr>
</table>

Introduction

The common integument is comprised of all tissues on the outside covering of the animal. This includes skin, hair, glands, nails, claws, hooves, horns, and antlers. The connective tissues that form the integument vary widely in appearance. We will consider some of the structures that accompany parts of the integument and their role in the life of the animal.

The phrase "**connective tissue**" is an umbrella term. It can refer to small areas of supportive material or to an entire class of structures. What they have in common is the presence of fibrous and/or ground substance. **Ground substance** refers to the scaffolding that contains specialized cells. For example, blood can be considered a connective tissue because it has a liquid base in which the active structures are carried and protected.

Connective tissue includes things like adipose (fat) tissue, mucous membrane, lymphoid tissue, cartilage, bone, and skin.

Skin

The anatomy of the skin can be referenced in Chapter 2, while here we will focus on the multiple functions of skin. Among them are **protection, thermoregulation**, and **maintenance of hydration**.

Protection

The skin is an organ in that it has a series of functions in common throughout its structure. It is, in fact, the largest organ of the mammalian body. The protective aspects of the skin become clear when there is a disease state or injury involving the skin. The many layers of the skin are designed to be a physical barrier to pathogens. Gaps in the skin allow bacteria and fungi to enter, as well as environmental dangers such as parasites. The **epidermis**, or outermost layer of skin, gets its strength from **keratin**. Keratin is a type of strong fibrous protein produced by **keratinocytes**. These specialized cells move up toward the superficial layers of the epidermis. As they move and age, they undergo **keratinization** or **cornification** where the cell slowly gives up its organelles and biological functions to be replaced by the keratin and form the strong outermost layers of the epidermis.

Another protective feature of the skin is regarding ultraviolet (UV) damage. The skin and fur, depending on the species, can help protect the body from UV radiation from the sun. This is done with **melanin**, a pigment produced by special cells in the skin called **melanocytes**. There are different types of melanin, along with some other pigment-inducing molecules, that give the wide variety of colors seen in the animal kingdom. Aside from producing color in the skin and coat, melanin can serve to provide protection against UV light. The melanocyte produces melanin at the cell body and then sends the

Anatomy and Physiology for Veterinary Technicians and Nurses: A Clinical Approach, Second Edition. Lori Asprea.
© 2026 John Wiley & Sons, Inc. Published 2026 by John Wiley & Sons, Inc.
Companion website: www.wiley.com/go/asprea/anatomy_vettech2e

pigment up into the fingerlike projections that reach into the more superficial layers of the epidermis. The type and quantity of melanin results in the amount of color or pigment developed.

Thermoregulation

Mammals are able to maintain a constant internal temperature, regardless of outside temperature. This type of animal is referred to as a **homeotherm**. The opposite would be a **poikilotherm**, an animal whose body temperature varies depending on its environment. The temperature range in which the mammal's internal organs work is called "**core temperature.**" As the name implies, the center of the body, heart, and brain must remain in this ideal temperature range. When temperature is measured, it must be remembered that the further away from the core of the body the temperature is assessed, the lower the temperature will be. Rectal temperature is closer to core temperature than is oral temperature, which is closer than axillary temperature (taken by simply placing the thermometer between the brachium and the axilla, occasionally done with very sick animals where an oral or rectal thermometer cannot be used). The rectal temperature level is easy to measure and is reasonably close to the core temperature, so it is used most commonly in clinical practice. However, where great precision in measuring body temperature is needed, such as during surgery, a thermometer can be temporarily placed within the body.

An important structure of the skin that participates in thermoregulation is the **sweat glands** or **sudoriferous glands**. Sweat glands form a fluid similar to saline that is discharged through a duct and either goes directly onto the skin surface or into the hair follicle, where it continues to the surface. Sweat glands that connect directly to the surface of the skin are **eccrine sweat glands**, whereas the sweat glands that connect to hair follicles are called **apocrine sweat glands**. The sweat approaches the surface of the epidermis and begins to evaporate. As it does, it cools the local area of the skin. The discharge of sweat is mediated by the **autonomic nervous system**. This is a series of neural commands that are delivered without conscious thought, but by automatic response to stimuli. There are also some sweat glands in hairless areas; these too are mediated by the autonomic nerves.

Water vapor is lost on exhalation. Panting is thus a useful activity to cause water evaporation. Cats generally do not pant to shed heat but use the other methods described to maintain body temperature. Evaporation is the main path to water loss as a method of temperature control in humans. In fact, when the ambient temperature rises to approach body temperature, evaporation is the most effective natural method of heat control. Cats and dogs generally only sweat through their paw pads.

Since sweating is not an extremely effective means of temperature control in our patient population, there are other mechanisms to help the animal thermoregulate. One of these is through **vasodilation** and **vasoconstriction**. Vasodilation means that the vessels are dilating or becoming wider in diameter. When vessels in the skin dilate, they allow more blood to come to the surface of the skin and come into contact with the ambient room temperature, which in most conditions is lower than the animal's body temperature. This allows for heat from the body to be more effectively "dropped off" and the blood to cool, thereby lowering the internal body temperature. The same mechanism is visible in humans that appear flushed when warm as a result of vasodilation bringing more blood to the surface of the skin. Opposite this is vasoconstriction in which the vessels close to the surface of the skin shrink down in diameter. This reduces the amount of blood that is in contact with the ambient temperature of the environment, preserving heat. It is for this reason that distal extremities can turn pale or blue in cold temperatures. The vessels constrict, decreasing blood flow and maintaining the core body temperature.

Another aspect of thermoregulation and the skin has to do with the concept of **convection**. When there is a significant difference between the air temperature and the temperature of the skin, with air temperature being cooler, air will flow away from the skin and lower its temperature. It is for this reason that puppies and kittens need to be kept in a warm area when newborns. Their internal mechanisms for temperature control, mediated by the brain, are not mature at birth. The body thus is not able to avoid losing heat in a colder environment by convection, and temperature control must be maintained by other means (such as a nest or the mother).

Along the same lines, animals can also "insulate" each other. Close proximity allows the skin to share heat with others. Puppies and kittens, or animals in a cold environment, will huddle together in an attempt to maintain a normal working body temperature.

The skin contains sensory receptors for local temperature. These convey information to the **hypothalamus**, as a special area in the brain that has temperature-sensitive neurons. Information is then communicated, mostly by way of the autonomic nervous system, to engage in activities like panting and shivering to help maintain core temperature.

The haircoat also plays a role in thermoregulation by way of trapping cool or warm air close to the skin. The **arrector pili muscles** found attached to hair follicles help raise the hairs, which enlarges the area in which air may be used as an insulating blanket. Once again, the arrector pili are mediated by the autonomic nervous system.

The **subcutaneous layer** of the skin is mainly composed of adipose tissue. Adipose tissue is an efficient insulator. Animals that live in cold climates, not surprisingly, have a thick layer of subcutaneous fat.

Another aspect of the thermoregulatory function of skin has to do with the concept of **conduction**. Skin in contact with, for example, a cold table or cold ground will lose heat. This is of particular importance if the patient is on a surgical table and under anesthesia. Most anesthetics slow the response of the central nervous system, including the activities relating to thermoregulation. With the ability of the body to regulate its internal temperature impaired, further loss by way of cooling of the skin is undesirable. As a result, most clinicians will place a warming device on the table or use a table with a built-in warming device when patients are under anesthesia. It is still necessary to assist with temperature control postsurgically until body temperature returns to normal.

Hydration

The adipose tissue of the body, particularly that of the subcutaneous layer, has an important function. It can hold a large supply of water. In the event that the animal is not drinking enough or is urinating too much, the animal may be in the position of losing too much fluid content. The water content of the subcutaneous fat can then be called upon. An animal that is clinically dehydrated may lose even this backup supply. When this happens, the skin loses **turgor**, the normal full, firm condition of the tissue. In addition, the mucous membranes, particularly those of the oral cavity, may become pale and dry.

In clinical practice, we pinch the skin of the scruff and see if the skin bounces back into position. If it stays in a tent shape, it has lost the firmness that the water content affords. This is a quick way to assess dehydration. Loss of water content in the tissues supporting the globe of the eye can cause it to appear sunken into the orbit. This only occurs when dehydration is severe.

Other Functions

There are other functions that the skin and integument can serve. This system is able to help excrete waste, like salts, through sweating. It is also an important sensory organ. The hair and skin both deliver important sensory information to the brain to help the animal best understand its surroundings. The haircoat has **tactile hairs** that, when touched, can send signals about touch without the skin actually being in contact with anything. Further, the skin has multiple sensory nerves throughout. The epidermis contains sensory cells called **Merkel cells and Merkel discs**, while the dermis contains **Meissner's corpuscles** and pain receptors. The subcutaneous layer, or hypodermis, contains **Pacinian corpuscles** which are sensory receptors to heavy pressure.

Another important feature of the integument is the synthesis of Vitamin D through the influence of sunlight. Vitamin D is critically important for a number of bodily processes like calcium absorption and bone strength along with promoting a healthy skin barrier.

Clinical Considerations

Other clinical indicators are provided by the skin and mucous membranes. Red blood cells contain a substance called **hemoglobin**. When a red blood cell dies, hemoglobin is converted to **bilirubin** within macrophages of the spleen and liver. In addition, there is a large store of bilirubin in the liver that normally is discharged by the gallbladder as a constituent of bile.

In cases of destruction of red blood cells within the body, or in some hepatic diseases, free-floating bilirubin will build up in the bloodstream. These excess levels of bilirubin impart a yellow color to the skin, usually most apparent on the inner surface of the **pinna, the sclera** (white connective tissue visible on the surface of the eyes), and the mucous membranes of the mouth. Noting this color in any or all of these areas is an indication of either **hemolytic disease** (destruction of blood cells) or severe hepatic dysfunction. The condition is referred to as **icterus**.

As discussed in Chapter 14, the hemoglobin in the red blood cell carries oxygen to all parts of the body. As oxygen is released from the hemoglobin, it actually takes on a slightly blue tinge. This is particularly evident in the mucous membranes, which have a vasculature very close to the surface. **Cyanosis** is a condition denoted by a blue color in the mucous membrane or lips. Generally, by the time the condition is evident, there has already been a severe decline in blood oxygen content.

Pigment changes in the skin can denote a clinical condition. Any newly developed area of pigmentation or depigmentation (loss of pigment in a previously pigmented area) should be explored diagnostically. Pigment changes can signal chronic inflammation, certain cancers like melanomas, or other neoplastic processes like leukemia. In fact, in dogs, a specific type of leukemia called **systemic lupus erythematosus (SLE)** can present with skin ulcerations, hair loss, and depigmentation, particularly on the nasal planum. There are normal changes to pigment and hair color as animals age, particularly from neonates to adults, and then again when they are geriatric. Consider the Dalmatian puppy; born completely white and then pigment changes occur, giving them the signature spotted coat. In geriatric animals, we can see increased pigment or spotting on the skin, as well as loss of pigment in the haircoat. These are generally normal, but anything outstanding should be investigated.

Glands

The sweat glands are divided into two types, as discussed above: apocrine and eccrine. In both cases, a rather thin fluid is discharged, having a large supply of sodium. In fact, there is a minor contribution to electrolyte balance made by the sweat glands in this regard.

The apocrine glands discharge a fluid with a high protein level directly into the hair follicle. They are scattered throughout the body. As is true for eccrine sweat glands, there are species differences in how the glands are distributed.

The eccrine glands are those associated with hairless (or relatively hairless) areas of the skin. Their excretion has a higher water content and plays less of a role in thermoregulation. There are many more apocrine glands than eccrine glands.

One other note, on a somewhat less scientific plane, concerns the degradation of sweat. Sweat in and of itself does not have a strong odor. What does happen is that the normal bacterial population of the superficial epidermis starts to degrade the sweat and then uses some of its constituents. This is what produces a strong, rather musty odor.

The other glands related to the integument are the **sebaceous glands**. The sebaceous glands produce a waxy material called **sebum**. Sebum contains dead cells and oily secretions. Sebaceous glands provide a lubricating function and offer some waterproofing. The characteristic odor of a wet dog can be related to the production of sebum.

The **circumoral glands** are located along the lips, particularly toward the caudal part of the mouth. They are well known in cats. Cats rubbing the side of their face against a person or an object are using circumoral gland secretions to mark territory.

Carpal glands are sebaceous glands present in the carpal area of the cat. The location is marked by a tuft of tactile hairs.

Dogs and cats have **tail glands**, which are sebaceous glands located on the dorsal surface of the tail. As their activity is much greater during the breeding season, they are thought to play a role in advertising reproductive status.

Circumanal sebaceous glands are present in certain carnivores, and omnivores such as dogs. It is most likely the secretions of these glands that draw dogs toward introducing themselves by sniffing under the tail.

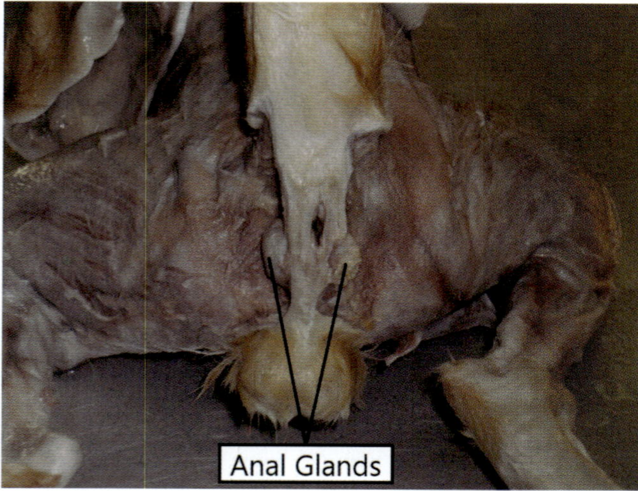

Figure 15.1 In the living animal, the anal glands appear as a pinhole-sized opening on either side of the anus. This animal was an intact male, indicated by the size of the scrotum (just above the words "anal glands" on the picture).

Sheep produce a substance from their sebaceous glands in cutaneous pouches that is processed for human use. These cutaneous pouches can be found in the inguinal area, the infraorbital area, and the interdigital area. This material is waterproof as well as lubricating and is occasionally used in cosmetics. It is known as **lanolin**. Musk deer produce a sebaceous product also called musk. This is used in perfumes for the human market.

The **anal glands** secrete a sebaceous material that lubricates and contains strong odors (see Figure 15.1). These odors serve as scent markers and are likely a functional analogue of the skunks' glands. In fact, when under severe stress, dogs and cats can actually expel the secretion toward the surrounding area. As noted before, the anal glands can become obstructed, leading to the phenomenon known as scooting. The animal is rubbing her hindquarters along the ground in response to the discomfort of the blocked gland. Anal glands can be "expressed" or emptied of their contents in the clinic. This provides instant relief for the animal. It does cause a strong, unpleasant odor, as anyone who has done the procedure will attest.

In addition, sebaceous glands assist the animal in scent marking by the production of pheromones. Pheromones are scents perceptible only to members of the same species (conspecifics). Pheromones are attractive odors and often have a calming effect. In addition, pheromones play a role in signaling reproductive status.

The **mammary gland** is actually a type of specialized sweat gland and will be discussed here. The gland has a complex series of ducts surrounded by fibrous connective tissue, the anatomy of which is discussed in Chapter 13. Eventually, the liquid content, to which fats and proteins have been added, exits via the teat.

It should also be noted that while males have mammary glands, they do not lactate. The teats of a male mark the location of their glands, but the glands do not enlarge unless there is some illness. While most male mammals have teats, rats do not.

In the first 24 hours or so after a puppy or kitten is born, the mother's milk is referred to as **colostrum**. This is because it contains a collection of maternal antibodies, protecting the infant from at least some infectious diseases until the young animal can make its own antibodies. This process is known as the conferral of **passive immunity**.

The flow of milk is governed by a number of factors. The nuzzling of a nursing newborn will set off a series of cues that alert the pituitary gland to release **oxytocin**. Oxytocin stimulates "**milk letdown**." This refers to the muscle contraction and ductile constriction that are associated with the passage of milk from the teat. Nursing (or milking by hand) also leads to the release of **prolactin**, which helps maintain lactation. **Growth hormone** is required for milk production. It was felt that giving dairy cows growth hormone would increase their output of milk; the administration of this hormone is controversial in that there is concern as to whether the growth hormone might affect humans drinking milk from these cattle.

Note that the production of milk actually begins before parturition (birth). The milk is stored in the alveoli. **Lactation**, which is the action of making the milk available to the newborn, occurs immediately before or during parturition. In fact, the presence of **progesterone** and **estrogen**, which are pregnancy-related hormones, actually inhibit lactation. When these factors no longer are present, lactation can proceed.

While milk letdown is usually stimulated by suckling, there are other ways to accomplish the discharge of milk from the mammary gland. The most familiar one is using manual pressure on the nipple, otherwise known as milking the animal.

Hair

The haircoat in most mammals sheds in whole or in part. The difference among them has to do with the time frame. In primates, shedding occurs throughout the year. In most domestic animals, shedding occurs at particular times of the year.

As a single hair begins to grow, the follicle will project it above the surface of the epidermis. At some point, as the season of shedding begins, the hair follicles will begin to atrophy. As they atrophy, the hair maintains its position. As a new follicle begins to grow again, the hair is pushed out of position and loses its connection to the follicle. In other words, it falls out. This does not happen all over the body at once. Similarly, birds molt in patches throughout the body and do not lose all of their feathers at the same time.

The phases of growth are called **anagen, catagen**, and **telogen**. Anagen is the growth phase, in which the **matrix** at the base of the hair follicle is rapidly producing cells that will keratinize and become hair. Once the maximum length is reached, the root of the hair will be clubbed off, and growing will stop. This phase is called catagen. Catagen is a relatively short phase that precedes telogen. Telogen is the rest phase, where the hair that is finished growing sits in the follicle until the new hair begins to grow under it, pushing it out to be shed.

In dogs and cats, the hairs that form the top layer of the coat are called **guard hairs** or **primary hairs**. They usually grow in long layers, with the occasional whorl or border. This factor facilitates the protective layer of the coat. For example, in the rain, the water will tend to "sheet" off the animal and thus provide some protection for it. Note that some species are bred to have different patterns of hair. While this may arguably improve their appearance, it actually does deprive them of some protection from the elements. So-called hairless breeds suffer not only from temperature extremes but also from damage related to extended exposure to UV rays or dampness.

As an aside, hair does not serve only to keep an animal warm. Haircoats can trap cool air as well, and in some breeds, leaving the haircoat on is more advantageous than shaving it off in hot weather.

The undercoat, made of so-called **wool hairs** or **secondary hairs**, is generally more contoured. Wool hairs are shorter than the guard hairs. As noted in Chapter 2, these are the hairs that shed when an animal is combed. Loose wool hairs can wrap around each other, particularly in long-haired dogs and cats, and cause painful knots known as "mats," short for matted hair. This matting is hopefully avoided by the shingled or scaled outermost layer of the hair called the **cuticle**.

The **tactile hairs** extend above the guard hairs and below the wool hair follicles. Some tactile hairs can be traced down to the level of the muscle. These follicles are surrounded by a venous sinus, or cuplike opening, lined with mechanical receptors that communicate with local nerve fibers. Thus, anything that touches the tactile hair will be perceived as movement and will command attention.

Whiskers are the classic example of tactile hairs, but there are others. For example, a cluster of tactile hairs marks the location of a sebaceous gland in the area of the caudal carpus in the cat. Whiskers are rarely shed and are quite hardy. The facial whiskers are known as **vibrissae**, most likely in recognition of their sensitivity to vibration. In fact, the vibrissae should never be trimmed except in cases of medical necessity, as this is quite bothersome to the patient.

The Pads

The pads of the paw are very thick, cornified epithelium. There is a thick layer of collagen and elastic fibers, combined with some adipose tissue that underlies this. The pads perform as a protective layer for the animals, regardless of the kind of surface upon which they move.

The stance of the animal determines which pads are in contact with the ground. The three stances in mammals are **plantigrade, digitigrade**, and **unguligrade**.

In the plantigrade stance, the entire palmar and plantar surfaces are in contact with the ground; that is, the paw, caudal metatarsal/metacarpal area, carpus, and tarsus are all in direct contact with the surface while the animal is moving around. The classic examples of this are rabbits and kangaroos. Thus, there are **digital pads, metacarpal/metatarsal pads**, and carpal or tarsal areas that meet the ground when the animal walks.

Dogs and cats have what is called a digitigrade stance. This means that the digital pads make contact with the ground. There is a single metacarpal pad on each forelimb, and a similar metatarsal pad, and these too contact the ground.

As previously mentioned, the pad contains, in its subdermal layer, a few sweat glands. The mark of a nervous cat in the examination room is the appearance of damp footprints as the animal walks across the table. These glands are more related to sympathetic nerve stimulation and territorial marking than they are to thermoregulation.

In ungulates, only the digital pad is in contact with the ground. In ruminants, the digital pad is called a **bulb**. In horses, it is called the **frog**. Given that the horse stands on one digit only, it is not surprising that the digital pad is quite stiff and complex in structure.

Claws, Nails, and Hooves

The claws are an important feature of the integument in most mammals. In cats, the claws are naturally retracted in a relaxed state. Using a series of muscles and tendons, the feline can extend their claws for use. These uses generally include climbing, hunting, and defense against predators or competitors. In dogs, claws function to help with traction on various types of ground. In birds, the nails or talons can be used for perching or prey depending on the species. Some species of birds have spines or spikes on their nails used in defense and fighting. Hooved animals have a nail-like substance that covers the hoof along with other important structures discussed in Chapter 2. All claws, nails, talons, and hooves need maintenance and medical attention. It is a critically important part of the physical exam to check the nails and nail beds of each animal being examined.

Antlers, Horns, and Beaks

Although we are primarily concerned with dogs and cats here, we would like to briefly discuss antlers, horns, and beaks. Both antlers and horns are composed of epidermis and have a dermal layer.

Antlers are outgrowths of the skull. As they protrude, they are covered with skin. The skin dies as it is stretched continually and is referred to as **velvet** due to its smooth appearance as it hangs from the prongs of the antler. The exposure of the bone to the elements causes it to die, and the antler falls off. The shedding of antlers, like the shedding of hair, is usually seasonal, responding to changes in temperature and length of day. Seasonal changes will incite the antler to grow again.

The horn grows from the **cornual process** on the skull. Horns grow continuously from the time they appear, which is shortly after birth. First, there are small button-like growths called **horn buds**, which are relatively easy to remove if there is some reason to dehorn the animal. Horns grow in length and width as the animal ages. In cattle, the interior of the horn is continuous with the frontal sinus, a hollow area rostral to the dorsal braincase. When animals are dehorned, it is particularly important to avoid any debris falling into the cavity and to use aseptic techniques to lessen the risk of sinus infection (Figure 15.2).

The beak is the external structure found in birds, turtles, octopi, platypuses, and some other animals. The beak is a bony projection of the mandible and maxilla, covered in a keratinized layer of epidermis called the **rhamphotheca**. The beak can be used for a multitude of functions including prehension of food, self-defense, preening or grooming, mating rituals, and navigation depending on the species. It is important to note that the keratinized material of the beak can overgrow and require trimming or filing. In owned animals, this can sometimes be achieved by using environmental enrichment tools that help to gently wear down the beak. This is similar to scratching posts for cats to help shed the layers of their nails.

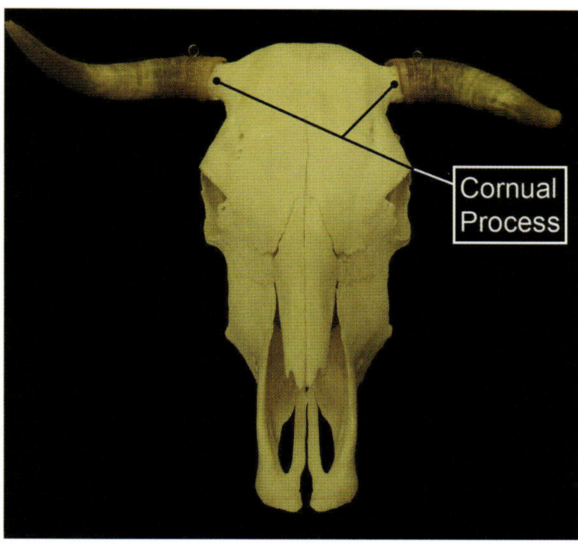

Figure 15.2 Horn grows out from the cornual process. In bovines, the interior of the process communicates with the interior of the skull.

Clinical Case Resolution: Sam

Upon physical exam it is noted that Sam has some ulceration on the nasal planum along with the owners described hair loss and depigmentation. The pattern suggested this patient may have SLE, and specialized blood work is performed to confirm the diagnosis.

SLE is more commonly seen in certain dog breeds, like Beagles, German Shepherds, and Poodles among others. It also tends to be overrepresented in male dogs. SLE is a complicated disease where the immune system attacks itself creating damage and inflammation that can manifest in many areas of the body.

Once it is confirmed that Sam has SLE, a treatment regimen is started that focuses on reducing inflammation and suppressing the immune system activity. Dogs with SLE are expected to need these medications for the remainder of their lives.

Review Questions

1 Which of the following are methods of <u>protection</u> provided by the integument?
   A Vasodilation
   B Blocking pathogens from entry
   C Vasoconstriction
   D Sudoriferous glands

2 Which of the following is used for scent marking, has a pungent foul odor and connects to the anus with a small duct?
   A Tail glands
   B Sweat glands
   C Cutaneous pouches
   D Anal glands

3 Define poikilotherm

4 Which of the following helps sweat and sebaceous material get pushed out and onto the skin?
 A Levator pili
 B Arrector pili
 C Eccrine gland
 D Cornual process

5 Which type of glands produce sweat directly only on the skin surface?
 A Sebaceous glands
 B Eccrine glands
 C Apocrine glands
 D Anal glands

6 If an animal has a decreased body temperature, what do we expect the skin vasculature response to be?
 A Vasoconstriction
 B Vasodilation
 C No response

7 Which cells are responsible for helping with UV protection in the skin?
 A Merkel cells
 B Pacinian corpuscles
 C Keratinocytes
 D Melanocytes

8 What is icterus?

9 True or False: Horns are shed seasonally.
 A True
 B False

10 What can it mean if an animal has decreased skin turgor?
 A The animal is overheating
 B The animal is dehydrated
 C The animal is cold
 D The animal is sweating

16

Sensory Physiology

<table>
<tr><td>Clinical Case: Cheeto, a 2-Year-Old Male Intact English Bulldog</td></tr>
<tr><td>

Cheeto is brought into the clinic for squinting in the right eye (OD) and rubbing his face. There appears to be some discharge and redness from the OD as well. The owners report that Cheeto began bothering with his eye 2 days ago, and they thought it was just allergies.

Unfortunately his condition seems persistent and progressive. The owners are concerned that something is stuck in his eye.

</td></tr>
</table>

Introduction

The sensory receptors are the cells that capture the stimuli from the outside world or elsewhere within the body and communicate them to nerve fibers. They are clustered within sense organs, specialized structures containing neural tissue that can be concentrated in a small area or spread along in a series of clusters, such as in the tactile system.

Receptors and Signals

Some receptors accept stimuli that come from a distance. For example, the visual system is designed to capture information from not only its immediate area but also from feet or even miles away. Contact sensory systems such as taste and touch are those that require proximity in order to function.

The sensory systems include the **visual, auditory (hearing), vestibular (balance), olfactory (smell), tactile (touch)**, and **gustatory (taste) receptors**. These systems take information in from outside the body. Each system includes the receptor cells and their surrounding tissue. While they vary greatly in structure, each gathers information and projects it toward the central nervous system, where the information is processed and acted upon.

There are also internal receptors, which give the central nervous system information about the workings of body systems and metabolism. These include **baroreceptors** and **chemoreceptors**, which will be discussed later.

The nature of sensory receptors governs how the information is processed. A given system may interpret any stimulation as if it belonged to the class of stimuli to which it is responsive. Applying pressure to the eye will often cause an impression of a visual image, even though there is no specific material to "see."

Receptors are classified according to the nature of the input to which they respond. They include **photoreceptors, auditory receptors, mechanical receptors, chemical receptors**, and **thermoreceptors**. Photoreceptors respond to light, auditory receptors to sound, mechanical receptors to physical contact, chemoreceptors to chemicals, and thermoreceptors to temperature. In fact, sensory organs have the ability to filter out information that they do not respond to. They also have a threshold; that is, stimuli have to reach a certain strength in order for the receptor to respond.

The thresholds for various stimuli vary by species. The auditory system of dogs and cats responds to a different range of sounds than that of primates. In turn, other species use completely different systems in order to carry out the same functions. Bats have minimal capacity to receive visual images. However, their refined auditory system serves the function of informing the central nervous system of the size and location of objects.

Anatomy and Physiology for Veterinary Technicians and Nurses: A Clinical Approach, Second Edition. Lori Asprea.
© 2026 John Wiley & Sons, Inc. Published 2026 by John Wiley & Sons, Inc.
Companion website: www.wiley.com/go/asprea/anatomy_vettech2e

In addition, most sensory systems are adaptive; that is, they have some method of coping with too much, or too little, information. For example, the mammalian eye can perform certain functions to limit the amount of light impinging on this sense organ so that it is not overwhelmed by constricting the pupil. Movement of the pinna can help amplify local sounds to make them easier to hear.

The sensory information that impinges on the receptor organ generates a response in local nerve fibers. This is known as **transduction**. An **action potential**, or neural signal, will be triggered when enough input from the fibers is received. This is called **integration**. The series of action potentials reflect the intensity of the input. If the input from the environment continues, the strength of the action potential will increase. If the input intensifies, the impulses usually will come more frequently.

If the stimulus continues past the ability of the receptor to keep up with it or if the stimulus is less startling as it continues, the response of the neural system decreases. This is known as **receptor adaptation**. A cat may respond strongly to the sound of an air conditioner being turned on. However, as the sound continues, his auditory system adapts, and the response lessens.

The Visual System

In the early stages of evolution, cells sensitive to light were present in various locations. In dogs and cats, those cells are now clustered in the eye, an organ that uses both neural and structural enhancements to accept visual input.

Structures of the Eye

In looking at the mammalian eye, we are struck by a number of complicated structures. From the outside, the most prominent feature is the **eyelid** or **palpebrum**. The upper and lower lids meet at a "corner" called the **lateral canthus** on the lateral side of the globe (eyeball) and the **medial canthus** near the nose. There is a "third eyelid," properly called the **nictitating membrane** (Figure 16.1), folded under the ventral palpebrum in the area of the medial canthus. It is made of stiff, fibrous material and will sometimes protrude if the animal is unwell. It contains a gland that helps produce tears. There is a duct at the medial canthus that conducts tears into the nasal passage. Blockage of the tear duct is not uncommon and can be tested by placing a dye into the duct at the medial canthus and seeing if the dye runs out of the nose.

The outermost part of the eye is the **cornea**, a transparent membrane covering the globe (see Figure 16.1). Between the cornea and the **iris** is the **anterior chamber**, which is filled with a thin fluid called **aqueous humor**. The white part of the eye is called the **sclera**. It is made of dense fibrous connective tissue. The iris is the colored part of the eye. In an animal which is an albino (lacking in the cells that make pigment, or color, for the connective tissues such as skin), the iris is usually pale pink. The opening through which light travels is the **pupil**. Immediately caudal to the iris is the **ciliary body**. This structure produces the aqueous humor and assists in focusing the lens.

Between the iris and the lens of the eye is the **posterior chamber**, also filled with aqueous humor. The lens is held in place by a number of suspensory ligaments called **zonules**.

Behind the lens is the **vitreous body**, a thick gelatinous material that helps the globe retain its shape. The part of the globe caudal to the lens is called the **vitreous chamber**. The vitreous humor also serves to press against the retina and hold it in place. On dissection, the vitreous humor appears as a puddle of viscous gel within the globe. The aqueous humor, on the other hand, will retain its watery appearance and volume.

The **retina** is a many-layered stack of cells that processes light so that the brain can attach meaning to the images. The retina contains the cells that distinguish light and dark and shades of color. Deep to the retina is the retinal pigmented epithelium, a layer of specialized cells. This, in turn, sits on the **choroid**, which is the vascular layer of the eye. The choroid contains the **tapetum lucidum**, which

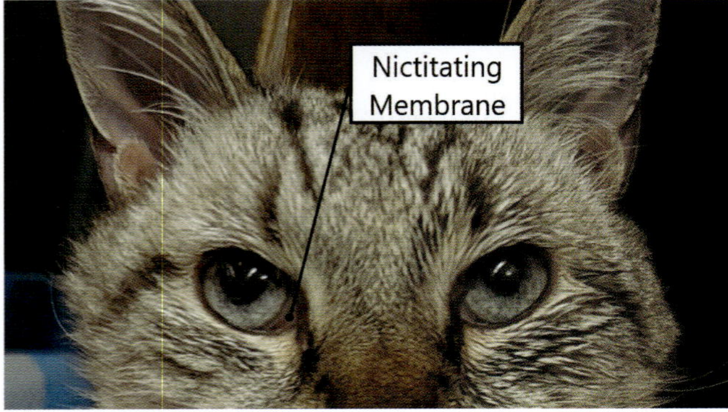

Figure 16.1 The nictitating membrane or "third eyelid" in a hospitalized cat.

in the living animal appears blue or green when one looks into the globe with an ophthalmoscope. On dissection, the tapetum often appears dark blue or green. Primates and swine do not have a tapetum lucidum. The glow of an animal's eyes when light is directed toward them in a dark room, or outdoors at night, is the reflection of the tapetum (Figure 16.2).

Function of the Eye

Muscle fibers in the iris are arranged both radially and circularly. This allows the pupil to allow in more or less light. This movement is controlled by the autonomic nervous system. During anesthesia, we can judge how much effect the drugs have had by looking at the dilation of the pupil. As the pupil comes down to a more normal size, we can infer how much the neurological system has recovered from the anesthetic agents.

There are also muscles caudal to the iris, in the ciliary body of the posterior chamber. These muscles help alter the conformation of the lens of the eye, allowing the animal to change its ability to focus. This accommodation allows for readjustment for near and far vision, where contraction of the muscles causes relaxation of the zonules, making the lens more round in shape. When attempting to process visual information at a distance, the ciliary muscles relax, which pulls the zonules tight, flattening the lens slightly.

The ciliary body has another important function. It participates in the production of aqueous humor. Under normal circumstances, the aqueous humor flows from the choroid through the pupil and into the anterior chamber. Aqueous humor is then drained out of the eye at the junction between the iris and the cornea. This location is called the **iridocorneal angle**. If the production of aqueous humor is abnormally high or the flow of the aqueous humor is blocked, the condition known as **glaucoma** results. This condition is an unrelieved increase in intraocular pressure caused by the larger than normal amount of fluid in the eye.

The retina has a number of layers. The **photoreceptor layers** are those that contain the cells called **rods** and **cones**. The rods are dedicated to responding to levels of light. The cones are sensitive to things like color and detail. As an aside, it is not true that dogs and cats are insensitive to color. The range of colors they see is most likely different from that of primates.

The tapetum lucidum reflects light strongly within the eye, helping to enhance the strength of the visual signal. The combination of the size and reflective quality of the tapetum, and the degree to which the pupil can open, makes some animals much better at distinguishing visual images in low light. Nocturnal animals demonstrate these qualities to a great degree.

The information gathered by the retina is transmitted by way of nerve fibers to the **optic disk**, which is where the fibers are gathered to form the **optic nerve (cranial nerve II)**. The optic nerve is unique in that its fibers are directed along its trunk in different directions. For example, some information from the medial portion of the retina of each eye follows the optic nerve as it crosses from right to left or left to right at the **optic chiasm**. However, information from the lateral part of each retina stays on the same side of the body as it travels along the optic nerve. This splitting of the fibers allows the visual cortex to make very precise calculations as to the position and strength of visual stimuli.

Another aspect of visual processing relates to the nature of the image. The visual image that the eye receives is inverted as it passes through the lens and the fluids of the eye. It passes through the optic nerve in this upside-down position and is not rotated to a "normal" position until it reaches the visual cortex of the brain.

There is a difference in the placement of the eye in predator and prey species. Most predators have eyes placed rostrally or at least close to the center of the muzzle. The fact that the eyes are relatively close together helps the animal focus and improves its depth perception. Prey animals tend to have eyes placed more laterally. This allows them to have a wider range of vision, including the ability to see more of the area to the side and even a little behind them. This is a clear advantage in sensing prey. However, it also means that the animal has much less depth perception and that it does not see well when it is approached directly from the front. Partly for this reason, it is best not to approach an animal like a horse directly from the front, so as not to startle it, unless one makes a noise or touches the animal or otherwise indicates one's presence.

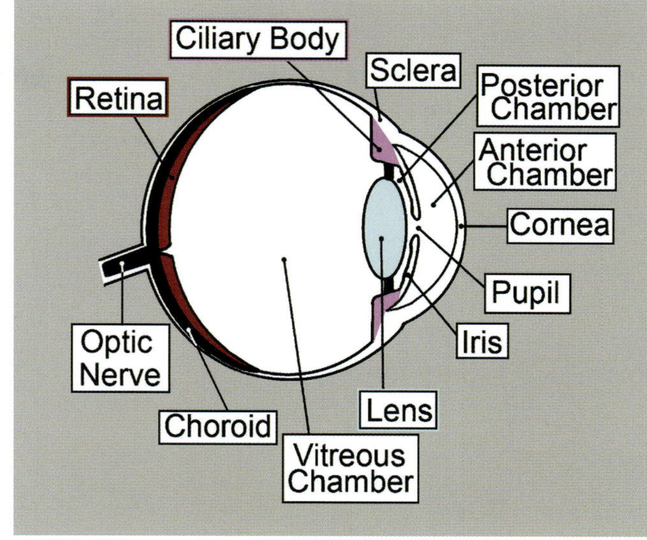

Figure 16.2 The parts of the eye. The anterior and posterior chambers are filled with aqueous humor and the vitreous chamber with a much thicker fluid called vitreous humor.

Other important structures integral to ophthalmic function exist around the eye. The eyelids have lashes to prevent debris from entering the eye. They also have **meibomian glands** which produce a waxy-like substance that helps to lubricate the eye along with tears. The **lacrimal apparatus** contains glands and ducts that produce tears and distribute them into the eye. Tears are a mix of water, electrolytes, and oils. A common affliction seen in dogs is a disease called **keratoconjunctivitis sicca** (KCS). This occurs when there is a deficiency of tear production, which results in dry eyes and an overproduction of mucous to compensate for the lack of tears. These animals present with thick mucoid ocular discharge and redness and irritation of the eye. KCS often predisposes animals to corneal ulceration or injury to the cornea. This can also be caused by trauma to the eye such as scratches or rubbing or eyelid abnormalities like **entropion** or **ectropion**, where the eyelids are abnormally folded in or out, respectively.

Proprioception and Equilibrium

Proprioception is the ability of the body to orient itself in space and to sense its direction of movement. Proprioception depends on the integration of information from a number of systems. Visual images and the relative expansion and contraction of muscle groups help the body to determine its position and the direction in which parts of it are oriented. The component of the system that is related only to the sense of balance is actually a part of the inner ear called the **vestibular apparatus**. It senses information regarding balance and position in space.

The **semicircular canals** and **vestibule** of the inner ear contain a viscous fluid called **endolymph**. At the terminal ends of the canals are patches of sensory epithelium called the **macula**. The macula contains ciliated cells and a gelatinous membrane that holds solid crystals called **otoliths**. As the body moves, the gelatinous matrix and otoliths move. This movement causes pressure on the ciliated cells. The mechanical act of the cilia being bent by the otoliths coming to rest on them triggers a response in the local nerve fibers, which lie at the opposite end of the ciliated cell. The macula allows the body to perceive linear movement. The fibers conduct the impulse as they gather together to form the vestibular part of the **vestibulocochlear nerve (cranial nerve VIII)**. The vestibular nerve meets the auditory part of the nerve, which exits from the cochlea, and they continue to the **auditory cortex** (located in the temporal lobe of the brain).

The semicircular canals all lie at a 90-degree angle to one another, filled with endolymph. At the ends of the semicircular canals is the **crista ampullaris** (Figure 16.3), which is responsible for perceiving rotary motion. The crista ampullaris has

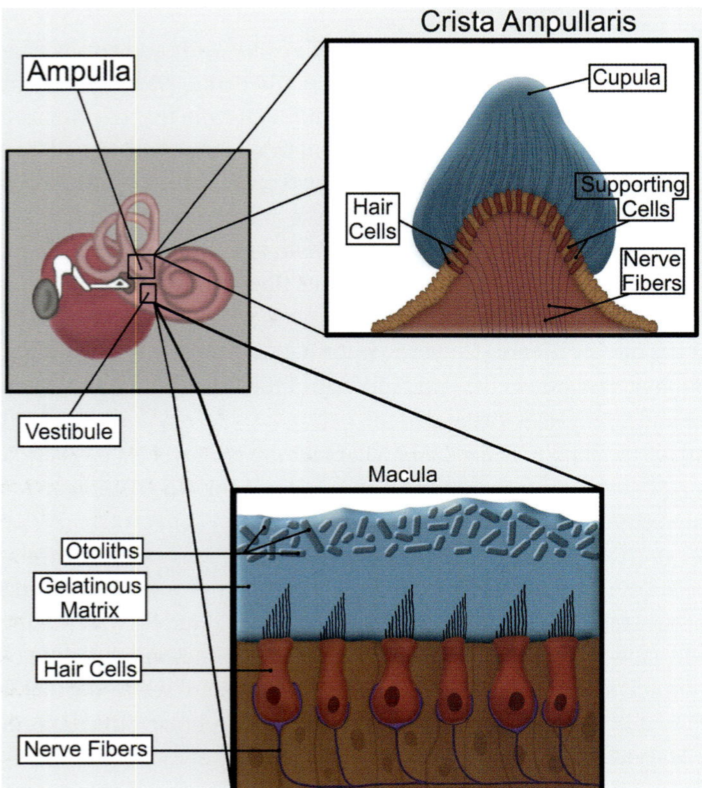

Figure 16.3 The macula and the cupula which participate in proprioception and equilibrium. Note these figures also appear in Chapter 3.

specialized ciliated hair cells that stick up into a gelatinous matrix, called the **cupula**, that is freely floating in the endolymph. As the body moves, the endolymph moves, causing the cupula to wave and bending the ciliated hair cells contained within it. Think of this as seaweed in the ocean, as the waves move, the seaweed sways back and forth. The bending of these cilia generates a signal to send to the central nervous system.

Infection or tumors of the inner ear or cranial nerve VIII can result in impaired function of the balance mechanism. The most common symptom of this problem is head tilt, where the animal is unable to keep its head in an upright position. The other symptom sometimes seen is **nystagmus**, which is a rapid side-to-side or up-and-down movement of the globe. It can be seen on gross examination of the living animal, particularly if the examiner tilts the patient's head back. The presence of nystagmus reflects the close association of the visual system and the inner ear in maintaining balance.

The Auditory System

The sense of hearing is facilitated by a number of anatomic, mechanical, and neurological features. It begins with the **pinna** in most mammals. In most dogs and cats, the pinna is not only relatively tall but is also somewhat mobile. In turning the pinna slightly from one side to another, sounds can be gathered in more directly. The pinna not only gathers the sound but also amplifies it, although very slightly. The length and width of the pinna relative to the size of the head is one factor in its amplifying capability. The "oversized" appearance of the pinnae of the bat contributes to the ability to sense and locate sound.

Sound is conducted from the pinna down the **external auditory canal** to the **tympanic membrane**. The strength of the auditory signal is reflected in the degree to which the tympanic membrane vibrates. The speed of the vibration of the sound waves, associated with whether the sound is low or high in pitch, is also transmitted in the movement of the tympanic membrane. The common name of the tympanic membrane is the eardrum, in deference to its similarity to the head of a drum.

The vibration of the tympanic membrane, in turn, sets off the vibration of the **ossicles**. This continues the transmission of the signal. The footplate (flat part) of the most medial ossicle, **the stapes**, sits in a membrane-covered opening called the **oval window**. This window is an opening into the **cochlea**, the part of the inner ear that has to do with hearing. The ossicles are housed within the **tympanic bulla**. Normally, the bulla does not contain any fluid. Infection in the nasal passages can enter the bulla by way of a tube connecting the nasal cavity with the bulla. This tube is called the **Eustachian tube**. Medial to the bulla is the cochlea, which looks like a snail shell. Most bacterial or yeast infections of the ear are in the external ear canal, with a few in the middle ear. An infection of the inner ear can only be called such when the infection is located within the cochlea or vestibular apparatus.

As the stapes vibrates, it sends a pressure wave through the fluid within the cochlea. This fluid wave sets off movement that leads to stimulation of the receptor cells within the cochlea called the **organ of Corti**. This organ has ciliated hair cells that gently rest against a gelatinous membrane called the **tectorial membrane**. As the fluid wave causes movement in the inner ear, the hair cells rub against the tectorial membrane, bending the sensory hairs and generating the nerve impulse to the brain. The action potential ends in the temporal lobes of the brain, where the information is processed.

The Olfactory System

Particularly for animals whose hearing and/or vision is not very acute, the sense of smell needs to be very keen. The olfactory system houses some receptor cells that are specialized, responding to a particular odor, and some that are general, responding to a variety of smells. Many olfactory cells are ciliated. Smell is a chemical sense very similar to taste, in which molecules dissolve and land on receptors to produce information.

Dogs and cats, among other animals, have a much higher number of olfactory cells as they have a much more developed sense of smell than humans. For example, dogs have hundreds of millions of olfactory receptors compared to the approximately five million in humans. Smells can come from one nostril or both. Animals are able to distinguish this and it helps them locate a smell depending on where it is entering the nose. When air carrying the smell enters the nose, the molecules dissolve in the moisture of the nasal cavity and land on receptors that create signals to be processed by the brain.

There are special receptors for **pheromones**, which are chemical substances that can be used for communication. Humans do not produce any known pheromones, but animals do. The importance of these species-specific olfactory

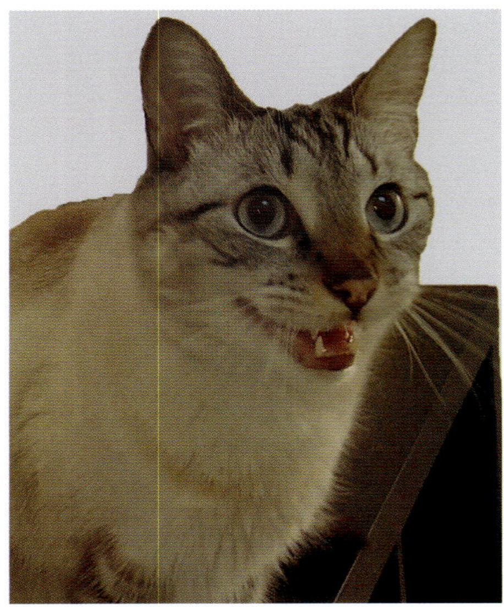

Figure 16.4 A cat having a Flehmen response when presented with an unfamiliar smell.

stimuli is reflected in the fact that they have their own receptors. Pheromones are particularly important in the reproductive cycle and in territoriality. A female in heat produces a particular pheromone to advertise her condition to others of her species. Males will often mark their territory with pheromones secreted by some sebaceous glands.

In felines, the **vomeronasal organ** presents an opportunity to enhance smells. The organ is a collection of soft tissue with receptor cells that is located near the nasal cavity. When air is drawn somewhat forcefully across this area, the **olfactory bulb** is stimulated. The reader may have observed a cat sniffing an object and then standing still with its mouth slightly open. What it is doing is drawing air across the vomeronasal organ to make the olfactory stimulus stronger. This is called the **Flehmen response** or vomeronasal response (Figure 16.4). It is thought that the vomeronasal organ in combination with the vast number of olfactory cells is what allows dogs to be used to smell and detect things like cancer cells, diabetic emergencies, and seizures before they happen among other skills.

Olfactory receptors are induced to produce an action potential when they are stimulated. These signals are brought directly to the olfactory bulbs, which are the rostral-most part of the cerebrum.

The Gustatory System

The tongue of most mammals is the primary sense organ for taste. Taste is a chemical sense that relies on taste buds and **gustatory cells**. When food or any material is ingested, the flavors dissolve and these chemicals enter the gustatory cells where the information can then be interpreted by the central nervous system. Specialized cells in the tongue respond to tastes such as sweet and sour. Some species respond only to very few tastes in that their taste receptors only categorize materials into a couple of general categories.

It is difficult to specify what tastes appeal to a given individual animal. For example, it is felt that cats do not have a strong response to sweet tastes. However, some felines clearly prefer sweet-tasting foods. How they interpret the taste is, of course, difficult to assess; what tastes sweet to us may taste sour to them. Unfortunately, the main chemical constituent of automotive antifreeze is ethylene glycol. This chemical appears to have a sweet taste to dogs and cats, and dogs will readily consume it if it is available. Ethylene glycol is very damaging to the kidneys and can be fatal.

The Tactile System

The distinguishing feature of the sense of touch is that it combines mechanical and neural signals to transmit information. **Stretch receptors** within the skin sense physical pressure, and **thermoreceptors** indicate changes in temperature. The ability to feel pain is referred to as **nociception** and is signaled by the inflammatory response. The latter refers to the fact that certain proteins and white blood cells are recruited when there is injury or infection. These materials also set off a cascade of neural responses that cause the central nervous system to interpret them as aversive.

Specialized Receptors

Throughout our discussion of physiology is the theme of feedback loops and self-monitoring of biological systems. Two receptor cell clusters that are linked to cardiovascular and respiratory functions deserve mention here. They are the baroreceptors which sense blood pressure and chemoreceptors that can detect levels of carbon dioxide. They will be discussed in greater depth as we go along. For now, it is important to note that sensory input occurs from within the body as well. The information obtained from these receptors is used by the nervous system to adjust the activities of the cardiovascular and respiratory systems.

Clinical Case Resolution: Cheeto

Examination of Cheeto reveals a slightly overweight animal in otherwise normal body condition. In order to assess the eye issue, a Schirmer Tear Test was performed to check the amount of tear production in both eyes. Fortunately for Cheeto, both eyes are producing tears at a normal amount, ruling out dry eye or KCS.

Next, fluorescein stain is dropped into both eyes. During this test, stain is placed into the eye, and any injuries to the cornea will hold the stain. It is revealed that Cheeto has a corneal ulceration in his OD. The left eye appears normal.

It should be noted that ophthalmic issues seem to be overrepresented in brachycephalic breeds. The altered conformation of the skull and related soft tissue leads to a number of medical issues, eyes included.

Cheeto is sent home on antibiotic ophthalmic ointment and a recheck is scheduled for 7 days from now, assuming symptoms improve.

Review Questions

1 If an animal is trying to look at something at a distance, what might you expect?
  A Ciliary muscle relaxation and zonule relaxation rounding the lens
  B Ciliary muscle contraction and zonule contraction rounding the lens
  C Ciliary muscle relaxation and zonule contraction flattening the lens
  D Ciliary muscle relaxation and zonule contraction flattening the lens

2 What does the macula in the vestibule contain?
  A Ciliated hair cells
  B Otolithic gelatinous membrane
  C Otoliths
  D All of the above

3 What generates nerve impulses to the brain to be interpreted as sound?
  A The bending of sensory hairs against the tectorial membrane
  B The vibration of perilymph
  C The stapes against the oval window
  D None of the above

4 Where are the photoreceptors located?
  A The nervous layer of the eye
  B The vascular layer of the eyes
  C The fibrous layer of the eye
  D The tectorial membrane

5 Where is the Organ of Corti found?
  A The external auditory canal
  B The vestibule
  C The semicircular canals
  D The cochlea

6 Where is the crista ampullaris found?
  A Semicircular canals
  B Cochlea
  C Perilymph
  D Gustatory cells

7 True or False: The gustatory sense is a mechanical sense
   A True
   B False

8 What organ can be used to smell pheromones?
   A The vomeronasal organ
   B The cochlea
   C The baroreceptors
   D The semicircular canals

9 What do Meibomian glands produce?
   A Oil into the ear
   B Watery tears onto the eye
   C Saliva onto the tongue
   D Oil onto the eyelids and eyes

10 Which receptors are responsible for sensing blood pressure?

17

Osteology

Clinical Case: Binx, a 13-Year-Old Male Neutered Siamese

Binx is referred to a specialty clinic because he has chronically lowered blood cell counts. On a Complete Blood Count (CBC), it is revealed that Binx has low levels of red blood cells, with no evidence of the body creating more, as well as low white blood cell levels and low platelet levels.

Introduction

The major bone groups of the mammalian body are the long bones, the short bones, the irregular bones, and the flat bones. The bony structure of the animal, the skeleton, does not serve only for support and protection of the interior organs. The skeleton also plays an important role in movement through its interaction with joints and serves as the site of blood cell production and mineral storage.

The Growth of Bones

All bones begin in utero as a hyaline cartilaginous model. The basic bone structure exists but has not yet formed into mature or compact bone. As the animal develops, special cells called **osteoblasts** infiltrate the cartilage and begin forming the outermost layer of the bone, the **periosteum**. Osteoblasts are the builders of bone. The cartilage center of the bone breaks down to form the **diaphysis**, or shaft. Once the diaphysis is fully infiltrated by osteoblasts, a **primary ossification center** is formed, which continues ossifying, or making into bone, through to the ends of the bones. Another set of specialized cells, called **osteoclasts**, are also used during bone development. Osteoclasts help to clean up any excess bony material and also get rid of any old or damaged bone cells.

Once the bony model is complete, it is time for the bones to lengthen through the animals' growing and maturation process. The lengthening of long bones, such as the femur, while the young animal grows, occurs at either end of the bone rather than in the middle. If the middle of the diaphysis of a long bone is marked, that mark will not move, even as the animal grows "taller." The growth area is in the **metaphysis**, caudal to the **articular surface** of the bone. In the young animal, a plate of cartilage is present at its border with the **epiphysis**. This **epiphyseal plate**, or growth plate, is gradually converted into mature bone by the action of osteoblasts.

It is important to note that the epiphyseal plate does not appear when bone is radiographed, as cartilage is mostly transparent to X-rays. A radiograph (X-ray image) of the long bone of a young animal will appear to have a separation between the ends of the bone and the diaphysis. This is sometimes mistaken for a fracture.

Bone cells do eventually get broken down by cells called osteoclasts. They need to be replaced, and so, while the bone does not get longer after a certain age, there continues to be growth within the bone itself. The activity within the metaphysis continues until adulthood. The material within the metaphysis is called the **cancellous bone**. It consists of softer materials like bone marrow. It has a spongy appearance. Flat and irregular bones have cancellous bone as well, although their growth patterns are different.

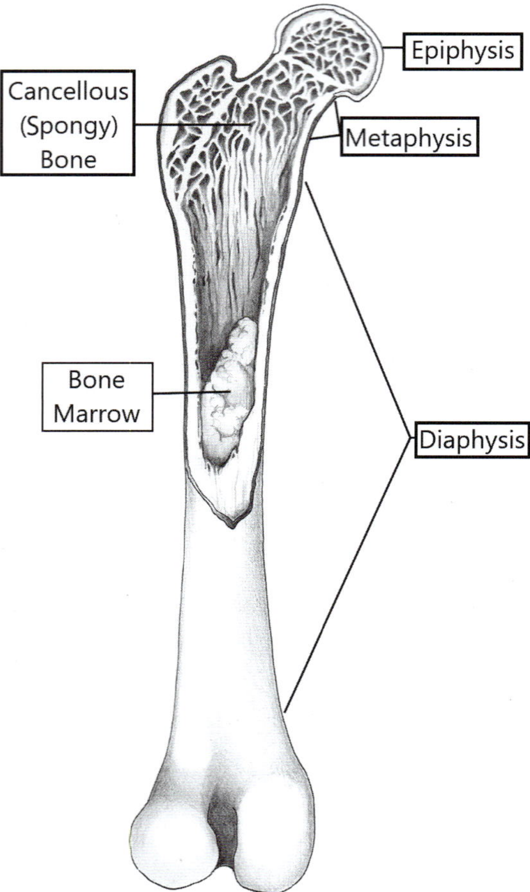

Figure 17.1 (1) Epiphysis, (2) metaphysis, (3) cortical bone, (4) endosteum, and (5) bone marrow.

The way bone grows is of particular concern when there is a fracture. As the bone rebuilds, the osteoblasts, the builders of new bone, start to repair the damage by creating woven, disorganized, immature bone first. The collection of this material is called a **callus**. The callus consists mostly of **fibrocartilage**, a relatively soft material. This will take a while to become mature bone. For this reason, severe fractures require immobilization of the area. Excessive movement will interrupt the building of the new bone.

Mature bone is called the **compact bone**. This is very durable and usually forms the outside wall of the bone. Compact bone is composed of a series of microscopic structures called **osteons**, which are a round series of layers with a central canal through which blood vessels flow. The osteons form a strong platform for the bony structure. Note that compact bone contains things like collagen and other proteins, and minerals like calcium and phosphorus. Cancellous bone does not have osteons but instead has a ladder-like series of intersecting cells. Cancellous bone is always covered by a thin layer of compact bone (see Figure 17.1).

The storage of calcium and phosphorus is important to the animal for use in energy production, and bone may be called upon to supply them if the usual stores of calcium and phosphorus are not sufficient. Calcium and phosphorus imbalance can be caused by dietary, endocrine, or renal problems.

In essence, the **parathyroid gland** is the part of the endocrine system that contributes to the balance of electrolytes – calcium and phosphorus. If the animal is hypocalcemic (low levels of calcium in the blood), **parathyroid hormone** (PTH) will be released by the parathyroid glands. PTH mobilizes calcium from the bones by inducing it to enter the bloodstream. Another hormone, **calcitonin**, encourages calcium to be stored in the bones. In this way, calcitonin stores excess calcium in the bone like a bank, and PTH can withdraw the calcium if the body needs it.

Note that **vitamin D** derivatives play a role in the activities of PTH. Vitamin D is important for other reasons as well. It is a key player in helping the gastrointestinal (GI) tract absorb calcium from the nutrients traveling through the tract. Some of that calcium goes to help build and maintain the bone.

Some animals undergo a **negative calcium balance**, meaning that they are losing more calcium than they are taking in. This can become a serious problem in milking cows. If they lose too much calcium in the milk they are excreting, they can develop hypocalcemia. The body is unable to mobilize enough calcium from its reserves to fill in the gaps, and the animal suffers severe weakness. The condition is fatal if not addressed promptly.

Bone Marrow

While there are small areas of marrow in other bones, the long bones contain the bulk of the bone marrow in mammals. Bone marrow is present in the **medullary cavity** of the bone. Bone marrow produces most of the blood cells the body uses. As the animal gets older, some of the marrow cells are replaced by fat cells and this becomes **yellow marrow**. The mature animal is still capable of producing new blood cells but at a reduced rate. The areas around the head of the humerus and the head of the femur continue to actively produce blood cells. It is for this reason that in cases of decreased white or red blood cell levels in the blood, we will usually check the bone marrow's ability to produce them by sampling from the humeral or femoral head.

Flat bones have marrow that continues to be active throughout life. Another place where bone marrow is sampled is from the ilium, for this reason. This is usually done in dogs only. In cats, the ilium is relatively thin and less sturdy, and it can fracture during the procedure.

The ability of the bone marrow to produce cells is dependent on a number of factors. There are regulating hormones, such as erythropoietin from the kidney, that tell the bone marrow to produce blood cells. If the kidneys are damaged, this hormone may not be produced, which leads to reduced red blood cell production. Alongside the body directing the bone marrow to create cells is having the appropriate materials to create the cells. In the case of red blood cells, adequate amounts of iron, folate, protein, and vitamin B12 are required. Chronic diseases can also cause a decrease in blood cell production, as they are a tax on all body systems. A lack of production of blood cells can come from missing instructions, like the lack of erythropoietin, a lack of building materials, like iron deficiency, or from bone marrow failure. If it is bone marrow failure, the factory may have the instructions and materials but cannot produce the cells. Animals that have depressed cell lines should be investigated for the causes behind this. Nutrient deficiencies or hormone imbalances can be the cause. If no overt cause is found in routine testing, sampling the bone marrow itself will potentially reveal the issue.

Cartilage

The difference between cartilage and bone is that cartilage, while it is a connective tissue, has no ossified material in it; that is, it does not have a hard matrix of osteons. It also does not have blood vessels or nerves running into it as bone does. Cartilage receives its nourishment not from the blood directly but from the diffusion of nutrients from local vessels through the interstitium into the cartilage.

There are three main types of cartilage: **hyaline, fibrocartilage**, and **elastic cartilage**. Hyaline cartilage is composed mostly of collagen, a protein common in the structure of connective tissues like bone and skin. It is the type of cartilage that lines the surface of bones where they meet a joint. Hyaline cartilage in the normal animal should have a smooth appearance and should be pink in color or slightly yellow in older animals. Hyaline cartilage is the most commonly occurring cartilage in the body and is responsible for the formation of articular cartilage. Articular cartilage is the cartilage found on the ends of bones that meet to create a joint. Excessive use and/or injury can cause the cartilage to wear down or tear, resulting eventually in inflammation and abnormal gait.

Fibrocartilage is a thick form of cartilage with strands of protein called **fibrin** running through it. Fibrocartilage is particularly strong. An example of fibrocartilage is the material that makes up the **articular labrum**, or the lip around a joint fossa. The labrum helps prevent friction as the femur moves. It can also be found in the intervertebral spaces, forming the intervertebral discs. Fibrocartilage has tremendous tensile strength. Subsequent to injury, fibrocartilage may replace hyaline cartilage.

Elastic cartilage bends freely. It provides shape but allows the tissue to be mobile as needed. The pinna of the ear is an example of elastic cartilage, where it has a defined shape but can easily be bent. Another example of elastic cartilage is the **epiglottis**, which covers the vocal cords and moves aside as needed to let sound and air escape.

Avians

Chapter 4 considered the concept of the pneumatized bones of the avian. The spaces within the bones are arranged such that the ossified (bony) parts run at angles to each other as well as in a parallel fashion. This provides a strong scaffold, particularly for the powerful muscles involved in flight. It also serves to lessen the animal's weight so that the bird can fly more successfully. Non-flighted birds also have pneumatized bones, although the bones may not be as completely pneumatized and thus may be heavier than those of flighted birds.

Other adaptations to flight include the presence of the air sacs (see Chapter 24), which allow efficient breathing while keeping the body weight low. The tibiotarsus is essentially one long piece, which provides greater stability when standing, given that the dorsal part of the animal weighs relatively little.

<table><tr><td>

Clinical Case Resolution: Binx

Binx undergoes a physical examination which reveals evidence of anemia by way of pale gums, increased heart rate, and increased respiratory rate. The owners note that he is slightly lethargic at home, with a mildly reduced appetite.

It is determined that Binx should have a bone marrow aspirate and biopsy to better understand if the bone marrow is working.

For this procedure, Binx will be sedated and a large-bore, specialized bone marrow needle will be introduced into the head of his humerus. A bone marrow sample will be obtained and sent for analysis.

If testing reveals that the bone marrow is not working, the treatment method will be based on why. For example, if it is due to infection, antibiotics may be used. If it is due to the immune system, immunosuppressants may be used.

</td></tr></table>

<table><tr><td>

Clinical Case Critical Thinking

Throughout the chapter, we discussed other reasons for the bone marrow to not be effective in its production of cells. What types of diseases would Binx have been screened for prior to bone marrow testing? If any of these issues were found, would a bone marrow test be necessary?

</td></tr></table>

Review Questions

1 True or False: The length of long bone growth occurs from the middle of the bone outward.
   A True
   B False

2 Which cells are responsible for cleaning up old or damaged bone?
   A Osteoblasts
   B Fibrocartilage
   C Osteoclasts
   D Erythropoietin

3 Which of the following is a common place for bone marrow aspirates in canines?
   A The head of the radius
   B The calcaneus
   C The wing of the ilium
   D The olecranon process

4 Which of the following is the dense mature bone?
   A Compact bone
   B Cancellous bone
   C Spongy bone
   D Medullary cavity

5 Which of the following describes the diaphysis?
   A The end part of a bone
   B The shaft or central part of a long bone
   C The growth plate
   D The outermost layer of the bone

6 True or False: All bones begin as a cartilaginous model.
   A True
   B False

7 Which is the most common type of cartilage?
- **A** Hyaline cartilage
- **B** Fibrocartilage
- **C** Elastic cartilage
- **D** All of the above

8 What hormone is responsible for instructing the bone marrow to produce red blood cells?
- **A** Vitamin D
- **B** Folate
- **C** Vitamin B12
- **D** Erythropoietin

9 What is endochondral ossification?
- **A** Replacement of fibrocartilage with bony tissue
- **B** Replacement of hyaline cartilage with bony tissue
- **C** Replacement of elastic cartilage with bony tissue
- **D** Replacement of medullary cavity with bony tissue

10 The production rate of bone marrow __________________ in older patients.
- **A** Increases
- **B** Decreases
- **C** Stays the same
- **D** Age has no impact on bone marrow production

18

Physiology of Joints

Clinical Case: Torpedo, a 16-Year-Old Female Spayed Persian

Torpedo is brought to the clinic for a routine examination. She has not been seen by a vet in many years, but the owner is concerned because she is older and wants to have her fully checked out.

In speaking with the owner, you learn that Torpedo has a normal appetite and is meal-fed. She regularly finishes her meals. The owner says she drinks from her water fountain and does not note any change in eating, drinking, or bathroom habits. When asked about her energy levels, the owner notes that Torpedo spends most of the day sleeping and resting, which the owner expects due to her age.

With further questioning, the owner mentions that Torpedo seems to be favoring her heated bed, as well as the litter box that is lower to the ground.

Introduction

Joints and their supporting features can be relatively simple or complex, depending on the role they play in the body. As discussed in Chapter 5, joints are made of two or more adjoining bones. Joints may be immovable, such as the suture joints in the skull, or highly mobile, such as the synovial joints found in the limbs. The movement, or lack thereof, of any joint is due to the way it is formed and the tissues involved in the joint.

The Immoveable Joints

The creation of immovable or limited mobility joints in the skeletal system is integral to its function. These joints are reserved for areas in which bones come together as one during development or where two bones come together in an articulation that functions to keep things in place rather than to serve as a point of flexion and extension.

The **fibrous joints** are generally immovable and involve dense connective tissues like collagen. In the skull, the **sutures** are a type of fibrous joint with no movement. In fetal development, the bones of the skull are formed as individuals. The skull can be developmentally divided into two parts: the **viscerocranium** and the **neurocranium**. The viscerocranium is the bones that make up the face, whereas the neurocranium is the bones that make up the surrounding case of the brain. Both areas are made up of a variety of bones, all of which slowly come together as the skull forms. During this formation, dense collagen tissue fibers bind the bones together. During development and through birth, these bony plates, although bound by collagen, allow for some movement. This aids in the animal passing through the birth canal. In the weeks shortly after birth, the spots between the bones will close and solidify into immovable suture joints. When the bones of the skull have openings, they are called **fontanelles**, and these can be persistent in some small and toy-breed dogs. In these cases, some of the openings on the skull remain throughout the animal's life, which is generally not problematic unless there is any traumatic injury to the head, as the brain is not fully protected.

Another relatively immovable fibrous joint is the **syndesmosis** joint. This is a joint that develops between two parallel bones that move together as one. This can be seen in between the radius and ulna in the thoracic limb, as well as the fibula

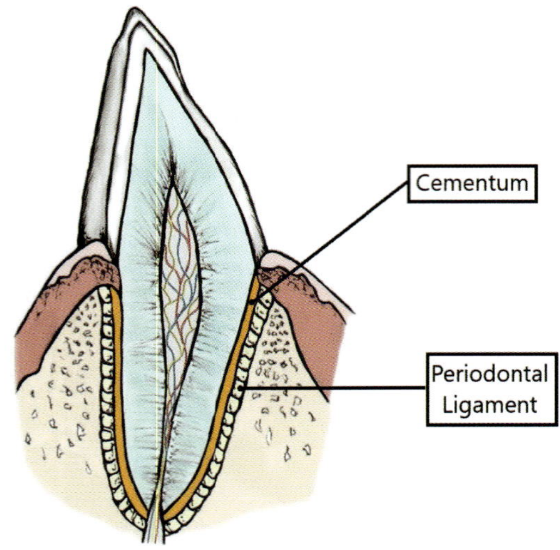

Figure 18.1 Gomphosis with the periodontal ligament identified.

and tibia in the pelvic limb. This connection forms using either **ligaments** or **intraosseous membranes**. Ligaments attach bone to bone and are found in a variety of different joints. An intraosseous membrane is a band of thick fibrous tissue that bridges the space between two bones. An example of an intraosseous membrane is the sheet of connective tissue between the radius and ulna.

The final relatively immovable fibrous joint is found in the oral cavity, called the **gomphosis**. This is the joint where the tooth is connected to the bony sockets in the jaw. Although a joint is typically defined as bones coming together in an articulation, here the joint is between bone and tooth, as a tooth is not technically a bone. In this joint, the **periodontal ligament** helps to attach the tooth root(s) to the space in the jaw. (Figure 18.1) The development of this ligament is critical in keeping the teeth positioned correctly in the mouth, but it can be slowly changed and moved by dental equipment like braces. Although braces aren't common in companion animals, they can be utilized to move the teeth in cases of severe orthodontic issues. It is important to understand that although the gomphosis is technically considered an immovable joint, there is a very small amount of movement, which is what allows for something like braces to slowly work to gently move teeth. It is also important to note these ligaments, as they must be accounted for and appropriately severed when a dental extraction is needed. Failure to do so adequately can result in a tooth fracture and a more difficult tooth extraction.

The next category of immovable joints are **cartilaginous joints**, which include the primary **synchondrosis joint** and the secondary **symphysis joint**. Cartilaginous joints are only peripherally vascularized, as cartilage is not considered vascular tissue. Surrounding blood supply helps to nourish the joint tissue. These joints are made of hyaline and fibrous cartilage. An example of synchondrosis is the epiphyseal plate, or growth plate. Recall from Chapter 17 that the growth plate, while active, is made of hyaline cartilage. Once the bone growth is completed, the hyaline growth plate undergoes ossification and becomes hard, compact bone in the adult animal. Another example is in the bones of the pelvis, where the ilium, ischium, and pubis are joined together with a synchondrosis.

The symphysis joint is formed by fibrocartilage between two bones. This joint is slightly more moveable than the others previously mentioned. There is the mandibular symphysis between the right and left sides of the mandible. There is also the pubic symphysis, where the right and left sides of the pelvis join at the pubic bone. The remaining symphysis joints exist in the vertebral column by way of the intervertebral discs. The intervertebral discs serve to separate each bony vertebrae, provide shock absorption for any impact on the spine, and allow for some flexibility when the spinal column moves.

The Moveable Joints

The synovial joints are the most moveable joints in the body. They are comprised of a number of anatomical features that vary depending on the specific joint. All synovial joints contain a joint capsule, a synovial cavity, and articular cartilage. They may also contain other supporting or cushioning elements, such as articular fat pads, articular disks, and bursae. These joints also contain tendons and ligaments.

Connective Tissues

Ligaments and **tendons** are made of connective tissue. Tendons are much thicker and, as a result, are supportive of a large range of movement. Tendons are both elastic and strong, which suits them to do the work of connecting bones across joints to muscles or other tissues. Tendons do not have great blood supply, and as a result, injuries to a tendon do not heal well as they are poorly supplied with materials to rebuild. Tendons are critically important to functional movement of the musculoskeletal system. It translates the contraction of muscles into the joint to allow for movement, while also maintaining shock-absorbing qualities.

Ligaments are fibrous tissue that connect bone to bone and generally serve to keep bones positioned together and provide stability to the joint. Ligaments have even less blood supply than tendons and therefore are even less positions to heal themselves when injured. When ligaments are stretched beyond their normal usage for extended periods, the ligament may be permanently damaged. This is evident in any ligament injury but is most apparent in joint dislocation. When the joint is dislocated from its original position, it stretches the ligaments. The longer it takes to reduce, or correct, the dislocation, the higher likelihood that the ligaments are permanently damaged.

The Synovial Joint

One of the key parts of the synovial joints is the joint capsule. This fibrous capsule creates the outer boundaries of the synovial cavity. The outer layer of the fibrous joint capsule helps to keep the adjoining bones together. The inner layer of the joint capsule is also called the **synovial membrane**. It is here that joint fluid, or **synovial fluid**, is produced.

The synovial membrane is lined with special cells that work to create joint fluid. This fluid is a mixture of plasma and other components like hyaluronic acid and lubricin, which help to lubricate the joint. Synovial fluid can be a diagnostic indicator in some cases and can be indicated when a patient has multiple effusive or swollen joints, shifting lameness, or a fever of unknown origin. In these patients, **arthrocentesis** is performed where a sterile needle is introduced into the joint to take a small sample for analysis. Normal joint fluid should appear clear to lightly straw-colored and viscous. If joint fluid is collected, it is generally submitted for microscopic analysis as well as cultured to check for bacterial growth.

Many of the structures contained within the synovial joint are intended to protect and limit damage to the joint. Remember that synovial joints are highly moveable and undergo consistent daily use. Synovial fluid works not only to provide lubrication but also to provide shock absorption and some nutrition to the joint.

Articular cartilage is the hyaline cartilage that lines the ends of the bones in the joint. It too serves to provide shock absorption and reduce friction between the opposing bones. A common illness in senior pets is linked to the loss of articular cartilage from wear and tear. **Osteoarthritis (OA)** is a degenerative disease of the joint where the cartilage and other supporting tissues breakdown, resulting in inflammation and pain. With the loss of articular cartilage comes bony changes to the epiphysis within the joint. This remodeling of bone is caused by inflammation and, unfortunately, creates worsening friction and pain for the patient. OA is often diagnosed on physical examination but is often paired with radiographs as well. All species are susceptible to OA, but there are some species and breeds in which it is overrepresented. Dogs that are known to have genetic joint diseases like hip dysplasia, elbow dysplasia, or patella luxation are more likely to develop osteoarthritis. Further, any joint that has sustained an injury in the past or is subjected to repetitive high-impact activities will also potentially suffer from OA in the future. Cats are unfortunately underdiagnosed with osteoarthritis. This is not because they do not develop the disease but because symptoms seem to be less obvious as elderly cats tend not to be as active as dogs, leading owners to be less likely to notice pain or stiffness. All animals presenting for a physical examination should have a thorough musculoskeletal examination that assesses for pain. A physical examination may reveal lameness, pain, or resistance to full extension or flexion of joints, and/or **crepitus**. Crepitus is the crunching or cracking sounds that can be heard when manipulating a joint. This can be representative of bones in the joint rubbing against one another, which is an abnormal finding consistent with osteoarthritis.

Beyond the items mentioned above that are found in every single synovial joint, there are other important features that can be discussed. Articular discs, sometimes called **menisci** (singular: meniscus), are pads of fibrocartilage that can be found in synovial joints. They allow for a more even distribution of forces within the joint and help to increase stability within the joint. **Articular fat pads** are deposits of adipose tissue that provide cushioning and protection to the articular cartilage. **Bursae** or **synovial bursae** are another item found in or around synovial joints that provide shock absorption and cushioning within the joint. They are small, sac-like structures filled with fluid that is very similar to synovial fluid. Bursae can be found subcutaneously, or under the skin, submuscular, or in between muscle and bone, or finally, subtendinous, or between tendon and bone. Synovial joints can also have **accessory ligaments**, which are fibrous bands that help the joint resist extreme movements during articulation.

There is also blood, lymphatic, and nervous supply to the synovial joints to be considered. The synovial joints are supplied with blood via the **periarticular plexus**, which is a network of vessels surrounding the joint. There are some blood vessels that enter the fibrous capsule of the joint which helps to supply the joint capsule and synovial membrane with necessary nutrients. The lymphatics in synovial joints are serviced by nearby lymph nodes or lymph nodes within the joints themselves.

Innervation to the synovial joints is complex and includes both **sensory** and **autonomic nerves**. The autonomic nerves are mostly from the sympathetic nervous system which relates to fight or flight. These nerves help communicate with the vessels in the area to control dilation or constriction, changing blood supply to the tissue. In times of sympathetic nervous system activation, or fight or flight, the nerves will send the signal for the vessels to dilate, allowing more efficient blood flow to the area.

The sensory nerve endings provide feedback regarding **proprioception**. Proprioception is the animals' understanding and perception of where the body is in regard to its surroundings. This information allows for the body to control its movement, balance and posture appropriately. **Nociceptors** or pain receptors are also found in the joint and can convey pain and inflammation to the central nervous system for pain perception.

Clinical Case Resolution: Torpedo

Torpedo has a physical examination performed. Unfortunately, due to patient temperament, the physical examination is slightly limited. It is noted that Torpedo has some mild muscle wasting in both hind limbs. It is also noted that Torpedo is resentful of hind limb manipulation. There is questionable crepitus felt in the right hind limb stifle, but manipulation of the joint was not repeatable due to patient being aggressive.

Radiographs are offered to the owners, but they have declined this diagnostic. They have approved routine senior bloodwork and urine analysis. The doctor shares concerns that Torpedo may be painful in her hind limbs and that it may be osteoarthritis. The owner then confirms that Torpedo is more hesitant to jump at home and is not climbing her cat tower as much as she used to.

Bloodwork results are all normal, and Torpedo is started on a regimen of joint supplements and pain medication to treat her presumptive osteoarthritis.

Clinical Case Critical Thinking

Consider the lifestyle of dogs and cats.

1) *Why is it more difficult to diagnose osteoarthritis in cats?*
2) *What part of the initial history might make a clinician consider that Torpedo is painful or uncomfortable?*
3) *What about a senior pet might make an owner not notice reduced physical capabilities?*

Review Questions

1 What are the small spaces in between skull bones called?
   A A gomphosis
   B A fontanelle
   C A bursae
   D A viscerocranium

2 What kind of joint is the coronal suture?
   A Cartilaginous
   B Synovial
   C Fibrous

3 Which type of connective tissue connects muscle to bone?
   A Tendons
   B Ligaments
   C Bursae
   D Fascia

4 Where might you find an example of syndesmosis?
   A In between bones of the skull
   B In the joint between the glenoid cavity and the humerus
   C The space between the tibia and fibula
   D The space between the tooth and the mandible

5 Which portion of the synovial joint secretes synovial fluid?
   A The outermost layer of the fibrous capsule
   B The meniscus
   C The articular cartilage
   D The inner layer of the joint capsule

6 Define crepitus.

7 Which joint begins as a cartilaginous joint and ends up as compact bone?
   A A symphysis
   B A syndesmosis
   C A synchondrosis
   D An intraosseous membrane

8 True or False: Ligaments are more richly supplied with blood vessels than tendons.
   A True
   B False

9 The degeneration of articular cartilage can lead to what disease process?
   A Dental fractures
   B Arthrocentesis
   C Anemia
   D Osteoarthritis

10 True or False: Nociceptors in the synovial joints help to create synovial fluid.
   A True
   B False

19

Muscle Physiology

> **Clinical Case: Soot, An 18-Year-Old Male Neutered Domestic Short Hair (DSH)**
>
> *Soot is brought in through the emergency room for lethargy and ataxia (uncoordinated gait). The owner says that Soot has lost weight and had a progressively decreasing appetite and energy for over a month now. The owner said he thinks this is just due to Soot getting much older, and he has not had Soot at the vet for approximately 3 years.*
>
> *When asked more questions about the way Soot has been feeling, the owner says he has noticed Soot is thirstier than ever before, and he has noticed him hovering over the water bowl in the last 2 days. Today he says that Soot's weakness and lethargy is significantly worsened.*

Introduction

Muscles are divided into three groups: **skeletal muscle, smooth muscle**, and **cardiac muscle**. Skeletal muscle can also be referred to as **voluntary striated muscle**, while smooth muscle can be called **involuntary non-striated muscle** and cardiac as **involuntary striated muscle**. This all has to do with the appearance of the tissue and how it functions. Both cardiac and skeletal muscle have a striated or striped/streaked appearance, while smooth muscle appears as one single sheet of tissue with no striations. Functionally, muscle is either voluntary, or under conscious control, like skeletal muscle, or involuntary, like cardiac and smooth muscle that operates without the need for conscious input. Here we will explore the mechanisms that make each of these muscle groups function.

Striated Muscle

The gross appearance of the skeletal muscles is an important part of a physical exam. Severe weight loss sometimes even affects the appearance of the muscles themselves; they will **atrophy**, or shrink, if they cannot sustain their normal energy level.

Recall that the structure of skeletal muscles, which provide the primary force for voluntary movement, includes bundles of fibers called **fasciculi**. Each muscle fiber is made up of contractile structures called **myofibrils**. Skeletal muscle cells have multiple nuclei.

The terminology regarding muscle cells is different. Structures may have different names, although they often serve the same function as the analogous parts in other cells. In striated muscle, which includes both cardiac and skeletal muscle, the cell membrane is called a **sarcolemma**, which receives signals for muscle contraction and regulates molecules moving in and out of the cell. The fluid part of the cell within its membrane is referred to as **sarcoplasm**, just as the interior of a somatic cell is called cytoplasm. In place of the endoplasmic reticulum of other cells, the phrase is **sarcoplasmic reticulum**, which is a storage organelle for calcium ions. These striated muscle cells also contain **transverse tubules** or **T-tubules**, which act as a highway for information and signals to travel through the cell (Figure 19.1).

Along with the cellular components, the muscle fiber is composed of a series of proteins called **myosin** and **actin**. Myosin is also referred to as **thick filament**, while actin can be referred to as **thin filament**. These proteins are stacked

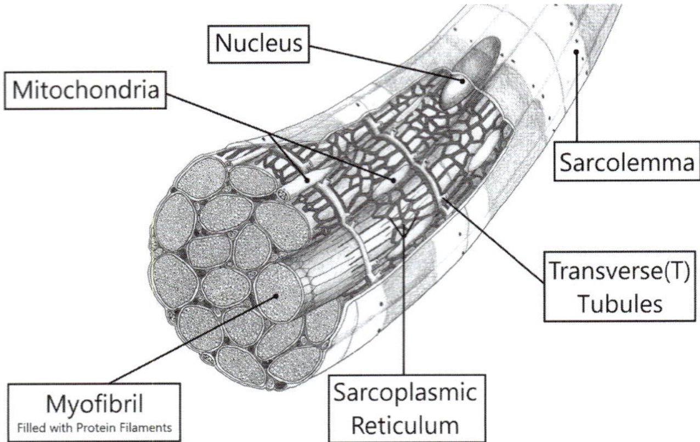

Figure 19.1 The skeletal muscle cell with organelles identified. Note the small openings on the sarcolemma, which allow information into the T-tubules.

parallel to one another in a repeating pattern in the cell called **sarcomeres**, which creates dark and light bands. Refer to Figure 6.3 for the anatomical features of the sarcomere. It is this alternate series of bands lying on top of one another that gives rise to the striated appearance of the muscle. Actin also contains some smaller proteins called **troponin** and **tropomyosin** which play a role in the contraction of muscle fiber, which will be discussed later.

The Generation of a Muscle Contraction

In Chapter 20, a full discussion of the neurological side of the stimulation of muscles is covered. The point at which the nerve meets the muscle is called the **neuromuscular junction**.

The nerve fibers that provoke skeletal muscle activity are called **motor neurons**. They contain the neurotransmitter acetylcholine (ACh). When a signal travels down the motor neuron, it hits the end point, or **terminal bouton**. This triggers the release of acetylcholine, which crosses the synapse to bind to the muscle fiber, specifically the sarcolemma. This generates an **action potential** that opens the channels to allow sodium and potassium to enter and leave the cell, respectively. At rest, sodium remains in the extracellular space, while potassium remains in the intracellular space. This creates a charge in which the inside of the cell is more negative than the outside, called a **polarized state**. When the muscle fiber is stimulated, the cell undergoes **depolarization**, in which sodium and potassium switch places. This exchange allows for changes in cell voltage that make the transmission of the nerve impulse possible.

The binding of acetylcholine to the sarcolemma and depolarization of the cell wall translates the signal from the nervous system to the muscle fiber. Next the T-tubules carry the impulse to the interior of the cell until it reaches the sarcoplasmic reticulum. The sarcoplasmic reticulum is an organelle that serves to store and release calcium ions when prompted. This signal from the T-tubules prompts the sarcoplasmic reticulum to release calcium, which plays an integral role in successful contraction. The released calcium binds to troponin.

Troponin is a protein that helps move tropomyosin in and out of the way during muscle contractions and relaxations. At rest, tropomyosin sits in the sarcomere, blocking binding sites on actin that allow for muscle contraction. When calcium binds to troponin, it pulls tropomyosin out of the way, revealing the actin-binding sites for contraction.

Once the binding site is exposed to actin, myosin can form **cross bridges** by connecting to actin. Cross bridging is where myosin, which has small arm-like projections, called **myosin heads** reach out and attach to the newly revealed binding sites on actin. Once the connection is made, the myosin heads pull the actin in, compressing the sarcomere, resulting in contraction. ATP provides the energy needed to both form and release these cross bridges that bind and release myosin from this site. It is important to understand that this is happening on a microscopic scale all over the muscle cell and throughout the muscle itself. This cycle, as described above, happens in very quick repeated cycles for any type of successful and sustained movement. Once the neurologic stimulus is over, the calcium is escorted back into the sarcoplasmic reticulum for storage, awaiting the next action potential (Figure 19.2).

Note that action potentials come along rapidly once they are started. The speed with which the exchange and movement of electrolytes, and the actin-myosin reaction, take place is enough to allow repeated movement of the muscle fiber. Until an enzyme breaks down the neurotransmitter completely, the neuron will continue to fire, and the muscle cells will respond. In the case of skeletal muscles, the enzyme **acetylcholinesterase** is used to break down acetylcholine. Therefore, two mechanisms are used to stop muscle contraction: depleting stores of ATP and interfering with the interface of the neurotransmitter with its receptors in the sarcolemma. There can be other interruptions in appropriate muscle contraction if there are serious electrolyte disturbances involving sodium, potassium, and calcium, as these are integral to muscle contraction.

There actually is always a low level of muscle tone, even in a stationary animal; that is, the majority of skeletal muscles are held in a "ready" state by being slightly contracted or extended. This is what allows animals to maintain a particular body position and to respond to any need for sudden movement.

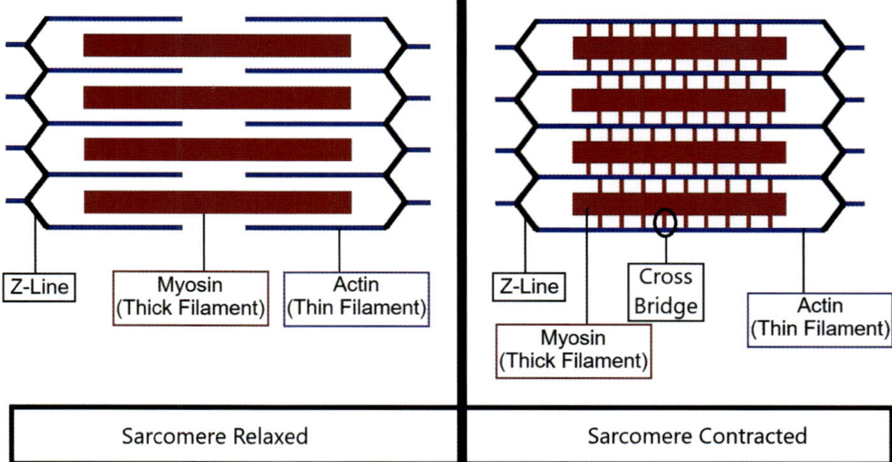

Figure 19.2 The sarcomere at rest and contracted. Note that in the contraction, there is the appearance of cross bridging from myosin heads connecting to binding sites on actin.

Skeletal Muscle versus Cardiac Muscle

Although skeletal muscle and cardiac muscle are both striated and share a large number of similarities, there are some key differences to consider. Skeletal muscle is innervated and controlled by a neurotransmitter, acetylcholine. This makes skeletal muscle **neurogenic** in that it only responds to a nervous system impulse. Cardiac muscle contraction is not generated by nervous system control but rather by itself. Cardiac muscle fibers are designed to create their own stimulus and are referred to as **myogenic**, as the signal originates from the muscle tissue, not the nervous system. The beginning of the cardiac conduction cycle is from the **sinoatrial (SA) node**, which is discussed in greater detail in Chapter 23. Another key difference is that cardiac muscle cells are connected by **intercalated discs**, which allow signal communication between cardiac muscle cells, allowing them to act in unison. This is necessary, as the heart must work in a constant synchronized state in order to sustain life.

Adenosine Triphosphate

The generation of **adenosine triphosphate** (ATP) is particularly important in the process of muscle contraction. ATP comes from a series of steps involving the oxidation of glucose and the processing of phosphates. A lack of glucose-containing nutrients will lead to abnormal muscle function. The lack of glucose, or abnormal glucose processing, can lead to twitching of muscles or **muscle fasciculations**. There is a particular risk of this in puppies and kittens, which do not have a mature glucose processing system. Note, however, that muscle can make energy from other sources as well if need be.

When ATP is utilized, the energy comes from one of the three phosphate groups being broken off. This results in one phosphate molecule being removed, creating **adenosine diphosphate** (ADP). A store of ATP is present in muscle cells, but it needs to be replenished once utilized. The major ways that muscles do this are by using the muscle cell's store of **creatine phosphate**, breaking down **glucose**, and **cellular oxidation** of nutrients. Creatine phosphate will give up its phosphate group to ADP to turn it back into ATP again, leaving creatine behind. Note that other important features are glucose and oxygen. Muscles can store glucose as **glycogen** and oxygen as **myoglobin**. These can be taken out of storage if necessary during sustained activity, but they too can be depleted. While the use of oxygen for processing is called **aerobic metabolism**, once oxygen availability and stores are empty, skeletal muscle can switch to **anaerobic metabolism**. Anaerobic metabolism in muscle is a short-term solution that causes the incomplete breakdown of glucose and a byproduct of **lactic acid**. Lactic acid is what causes the burning sensation and soreness in muscles during and after prolonged use.

The issue of creatine phosphate is also clinically significant. An animal that is losing a significant amount of weight will have some damage or atrophy to the larger muscles, usually those of the trunk at first. High blood levels of an enzyme called **creatine kinase** are associated with muscle damage and/or significant weight loss. This can be useful, particularly when a client is not sure how long the animal has been losing weight. If a client is new to the clinic, there may be no record of the animal's prior weight. The combination of an increase in the creatine kinase level in the blood and evidence of muscle atrophy is reflected in the **body condition score** (BCS).

A dog or a cat in good body condition will have a slight waist, ribs that are not easily visible but are palpated easily, and no large areas of fat deposits unless part of the animal's breed characteristics. Here, consider an Italian Greyhound versus an English Bulldog. BCS is graded on a scale, generally 1–5 or 1–9. An animal in perfect condition would be given a score of 3 out of 5 (written 3/5) or 5 out of 9 (5/9) depending on the scale. The higher the number, the more overweight the animal is. The lower the number, the more underweight the animal is. The condition called **cachexia** refers to a person or an animal that is severely underweight. This body condition is usually associated with cancer or severe chronic illness. We would judge an animal appearing like this as having a 1/5 or 1/9 BCS. Keeping track of these scores each time the animal gets a physical exam will help the examiner recall what the animal looked like before. Along with BCS is the **muscle condition score** (MCS), which allows us to specifically point to the condition of the muscling regardless of the fat content of the animal. There are chronic disease processes in which the animal will have muscle wasting or atrophy but still maintain a somewhat normal fat content. Similar to BCS, MCS has a numerical scoring chart, usually 0–3, where 0 is severe muscle loss and 3 is normal muscle mass. A healthy pet should be a 3/3 MCS.

The Basis of Speed

Muscle fibers can be described as either "**slow twitch**" or "**fast twitch**." Slow-twitch fibers are also known as "red" muscle as a result of their high level of myoglobin. Fast-twitch fibers are correspondingly lower in myoglobin and are referred to as "white" muscle. The reason the terms slow and fast are used is that the neurons that innervate these muscles are either of small diameter or large diameter. Small-diameter neurons have a slower transmission of the action potential and larger-diameter neurons a faster transmission.

This has a bearing on our clinical practice in that it helps us understand why some animals can maintain a high level of activity for a short period of time or a lower level of activity for a longer time. The slow-twitch muscles are best for endurance; they produce a sustained level of energy, albeit at a slower pace. This kind of muscle serves a bird in flight quite well. Avian flight can cover very long distances without fatigue because the muscles are not being asked to come up with a sustained rapid pace.

A strong release of high-energy movement that lasts only a short time utilizes the fast-twitch fibers. Watching a lion hunt down prey will reveal this pattern. The lion can put on a tremendous explosion of energy, running quickly and covering a great deal of ground. However, the lion cannot keep that up for too long. If the prey can stay away from the predator long enough, the predator will have to stop to rest, and the prey can move further away.

Non-Striated Muscle

The lack of striations in the outward appearance of smooth muscle reflects the fact that these muscle fibers are shaped like a spindle rather than straight lines. They do have thick and thin filaments, as do striated muscle fibers, but the arrangement of these proteins is different. Smooth muscle cells also contain **dense bodies**, which serve to anchor actin. They also contain **intermediate** filaments, along with the thick and thin filaments. Due to the different organization of contractile filaments in smooth muscle, when contraction occurs, it acts like a net over the cell, pulling it all in to shorten on contract. Despite this, the mechanism of actin–myosin interaction is similar in that they form cross bridges to contract. The series of steps that are involved in this cycle go at a much slower rate. This slower rate consumes energy at a much lower level.

As a result, smooth muscle can maintain a constant or slowly changing state of relaxation or contraction. This serves an important function: smooth muscles are associated with actions like changes in the diameter of blood vessels and contraction of muscles associated with the gastrointestinal (GI) tract. These are functions that go on constantly or intermittently throughout each day. Unlike skeletal muscles, which are only called upon during voluntary movement, smooth muscles require continued activity. In fact, many smooth muscles are called into action while the animal is asleep or relatively inactive. They maintain a constant tone or low-level activity on a much greater level than skeletal muscle does. The gastrocnemius muscle is only active at times when the animal is moving the pelvic limb. The muscles controlling the walls of the saphenous veins go into and out of function regardless of the animal's state and without the animal's conscious awareness.

Smooth muscles do not rely strictly on motor neuron circuits. The **autonomic nervous system** has a primary role in the contraction or relaxation of smooth muscles, using different neurotransmitters to stimulate motor movement. These neurotransmitters include **norepinephrine** and acetylcholine and chemical messengers like **nitric oxide**. Ongoing research into the function of nitric oxide as a messenger is the basis of research into current and potential pharmacological treatment of disease.

Hormones have a direct influence on the function of smooth muscles. For example, the reproductive system responds to the pituitary hormone **oxytocin**. Oxytocin causes contraction of the smooth muscles associated with the uterus, as well as the mammary glands.

Other chemical messengers play a role. The substance **histamine**, an inflammatory chemical carried by **basophils** (a type of white blood cell) and by **mast cells** (another inflammatory cell), will be released in the presence of allergens. Another type of white blood cell called an **eosinophil** is able to cause the release of histamine. Histamine causes contraction of the smooth muscles of the respiratory tract.

It should be noted that there are areas of smooth muscle within the heart. The smooth muscle components, with their sustained capacity for work, are important in a muscle that absolutely must keep functioning for the animal to live. They help regulate blood flow and blood pressure, which are necessary for cardiac function. On the other hand, the ability to provide very forceful contractions, with bursts of energy as needed in emergencies, requires the efficient use of large amounts of energy associated with striated muscle.

Innervation

The number of muscle cells stimulated by a single neuron, based on the number of dendrites it has, is called a **motor unit**. In some cases, a single neuron may stimulate a very small number of muscle fibers. In others, a neuron may cause a large section of a muscle cell to stretch or contract. The fewer muscle fibers a single neuron connects to, the more specific the muscle response; that is, if a single neuron controls a single fiber, very fine control over the movement of that muscle is possible.

As discussed above, the motor units that control the function of skeletal muscle are nerves that release acetylcholine to stimulate contractions. In smooth muscles, there are nerves that control movement, but they are not under conscious control. This is all controlled via the autonomic nervous system and is in response to neurotransmitters. Innervation to smooth muscle can be **single-unit** or **multiunit**. The single-unit innervation of smooth muscle means that there is one nerve controlling a sheet of organized smooth muscle. This is true in areas like the GI tract, where waves of peristalsis are orchestrated by one signal. Multiunit innervation of smooth muscle means that there are smooth muscle cells that function more independently. These cells are not organized into sheets and tend to have more nerve input. Multiunit smooth muscle is capable of very delicate movements like those in the iris of the eye.

While the heart generates its own action potential, it is also governed to some extent by the autonomic nervous system. The effect is to ramp up or dampen the ongoing strength of contraction as needed (e.g., to step up the rate and force of the heartbeat if a predator on the hunt occurs). This will be discussed further in Chapter 23.

Clinical Case Resolution: Soot

Upon examination, it is revealed that Soot is very weak and lethargic, with a BCS of 3/9 and an MCS of 1/3. These findings indicate an underlying chronic disease process. Along with this, it is noted that Soot has pale mucous membranes and is dehydrated, and a cardiac arrhythmia (abnormal heartbeat) and heart murmur is auscultated.

Because Soot is in a concerning medical state, it is decided that bloodwork will be performed in the clinic to get rapid results.

Blood work reveals severely elevated kidney values (BUN and Creatinine—not to be confused with creatine), low levels of red blood cells (anemia), and severe hypokalemia (low blood potassium). Recall the importance of oxygen delivered by red blood cells, and electrolytes needed in the contraction of muscle when considering how this patient is affected.

Soot is admitted to the hospital in an effort to rehydrate him, reduce the elevated kidney values, and correct the electrolyte imbalances. A blood transfusion may be considered as well.

Clinical Case Critical Thinking

1) *Which part of Soot's bloodwork results is most likely leading to his profound muscle weakness?*
2) *Review hematology in Chapter 14 and renal physiology in Chapter 22:*
   a) *Why are BUN and creatinine elevated in this patient?*
   b) *Why is potassium so low?*
   c) *Why is this patient anemic?*
3) *How can the findings on Soot be related to his arrhythmia and murmur?*

Review Questions

1 Where would we expect to find dense bodies?
   A Striated involuntary muscle
   B Non-striated involuntary muscle
   C Striated voluntary muscle
   D Non-striated voluntary muscle

2 Where would we expect to find multiunit smooth muscle?
   A The stomach
   B The colon
   C The leg
   D The eye

3 What connects one cardiac muscle cell with the next?

4 What part of the muscle cell is the storage center for calcium ions?
   A Sarcolemma
   B Sarcoplasm
   C Sarcoplasmic reticulum
   D Mitochondria

5 What neurotransmitter is released from motor nerve fibers innervated skeletal muscle to stimulate contraction?
   A Acetylcholine
   B Troponin
   C Epinephrine
   D Norepinephrine

6 What is the byproduct of anaerobic metabolism?
   A Oxygen
   B Carbon dioxide
   C Glycogen
   D Lactic acid

7 When an impulse travels into a muscle cell and reaches the sarcoplasmic reticulum, what is released from the sarcoplasmic reticulum?
   A Acetylcholine
   B Calcium
   C Sodium
   D Potassium

8 True or False: ATP is needed for both muscle contraction and muscle relaxation
   A True
   B False

9 What does calcium bind to in order to allow cross-bridging?
   A Troponin
   B Tropomyosin
   C Creatine phosphate
   D Myosin

10 Which chemical found in muscle fibers is used to "recharge" ATP?
   A Creatine kinase
   B Lactic acid
   C Creatine phosphate
   D Adenosine diphosphate

20

Neurophysiology

Clinical Case: Boots, a 4-Year-Old Male Neutered DSH

Boots is presented to the emergency room for drooling, vomiting, trembling, muscle twitching/tremors, and depression. The owner notes that these symptoms have been progressive over the last 36 hours.

Boots has always been a healthy cat and is up to date on his vaccines. He is an indoor/outdoor cat as the owners have a barn and Boots is an excellent mouser. He is one of two cats in the home, but the other is elderly and no longer goes outside. The other cat in the home appears asymptomatic. Boots was separated from the other cat as soon as he appeared to be sick with vomiting.

Boots tends to stick near the property, as far as the owners know, but there is not much around them except for farmland.

Introduction

To maintain homeostasis, the body must be able to "read" its status with regard to every organ and body system, including the brain itself. Neurological physiology involves the propagation of a signal along each nerve cell, bringing information to or taking information from cells or groups of cells throughout the body. Along with hormones, nerve impulses are mediators of metabolism. From the management of cardiac and respiratory functions to the governance of the olfactory sense to the ability to play catch, the nervous system is crucial.

Information from outside the body must be gathered, delivered to the central nervous system (CNS), which consists of the spinal cord and the brain, and then acted upon.

The Neuron

The **neuron**, or nerve cell, is composed of a cell body, projections called **dendrites**, and a relatively long extension called an **axon** (see Figure 20.1; this illustration also appears earlier in this text). Neurons can deliver information directly to each other but more commonly communicate with cells outside the neurological system. An average mammalian vertebrate has 10 billion neurons. In large animals, a single axon can be 1 m long.

Note that the neuron itself needs energy in order to function. It depends strictly on glucose (e.g., as opposed to lipids) in order to generate energy. The use of glucose to produce energy requires the presence of oxygen. As has been discussed, the CNS cannot use anaerobic energy systems. This is why oxygen deprivation has such a catastrophic effect on the nervous system. It is also the reason that hypoglycemia (low blood glucose level) affects the nervous system.

Energy created by variations in electric charge propagates along the axon, like ripples in a pond, until it can be handed off to the next cell. The stimulation of this energy pulse is what provides the platform for launching the activity of the destination cell.

The **soma** is the body of the nerve cell and the axon the long projection coming from it. The thicker the axon, the faster the nerve impulse can travel. Some axons have a sheath of fatty tissue called **myelin**, which insulates the axon.

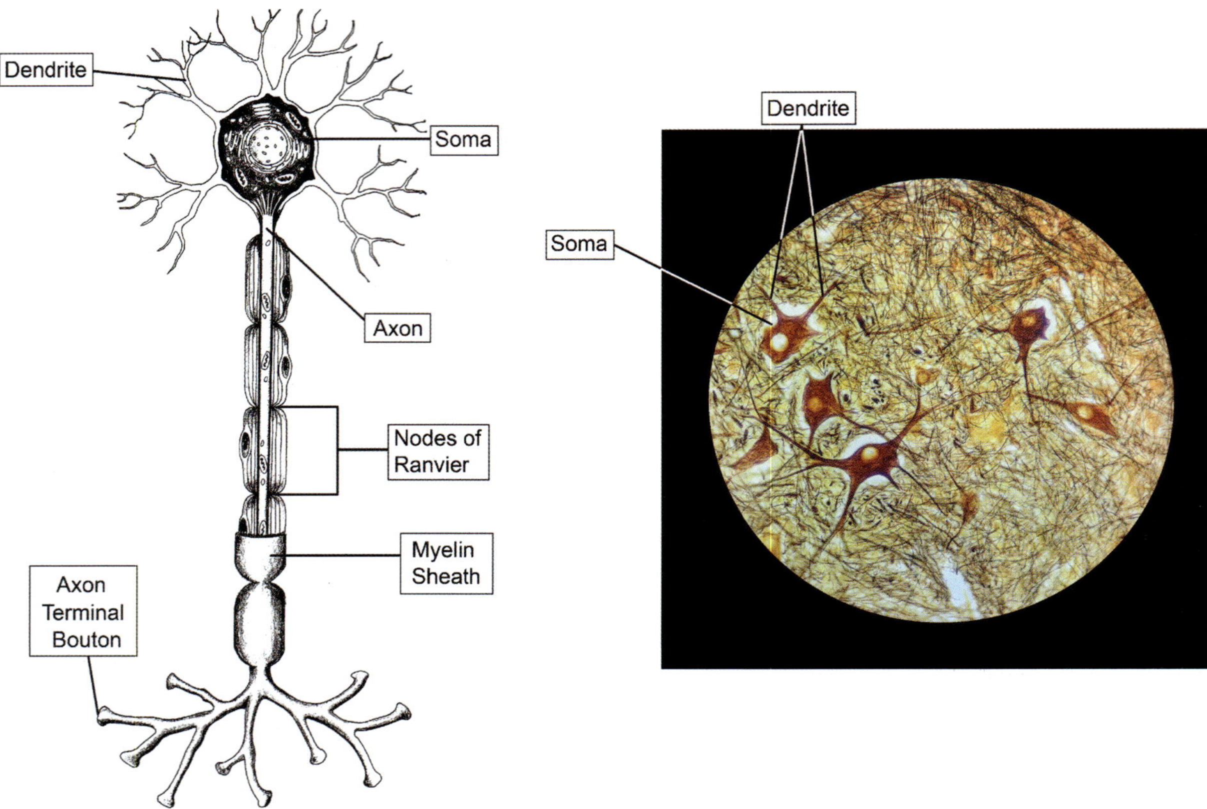

Figure 20.1 The neuron schematic as well as a microscopic view of the neuron cell bodies in the spinal cord. Not all neurons have myelin. The nodes of Ranvier are locations where there is no insulation covering the nerve fiber itself.

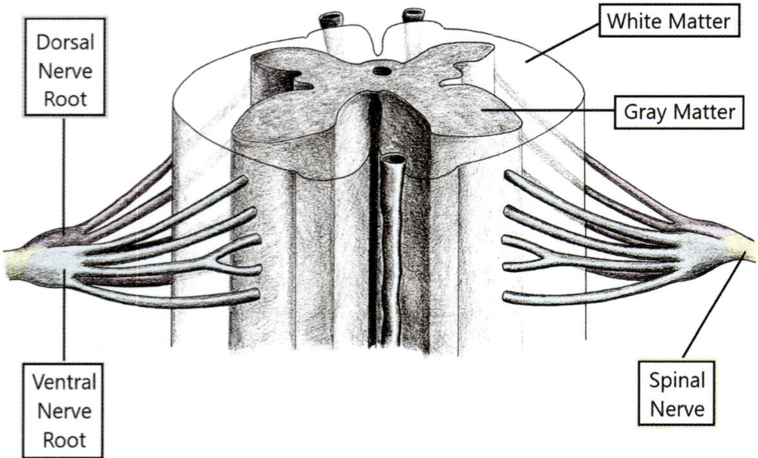

Figure 20.2 The sections of the spinal cord schematic.

Note that **afferent signals** are the ones that bring sensory information from the rest of the body, or from outside the body, into the CNS; **efferent signals** are those heading from the CNS to another destination. In the spinal cord, neurons conducting afferent signals have their soma in the **dorsal root ganglion** of the spinal nerves (Figure 20.2). Efferent fibers, some called motor neurons, usually have a soma in the CNS, with axons going out to the muscles, glands, or other organs. As will be noted below, the architecture of the autonomic nervous system is somewhat different (Figure 20.3).

When a nerve impulse, called an **action potential**, arrives at the soma, it can produce another action potential, which travels along its axon to propagate the message. The distal end of the axon is known as the **axon terminal**, or the

terminal bouton. The axon terminal can direct its energy to another axon, a dendrite, or a cell in the organ or tissue being stimulated, known as the **target tissue**. For example, if the trigeminal nerve (cranial nerve V) is bringing a signal to the muscles of the jaw, those muscles would be the target of that nerve. Where the nerve ending communicates with the target tissue, there is a small space called the **synapse**.

Transmission across the synapse can be chemical or electrical. In mammals, the vast majority of transmitters are chemical. In other words, the axon terminal releases a chemical across the synapse when the nerve is stimulated. The **presynaptic membrane or terminal** is the nerve tissue before the synapse. This chemical information travels across the synapse, arrives at the **postsynaptic membrane** (i.e., the next cell in the chain), and stimulates an activity that varies depending on the nature of the target. These chemical messengers are called **neurotransmitters**.

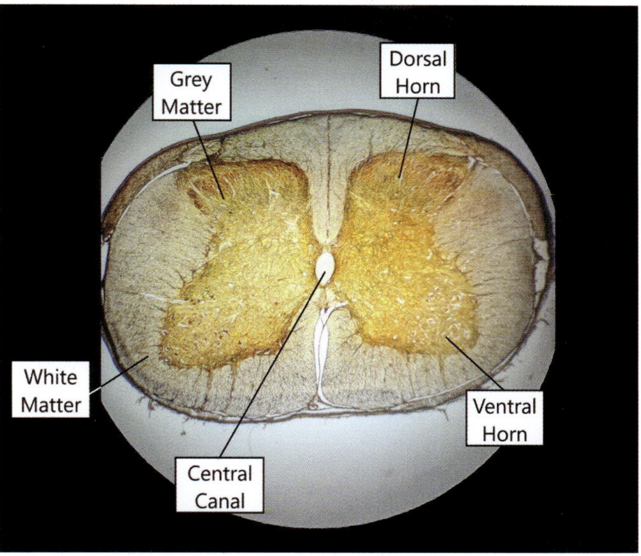

Figure 20.3 The sections of the preserved spinal cord as seen through the microscope.

The Action Potential

The action potential is the wave of electrical energy that is propagated along the axon and causes the release of the neurotransmitter. It is particularly dependent on certain electrolytes: sodium and potassium. Disease states that disrupt the levels of these ions can seriously impact neurological function. In addition, potassium is the basis of some of our euthanasia drugs; an excess of potassium will fatally interrupt nerve impulses and muscle function, causing the heart to stop.

The **resting potential** of a neuron is the electrical charge within the cell relative to the electrical charge in the tissue around it. The area around the cell is relatively more positively charged. The slightly negative charge within the cell is referred to as its '**resting potential**." In domestic mammals, that charge is -75 mV.

The extracellular area contains less potassium and more sodium than the intracellular area. Using the energy of ATP within the cell, potassium can be pumped outside of the cell, bringing sodium in. The reverse can also occur. The process is called the **Na+/K+-ATPase pump**.

Depolarization is the change in the cell's electrical charge and occurs when this ion exchange makes the interior of the cell less negative. The use of the phrase "less negative" is deliberate; the charge may rise to -50 mV, for example, which is still negative, but less so than -75 mV. When it returns to its resting (usual) potential, the process is called **repolarization**.

A neuron at rest has a minute electrical charge. The charge changes when the neuron is stimulated by another neuron or by chemical interchange. When this happens, channels will open within the axon.

Sodium in the surrounding tissue takes advantage of this to rush into the neuron. As sodium is a positive ion, the amount of negative charge decreases. Once all the channels open, there will be a large surge of electrical energy, kicking off the response along the rest of the axon. However, with all the channels open, potassium, which is also a positively charged ion, goes out of the cell. Since there is usually less potassium surrounding the cell than in it, the potassium within the cell is drawn to an area where it has more room.

In short, the neuron uses glucose as a fuel to produce energy. That energy kicks off an exchange of sodium and potassium that changes the electrical charge of the cell.

As the neuron returns to its resting potential, it usually "overshoots" the mark. In other words, instead of returning to the resting level of -75 mV, it will go to an even more negative level, say, -95 mV. This overshoot is referred to as **hyperpolarization**. The amount of time it takes to get back to the resting level is known as the **refractory period**. The refractory period can be broken down into two parts: the **absolute refractory period** and the **relative refractory period**. During the absolute refractory period, the neuron cannot respond to another stimulus even if it receives one. This is because the

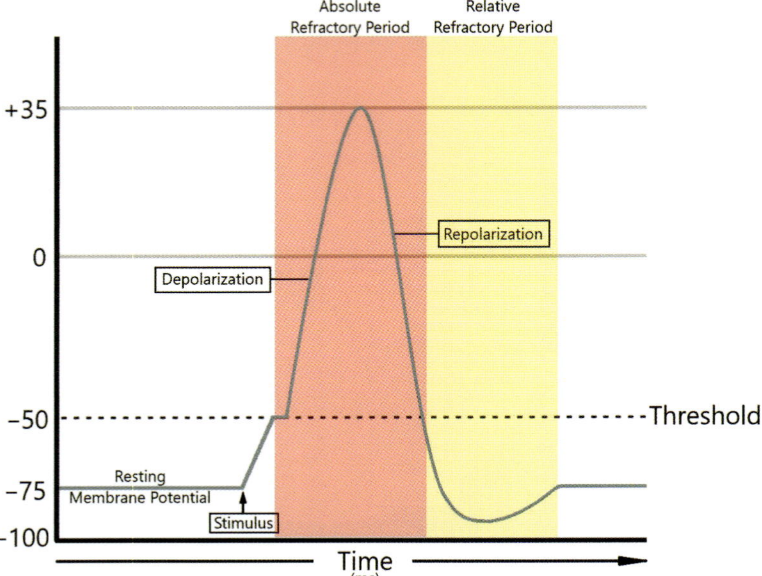

Figure 20.4 The wave of depolarization with the absolute and relative refractory periods highlighted.

sodium channels are not active and therefore cannot generate a new impulse. During the relative refractory period, the neuron *might* be able to depolarize again if the stimulus is strong enough to reach the threshold. As a result of the refractory periods, not all neurons fire at the same time (Figure 20.4).

Nerve impulses vary in both the speed and the frequency at which they travel. In mammals, the flowing series of electrical changes can travel at 20–100 m/s, and there can be more than 100 impulses/s.

As mentioned earlier, the axon of neurons can be myelinated or covered in specialized fatty cells. Myelin is formed by **glial cells** called **oligodendrocytes** within the CNS and **Schwann cells** within the **peripheral nervous system (PNS)**. The spaces in between the myelin are called the **nodes of Ranvier**. As with a bare wire, the electrical charge can jump across those areas rather quickly, and this process is called **saltatory conduction**. This forms an efficient way of propagating the action potential. Diseases that cause demyelination, or the destruction or lack of the myelin sheath, cause severe neurological abnormalities. Demyelinating disease in dogs is quite rare. In humans, perhaps the most familiar one is multiple sclerosis (MS).

The generation of the **excitatory potential**, or stimulating a neural response, will set off a cascade of ion exchange along the length of the axon until it reaches the end. Bear in mind that nerve impulses can be **inhibitory** as well; they can slow down or interrupt a message or body function.

The distal-most part of the terminal bouton is called the **synaptic terminal**. The axon from which the signal comes is the presynaptic membrane, and the cell that receives it is designated as the postsynaptic membrane. In discussing the function of the autonomic nervous system later in this chapter, the question of presynaptic and postsynaptic fibers will assume particular significance.

As mentioned before, the axon of the neuron is a projection of the cell itself. Among other things, this means that its cytoplasm is the same material as that in the soma. In addition, it means that its membrane surrounds not just the terminal bouton but also the entire neuron.

Signal Transmission

Neurotransmitters are chemicals that transmit messages to the postsynaptic neuron, allowing it to undergo depolarization. The number and types of neurotransmitters vary tremendously; only some of them will be discussed here. The use of neurotransmitters, natural or synthetic, to control nerve impulses is an area of intense interest and research in searching for new medications. Drugs that can mediate these reactions can help control the metabolism to an impressive degree.

Once neurotransmitters, such as acetylcholine, cross the synapse, they impinge on the cell membrane of the postsynaptic neuron. These neurotransmitters stimulate small openings to emerge at various places along the membrane. These openings are called **channels**.

The specific cause of channel opening depends on the type of channel it is. **Voltage-gated channels** are those that open in response to voltage change. This reaction causes the channel to open and accept charged particles, such as sodium. This allows the ion exchange that triggers the next action potential. The entire reaction is based on the voltage on either side of the membrane. Ionotropic channels form the basis of the action potential propagation along the axon.

Another type of receptor is known as the **ligand-gated channel**. These channels are paired with a large molecule receptor that functions as a dock or receiving area. The receptor has a particular size and shape. Thus, only a certain transmitter can link up with this channel, by way of the receptor, like a lock-and-key mechanism. The binding of the neurotransmitter to the receptor forces open the channel and allows ion exchange. Unlike a voltage-gated channel, ligand-gated channels do not depend solely on voltage differential. If enough neurotransmitter comes along, it will bind to the ligand and gain entry into the cell. More neurotransmitters will cause more channels to open. These channels are found in large numbers at the postsynaptic axonal membrane.

Having crossed the synapse and caused the channels to open on the postsynaptic membrane, the neurotransmitter will either be broken down by enzymes or returned to the point of origin. For example, the enzyme that breaks down acetylcholine is **acetylcholinesterase**. If the neurotransmitter were to stay in the synapse, the target cell would be constantly bombarded with energy and would not be able to "turn off." This can be advantageous in designing medications for use in neurological or neuromuscular disorders.

Central and Peripheral Functions

From a functional standpoint, the nervous system is divided into two parts. The CNS is composed of the brain and the spinal cord. The PNS is, essentially, all the other nerve fibers (neurons). In general, peripheral nerves carry information toward and away from the CNS. There are, of course, blood vessels and supporting tissue affiliated with both sections of the nervous system.

Some transactions involve sending information to and from the spinal cord and not to the brain. In particular, responses called **reflexes** often are mediated by the spinal cord alone. The **patellar reflex** is a type of **myotatic reflex**, in which the stretch of a muscle causes a reflex reaction. It is commonly assessed to investigate suspected neurological damage affecting the pelvic limb. A sharp tap of the patellar tendon generates a nerve impulse that travels to the spinal cord. The spinal cord, in turn, sends a message to the limb, causing the stifle joint to flex. The brain is not involved in this activity. The brain can be functioning perfectly, but damage to the spinal cord may prevent the reflex from occurring. In fact, we use this information to help determine if signs of neurological disease are related to problems in the brain, the spinal cord, or peripheral nerves.

The CNS has an integrative function; it takes input from various sources and systems and generates a response. For example, information from the auditory and visual nerves can be analyzed. If the result of the analysis is that a bear is coming after the dog, the brain can send the motor neurons into action, stimulating the dog to, say, run away.

Much of the animal's sensory input (sound, taste, visual images, odors, and tactile sensations) travels to the brain stem and is then projected on to the **hypothalamus**. The hypothalamus is a center in the brain that can exert control over the autonomic nervous system. It can direct the activities associated with thermoregulation, systemic blood pressure, stress responses, reproductive hormones, and the digestive system. Many of these functions involve the endocrine system, which is discussed in Chapter 21.

The hypothalamus has other functions as well. For example, it senses levels of electrolytes (sodium, potassium, and calcium) and induces the pituitary and adrenal glands to help control these levels. It also helps monitor blood glucose. Using information from the eye, it helps control the circadian rhythms. The circadian rhythms are a type of internal clockwork that uses the 24-hour day as a base. Cycles like temperature regulation and the sleep/wake cycle depend, in part, on the function of this part of the brain.

The Brain

The **brain** itself can be described in a number of ways. A common way of approaching the subject is to divide it into three parts. These are functional divisions, not physical ones.

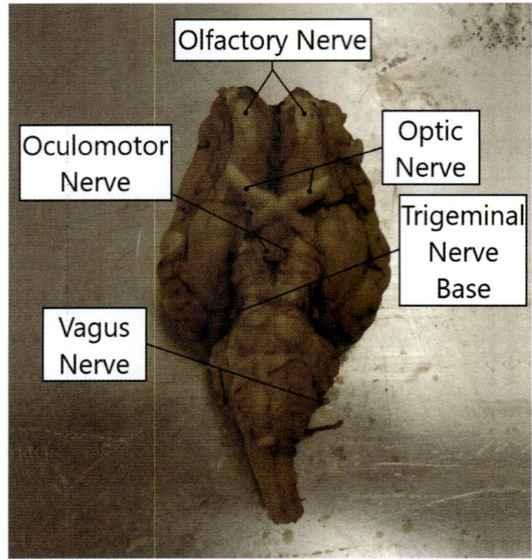

Figure 20.5 The vagus and trigeminal nerves exit the brain stem. The optic nerve comes from each side of the head and crosses at the optic chiasm. The rostral-most parts of the ventral brain are the olfactory bulbs.

The **forebrain** includes the **cerebrum**, which is the largest part of the brain in domestic animals. It oversees higher-order behaviors like reasoning and intelligence. The cerebrum also helps deal with voluntary nerve impulses sent to skeletal muscle, communication, emotional responses, memory, and recall. It contains the **thalamus** and the hypothalamus. The thalamus serves as a relay station for sensory input that will enter the cerebrum, while the hypothalamus is the part responsible for maintaining communication between the nervous system and the endocrine system. It also includes the **hippocampus**, a part of the brain devoted to learning and memory, and the **limbic system**, where emotions are processed.

The hindbrain includes the **cerebellum**, which is the second largest portion of the brain. The cerebellum governs coordination, fine motor movement, and the autonomic nervous system. Kittens exposed to the virus-causing panleukopenia prior to birth (in other words, if the mother is infected) often develop **cerebellar hypoplasia**. This literally means that the cerebellum is undersized and abnormally shaped. These kittens walk abnormally and may have other neurological signs.

The **midbrain** is a region at the cranial brainstem and helps to connect the forebrain and hind brain. It helps to process all of the sensory integration areas within the brain. These are the areas where sound, light, and tactile information are processed.

The **cranial nerves** are those that emanate as a trunk (large collection of nerve fibers) from the brain and travel directly to the target of interest. See Appendix 2 for their names, numbers, and functions (Figure 20.5).

The Autonomic Nervous System

The peripheral nervous system itself is divided into two parts. One is the **somatic system**, which is involved with voluntary responses such as skeletal muscle movement. The other is the **autonomic nervous system**. In its resemblance to the word "automatic," it may be apparent that the autonomic nervous system relates to activities of the body that do not require conscious thought. This covers functions of the smooth muscle, such as is present in the blood vessels, various glands, and the cardiovascular and respiratory systems.

The autonomic system is further divided into the **sympathetic** and **parasympathetic** systems. They have opposing functions under most conditions; one speeds things up while the other slows them down. See Table 20.1 for more information.

Most efferent autonomic nerve fibers originate in the hypothalamus. As they travel along, they exit the CNS and head toward their destination. The part of the nerve that exits the CNS is called a **preganglionic fiber**.

Table 20.1 The effects of each side of the autonomic nervous system.

The autonomic nervous system	
Sympathetic nervous system effects	**Parasympathetic nervous system effects**
Dilate bronchi	Return bronchi to normal diameter
Increase heart rate	Decrease heart rate
Increase respiratory rate	Decrease respiratory rate
Widen pupils	Constrict pupils
Constrict sphincter muscles	Relax sphincter muscles
Dilate or constrict blood vessels	Normalize blood vessel diameter

Once the nerve fiber reaches the **ganglion**, it stimulates a soma. A ganglion (plural: ganglia) is a group of cell bodies that can act as a relay station to multiple other points in the nervous system. Axons go out from the ganglia to the target tissues or organs. These latter fibers are called **postganglionic**. The distance of the ganglion from the origin of the fiber is different for the sympathetic and the parasympathetic systems, but the concept of the structure is similar.

The sympathetic nervous system is often called the "**flight or fight**" system, or the **thoracolumbar nervous system**, based on where the nerves emerge from the spinal cord (in the thoracic and lumbar regions). When an animal is startled, stressed, or otherwise exposed to a strong stimulus, it will either run away or confront the source of the stimulation. The ability to do this requires a number of responses. There will be an increased heart rate to bring more circulating blood to the organs that are now in need of great amounts of energy. The bronchi expand to allow in more oxygen. The functioning of the urinary and intestinal systems is changed so that they are less active; wasting energy on urinating or digesting while trying to escape a predator is less than convenient.

The parasympathetic system is known by the phrase "**rest and digest**," or the **craniosacral nervous system** based on the nerves emerging from the head and sacrum. When the animal needs to rest, the parasympathetic nervous system brings the heart rate back to normal or even slows it. When the animal is at rest, the digestive system is at the ready when food is available.

The sympathetic nervous system relies mostly on **norepinephrine** and **epinephrine** to carry messages from one nerve fiber to another. Nerve fibers that use norepinephrine as a neurotransmitter are referred to as **adrenergic** neurons. Areas that receive their neurotransmitters are called **adrenergic receptors**. Adrenergic receptors are divided into different types and subtypes. The main categories we will discuss are $\alpha 1$, $\alpha 2$, $\beta 1$, and $\beta 2$. These receptors are found in various locations and, when stimulated in those areas, produce a variety of effects, as seen below.

- $\alpha 1$ receptors, when stimulated, help to control smooth muscle contractions, vessel constriction in the mucosa, skin, and abdominal organs, as well as sphincters in the urinary and GI tracts.
- $\alpha 2$ receptors, when stimulated, work to inhibit norepinephrine release like a negative feedback loop. They also contribute to vessel constriction in the veins and decrease heart rate. **$\alpha 2$ agonist drugs**, or drugs that stimulate the $\alpha 2$ receptors, are used frequently in anesthesia, as they produce sedation.
- $\beta 1$ receptors, when stimulated, work to increase the heart rate, cardiac contractility, and force of cardiac contractions.
- $\beta 2$ receptors, when stimulated, help to relax smooth muscle, such as in the respiratory tract, causing bronchodilation.

Many of the drugs we use, particularly in the cardiovascular system, have to do with blocking or enhancing the function of these receptors.

The parasympathetic system, as mentioned a moment ago, uses acetylcholine to transmit information from one nerve fiber to another. **Cholinergic neurons** are neurons that release acetylcholine which can bind to one of two types of receptors: **nicotinic** or **muscarinic**. The muscles have many **nicotinic receptors**. People who smoke nicotine are well aware of the relationship between nicotine and involuntary muscle tremors. **Muscarinic receptors** are present throughout the parasympathetic nervous system. They are present in large numbers in the heart and help to slow the heart rate down. They are also present in the digestive system to stimulate intestinal motility and in the eyes to control pupil constriction.

The urinary bladder has both sympathetic and parasympathetic innervation. When the sympathetic system is not actively engaged, the parasympathetic system will respond to the expansion of the urinary bladder as it fills with urine and will contract to expel the urine. Recall that there is skeletal muscle (voluntary) control of the exit of urine as well; this is what allows an animal to urinate only in certain places or under certain conditions, such as going out for a walk with a human.

Clinical Case Resolution: Boots

Boots undergoes a full physical examination which, along with the presenting complaints, reveals miosis (constricted pupils) and ataxia. Boots' presentation is concerning for some type of acute toxicity.

A rapid urine drug test reveals no exposure to any substances like methamphetamines, barbiturates, opiates, or marijuana. While the owner is asked more details, a coagulation test is run to ensure there is no evidence of rodent poison ingestion. This test is normal and rules this out.

The owner said that they have not changed anything in the home, and the cats do not have access to any cleaning products or other chemicals. They did note that, earlier this week, the farm nearby had the crops sprayed for insect control.

After hearing this, the primary suspect for Boots, based on history and presentation, is organophosphate toxicity. Organophosphates are used as insecticides and can be toxic depending on the dose/rate of exposure. They cause toxicity by inhibiting acetylcholinesterase, leading to the variety of signs described above.

In order to treat Boots, a number of steps are taken. Atropine, an anticholinergic agent, is administered along with another drug called pralidoxime. Pralidoxime works to reactivate acetylcholinesterase. After receiving doses of both drugs, Boots is given a gentle warm water and soap bath to remove any remaining toxin from the coat and skin. Special care is taken to avoid irritating the skin with scrubbing. Boots will be hospitalized on supportive care and continued treatment until symptoms of toxicity subside. Activated charcoal will also be administered, as it may help absorb any ingested toxins.

Clinical Case Critical Thinking

1) *Consider obtaining a patient history with animals that have free roaming access to outdoor or unknown areas. What complications may occur when trying to get an accurate history?*
2) *Consider the possible routes of organophosphate toxicity for Boots. Was it helpful that the owners separated him from the other cat in the home? How could that cat also have possibly gotten sick?*
3) *Why does blocking acetylcholinesterase cause all the signs seen above? Consider each of the receptors discussed and their effects when stimulated.*
4) *Why did we use atropine to treat this toxicity?*

Review Questions

1 Which type of signals bring information into the central nervous system?
  A Afferent signals
  B Efferent signals
  C Motor signals
  D Depolarization signals

2 Where does the neurotransmitter get released from?
  A The soma
  B The presynaptic nerve
  C The postsynaptic nerve
  D The dendrites

3 The resting potential of nerve cells results in the interior of the cell being slightly more ______________ than the inside.
  A Positive
  B Neutral
  C Saline
  D Negative

4 True or False: Reflexes can only occur if the brain is involved.
  A True
  B False

5 Which feature allows for saltatory conduction?
  A The soma
  B The motor neuron
  C The myelin sheath
  D The adrenergic receptors

6 When depolarization occurs, two ions switch places with the help of ATP. These two ions are:
   A Calcium and magnesium
   B Sodium and potassium
   C Potassium and calcium
   D Calcium and sodium

7 When the sympathetic nervous system is stimulated, we expect the body to be responding to which main neurotransmitter?
   A Epinephrine
   B Serotonin
   C Schwann cells
   D Atropine

8 True or False: No stimulus can create another action potential if the cell is in its absolute refractory period.
   A True
   B False

9 If the animal is experiencing lowered heart rate, lowered respiratory rate, and increased GI motility, it can be said that they are in the _____________________ state.
   A Adrenergic
   B Sympathetic
   C Fight or flight
   D Rest and Digest

10 Which part of the brain acts as a relay station for sensory input into the cerebrum?
   A Thalamus
   B Cerebellum
   C Hippocampus
   D Limbic system

21

Endocrine Physiology

Clinical Case: Cooper, a 10-Year-Old Male Golden Retriever

Cooper is brought in for an appointment because the owner has noted some changes at home. Cooper appears to be drinking much more water, and as a result, is urinating much more frequently. He is also losing hair on either side of his body along the spine. They also note that Cooper seems to be panting more frequently, but they think that may be because he seems to have gained weignt. When asking more about this, they point out his pot-bellied appearance and increased appetite.

Introduction

The various systems that control the metabolism of the animal are as intricate as they are interdependent. Careful study of even one system can be exhausting, and there are literally volumes written on each. In particular, the endocrine and neurological systems are so intertwined in their function that they are often referred to as a single unit, the **neuroendocrine system**. In the interest of making the material manageable, we will consider the endocrine system as a unit here. Bear in mind, however, that the functions of the endocrine and neurological systems are very closely related.

Endocrine Glands

The **endocrine glands** are distinguished from other glands in the body in that they are ductless or without tubes to carry their products out to the body. The endocrine glands usually deliver their products directly into the bloodstream. The products of endocrine function are called **hormones**. They have the ability to initiate or catalyze reactions involving changes in the metabolic rate, the autonomic nervous system, and the limbic system. There are **discrete endocrine glands**, organs that contain hormone-producing clusters of cells, or organs that have only patches of endocrine cells within them. Disorders of the endocrine system are among those most commonly encountered in small animal practice; these include over- or underproduction of hormones. The most common issues in small animal practice usually involve the thyroid hormone, adrenal gland hormones, and manufacturing of insufficient or poor-quality insulin by the pancreas.

Hormones can be carried rapidly throughout the system and are able to cause significant change even in very small amounts. Certain cells in the body have specific receptors, or lock and key mechanisms, for a given hormone. The more receptors a cell has, the more sensitive it is to that hormone. By the same token, cells that do not have a receptor for, say, estrogen, will not be affected by it. Receptor cells for a given hormone may be grouped in one location or spread all over the body.

Regulation of Hormones

Hormones are regulated by **feedback loops**. Feedback loops are either called **negative feedback loops** or **positive feedback loops**. Negative feedback loops work similarly to the thermostat in the home. The body has a set point of how much hormone should be active in the body at any given time. Under the influence of the central nervous system, the

Anatomy and Physiology for Veterinary Technicians and Nurses: A Clinical Approach, Second Edition. Lori Asprea.
© 2026 John Wiley & Sons, Inc. Published 2026 by John Wiley & Sons, Inc.
Companion website: www.wiley.com/go/asprea/anatomy_vettech2e

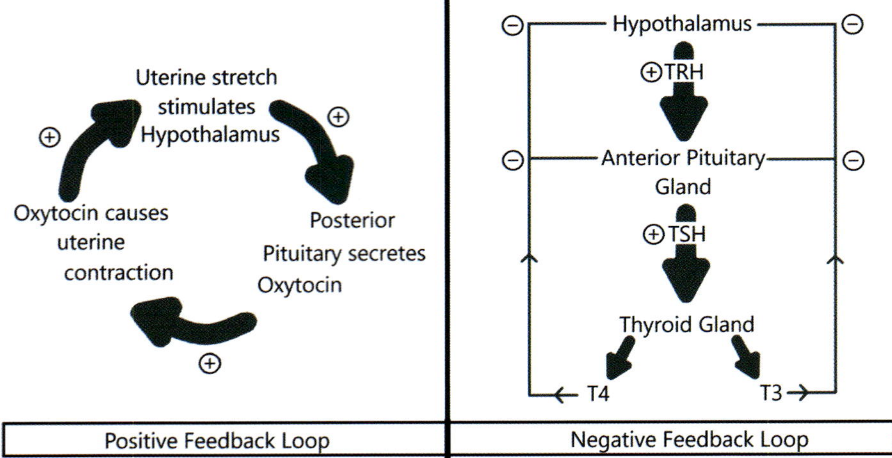

Figure 21.1 Examples of positive and negative feedback loops. In the positive feedback loop, each action stimulates more of the same in a cycle. In the negative feedback loop, once the body reaches the desired set point of thyroid hormones (T3 and T4), they will have a negative impact on both the hypothalamus' production of TRH (thyroid-releasing hormone) and the anterior pituitary production of TSH (thyroid-stimulating hormone) thereby shutting the system.

endocrine gland will produce hormones until that level is reached. Once it is reached, the hormone being produced communicates with the central nervous system to let it know that enough hormone has been produced, and the cycle shuts off. Once the levels of hormone in the body drop below what is required at the time, the central nervous system will then begin to stimulate the endocrine gland again, until adequate levels are achieved, and the system shuts off again. This is the most common method of control in the endocrine system.

Positive feedback loops work to increase or amplify the changes occurring. The most common example of this is in parturition, or birth, when oxytocin stimulates uterine contractions, and the contracting myometrium stimulates the production of more oxytocin, which in turn stimulates more uterine contractions (Figure 21.1).

Hormone Types

Hormones can be broken down into three main groups: **steroid hormones, peptide hormones**, and **monoamine hormones**. These groups reflect the chemical composition of each and give us information about how they will interact with the body.

Steroid hormones are made with lipids, or fats, that have been synthesized from cholesterol. They are generally named with the ending of "-ol" or "-one", like estradiol or testosterone, both of which are sex hormones. This cholesterol derivation makes them hydrophobic, or not able to mix easily with water. Since hormones must travel through the blood which has a high water content, steroid hormones must bind to hydrophilic transporters, or transporters that pass easily through water, for effective travel. Hormones that use protein carriers can either be **bound** or **unbound/free**. When the hormone is bound, or tied to, the carrier protein, it can travel through the bloodstream but cannot interact with cell receptors. As a result, hormones can be stored in the blood, bound to carrier proteins until needed. Unbound or free hormones have arrived at their destination and have been released from the carrier protein, allowing them to interact with the receptor. As a result, unbound or free hormones are considered active. Once the steroid hormone arrives at its target cell, its lipid makeup allows it to travel through the phospholipid cell membrane with ease. As a result, receptors for steroid hormones are found inside the cell in either the cytoplasm or nucleus.

Peptide hormones are made of long chains of amino acids or polypeptide chains. They are hydrophilic, and therefore travel·easily in plasma, and do not have a need for a carrier protein, like steroid hormones. Although it can travel easily, it cannot get through the phospholipid membrane easily, which results in having receptors on the cell wall, instead of inside like steroid hormones.

Monoamine hormones get their name as they are formed from amino acids and retain a single amine group. These hormones generally end in "-ine" like thyroxine, a thyroid hormone, and epinephrine, which is considered both a neurotransmitter and hormone. Recall how intertwined the endocrine and nervous systems are. Monoamine hormones can be further broken down into two groups: **catecholamines** and **thyroid hormones**. Catecholamines are monoamines that are hydrophilic and thus able to travel through plasma easily and receptors for catecholamines are found on the cell membrane. This is similar to peptide hormones. Thyroid hormones are hydrophobic, limiting their ability to travel through plasma and require transport protein and receptors for thyroid hormones are found inside the cell in the nucleus or cytoplasm. This is similar to steroid hormones.

Hypothalamus and Pituitary Gland

The **hypothalamus** is an area in the brain which controls many important nervous system functions like body temperature, appetite, emotions, sex drive, and sleep–wake cycles. While all of these are integral to life, here, we will discuss another critical function: hormone production control. The hypothalamus is responsible for orchestrating hormone production and acts as a bridge between the nervous and endocrine systems.

The hypothalamus produces hormones that interact with the **pituitary gland**. The pituitary is a small but very powerful gland immediately ventral to the hypothalamus. It is often referred to as the "master endocrine gland". Although it appears to be one gland, it is bilobed and works as two: **the anterior pituitary** and the **posterior pituitary**. The anterior pituitary, or **adenohypophysis**, is connected to the hypothalamus by a complex series of blood vessels called the **hypophyseal portal system**. The posterior pituitary, or **neurohypophysis**, connects to the hypothalamus via the **pituitary stalk** made of nerve tissue.

On the anterior pituitary control side, the hypothalamus creates mainly **releasing hormones** or occasionally **inhibiting hormones**. These hormones travel through the hypophyseal portal system to the anterior pituitary to give instructions. Releasing hormones stimulate the production of more hormones, while inhibiting hormones suppress the release of more hormones. We will discuss specific releasing and inhibiting hormones shortly.

On the posterior pituitary side control side, the hypothalamus produces two main hormones called **oxytocin** and **vasopressin**. These are delivered to the posterior pituitary via the pituitary stalk and stored in the posterior pituitary until the hypothalamus directs the posterior pituitary to release them when needed.

The Anterior Pituitary

The anterior pituitary produces seven hormones in response to instructions by the hypothalamus. These hormones are **adrenocorticotropic hormone (ACTH), growth hormone (GH), thyroid-stimulating hormone (TSH), prolactin, follicle-stimulating hormone (FSH), luteinizing hormone (LH),** and **melanocyte-stimulating hormone (MSH)**. MSH is actually produced by the intermediate pituitary; however, since this is very small, it is often considered as a part of the anterior pituitary. See Table 21.1 for how the hypothalamus controls each hormone, and what they do.

In viewing Table 21.1 we can see that the hypothalamus has specific hormones that communicate specific messages to the anterior pituitary, resulting in specific actions. It is important to note that the hypothalamus and anterior pituitary, among the remainder of the endocrine glands, are able to produce multiple hormones at once. The hypothalamus also produces **somatostatin**, which is an inhibitor (Table 21.2).

When ACTH is released from the anterior pituitary, it travels to the adrenal glands to stimulate them to produce their hormones, which will be discussed later in the chapter. Growth hormone (GH) is released from the anterior pituitary to have effects throughout the body. Aside from encouraging growth, it also works on the health of the whole body at a cellular level. GH encourages the **anabolism** of proteins, or the building of large molecules from small building blocks. GH also stimulates stored fats to be **catabolized**, or broken down as a primary energy source, while discouraging the use of carbohydrates as a primary energy source. This function can cause a rise in blood sugar, as carbohydrates are broken down into simple sugars, and if not used, remain in circulation.

TSH stimulates the thyroid to produce hormones that are used to regulate the body's metabolism. There is an additional hormone from the thyroid that is not under the control of TSH. These hormones and their functions will be discussed in the thyroid section. Prolactin works to help develop mammary glands and milk-secreting cells, and milk production. Teat stimulation by suckling sends a message to the hypothalamus to continue stimulating the production of prolactin in order to keep milk production high. In most mammalian species, when the young wean, the teat stimulation diminishes, and the milk production slows as a result of lowered prolactin production. Interestingly, dairy cows have been bred to be high milk

Table 21.1 Column 1 shows what the hypothalamus produces to influence the release or inhibition of hormones from the anterior pituitary, Column 2, while Column 3 shows what each of the anterior pituitary hormones primarily do.

Hypothalamus creates:	Anterior pituitary:	Result:
Corticotropin-releasing hormone (CRH)	Adrenocorticotropic hormone (ACTH)	Stimulates the adrenal glands to produce their hormones
Growth-hormone-releasing hormone (GHRH)	Growth hormone (GH)	Promotes growth in young animals Regulates the metabolism of proteins, carbohydrates and lipids
Somatostatin		Somatostatin inhibits the release of GH
Thyrotropin-releasing hormone (TRH)	Thyroid-stimulating hormone (TSH)	Stimulates the thyroid to produce thyroid hormones
Dopamine	Prolactin	Stimulates milk production and lactation
Gonadotropin-releasing hormone (GnRH)	Follicle-stimulating hormone (FSH)	Stimulated testes to produce sperm Stimulates ovaries to form the follicle and begin maturation of the egg
	Luteinizing hormone (LH)	Stimulates testes to produce testosterone Stimulates hormone production from ovaries, helps finish maturing oocyte, and helps create the corpus luteum

producers and need much lower levels of prolactin to continue producing milk. Prolactin plays other roles in the body, including being involved in immune system signaling and molting of feathers in some birds. In fish, prolactin helps regulate the water and salt balance in the body.

FSH has different roles in the body depending on the sex of the animal. In both the male and the female, it is considered the main hormone of sexual maturity, as it stimulates gonadal maturation. In the mature female, it works to develop the **follicle** around the oocyte, which acts as an incubator for the maturing egg and will later play an important role in maintaining pregnancy as the follicle becomes the **corpus luteum**. FSH also works to stimulate the follicle to produce estrogens. In the mature male, FSH stimulates the production of spermatozoa. In the female, LH helps to finish the maturation of the egg and leads to ovulation. It also promotes the secretion of progesterone through the creation of corpus luteum. LH is also called **interstitial cell-stimulating hormone (ICSH)** because in the male, it stimulated interstitial cells in the testicle to produce testosterone.

The Posterior Pituitary

The posterior pituitary gland receives oxytocin and vasopressin from the hypothalamus and stores it until it is needed by the body. Oxytocin has many roles, including stimulating uterine contractions during birth, assisting in lactation through milk let down, sexual arousal, and bonding. Vasopressin is also called **anti-diuretic hormone (ADH)**, which regulates the control of the body's water levels which affect hydration, urine output, and blood pressure.

The Thyroid Gland

The thyroid gland produces three major hormones: **triiodothyronine (T3), tetraiodothyronine (T4)**, or **thyroxine**, and **calcitonin**. T3 and T4 have a wide range of activities that together control much of the body's metabolic rate. The other, calcitonin, is a more specific hormone that has to do with calcium levels in the body.

The thyroid gland contains groups of cells called follicles. They help produce **thyroglobulin**, which is the base from which the hormones thyroxine (T4) and triiodothyronine (T3) are manufactured. This process is not possible without the presence of iodine. In fact, the mammalian body needs iodine as part of its diet in order to effectively create these thyroid hormones. As you may have guessed, triiodothyronine has three iodine molecules, while tetraiodothyronine has four. The initiation of T3 and T4 production begins with the hypothalamus thyrotropin-releasing hormone (TRH) communicating with the anterior pituitary, which then communicates TSH with the thyroid to produce T3 and T4. See Figure 22.1 for a diagram of the feedback loop involved.

Table 21.2 See below for a summary of each endocrine gland, what it produces and what effects the hormones have.

Endocrine gland	Hormone	Effect
Anterior pituitary	Adrenocorticotropic hormone (ACTH)	Stimulates the adrenal glands
	Growth hormone (GH)	Promotes growth in young animals
		Regulates the metabolism of proteins, carbohydrates, and lipids
	Thyroid-stimulating hormone (TSH)	Stimulates the thyroid
	Prolactin	Stimulates milk production and lactation
	Follicle-stimulating hormone (FSH)	Stimulated testes to produce sperm
		Stimulates ovaries to form the follicle and begin maturation of the egg
	Luteinizing hormone (LH)	Stimulates testes to produce testosterone
		Stimulates hormone production from ovaries, helps finish maturing oocyte, and helps create the corpus luteum
Posterior pituitary (created by the hypothalamus)	Vasopressin	Regulates water in the body
	Oxytocin	Stimulates uterine contractions, milk let down, arousal, and bonding
Thyroid	T4 (tetraiodothyronine)	Inactive form of hormone
	T3 (triiodothyronine)	Active hormone – regulated metabolism of all cells
	Calcitonin	Manages calcium levels by driving excess calcium into bones
Parathyroid	Parathyroid hormone/Parathormone	Manages calcium levels by withdrawing calcium from bones, kidneys, and gut into blood
Adrenal cortex	Glucocorticoids (cortisol, etc.)	Increase glucose, help deal with stress
	Mineralocorticoids (aldosterone)	Regulate sodium, potassium, and hydrogen
	Sex hormones	Minimal effect – primary: gonads
Adrenal medulla	Catecholamines (Norepinephrine, epinephrine)	Activate sympathetic nervous system. Increase, HR, RR, etc.
Pancreas	α – Glucagon	Increases blood sugar
	β – Insulin	Allows cells to use glucose
	δ – Somatostatin	Inhibits GH, insulin, and glucagon
Kidney	Erythropoietin	Stimulated bone marrow to produce red blood cells
	Renin	Initiates the RAA system to increase blood pressure
Stomach	Gastrin	Stimulates production of stomach acid and digestive enzymes
Small intestine	Secretin	Stimulates the pancreas to produce bicarbonate
		Stimulates the gallbladder to contract
		Decreases stomach acid production
		Slows gastric motility
	Cholecystokinin	Stimulates the pancreas to produce digestive enzymes
		Stimulates the gallbladder to contract
		Decreases stomach acid production
		Slows gastric motility

The presence of feedback loops is an important part of the function of the endocrine system. The thyroid provides a good example of this. TSH is sent to the thyroid, which causes it to produce T3 and T4. Much of the T4 is converted to T3 during metabolism. When blood levels of thyroid hormone rise to a certain point, this will be noticed by the pituitary gland and hypothalamus. The hypothalamus and pituitary then suppress the production of TRH and TSH, respectively, which, in turn, ensures that less thyroid hormone is sent out into the system. This suppression is the "negative" from negative feedback loop. It is important to note that with the thyroid, or any other endocrine organ, illness resulting from too much or too little hormone can be due to a misfire or issue at any point in the negative feedback loop. In other words, if the thyroid is producing too much hormone, it may be because the hypothalamus has an issue and is overproducing

TRH, or the anterior pituitary has an issue and is overproducing TSH, or finally, the thyroid has an issue and despite instructions, will overproduce T3 and T4.

Most thyroid hormones are circulating in the bloodstream bound to proteins. A very small amount of T4 (and even less T3) is unbound or "free". It is the free form that actually enters the cells to regulate the metabolic rate at a cellular level. When more hormone is needed by the cells, the hormone is released from the blood proteins so that they are available for uptake. In fact, the level of free T4 is one measure the pituitary uses to direct the feedback loop. We take advantage of this system when we test animals for hyperthyroidism and hypothyroidism. The amount of T4 circulating in the bloodstream is a good indicator of thyroid function. Measurement of free T4 is even more specific.

A normal thyroid gland releases mostly the T4 form into the bloodstream. The T4 molecule is converted to T3 by a change in the iodine content of the molecule. Certain changes will create a T3 that upregulates (increases) the level of cellular activity. Other changes lead to a type of T3 that decreases the activity in a cell. Thus, the thyroid is very much like the accelerator of a car; it can speed up or slow down the production of energy in cells in the kidney, heart, and so on, to increase or decrease their activity. T4 is considered the inactive form of thyroid hormone, while T3 is the more potent and active form. This is why the body converts T4 to T3 when needed.

The phenomenon of "**sick euthyroid**" laboratory findings is a reflection of the complexity of these relationships. Under ordinary circumstances, a healthy animal produces a certain amount of thyroid hormone. In an animal with chronic illness, however, thyroid hormone levels may be low without any thyroid disease. The condition is not clearly understood; theories include decreased release of TSH or failure of the T4 and/or T3 to bind to proteins in the blood in a normal manner.

The thyroid hormones have effects on all body cells. They create a **calorigenic effect** or an increase in the body's metabolic rate. The properties of thyroid hormone are similar to GH in that they encourage protein anabolism, lipid catabolism, and carbohydrate metabolism. Differing from GH, thyroid hormones can change their effect on proteins in times of need. If an animal is malnourished, thyroid hormone can switch to protein **catabolism** or a breakdown of proteins as a main energy source. In young animals, the thyroid hormone influences the development of the muscles, bones, and central nervous system.

As stated before, the creation of T3 and T4 relies on iodine. The thyroid is the only organ in the body that picks up any iodine that enters the system. The body does this naturally; however, we can use it to our advantage in treatments. One of the methods to treat **hyperthyroidism**, or an overproduction of thyroid hormone from the thyroid, is to use **radioactive iodine (I131)**. In order to treat hyperthyroidism so that the client does not have to administer medication at home, radioactive iodine is administered. It goes directly to the thyroid and ablates or destroys abnormal parts of the gland, reducing its ability to produce as much thyroid hormone and eliminating the need for medication to control the overproduction of the hormones.

Hyperthyroidism is commonly seen in senior cats and, as mentioned above, is an overproduction of thyroid hormone. This can be from any organ in the negative feedback loop. As expected, since thyroid hormone controls metabolism, an overproduction of this hormone affects all body systems. A highly increased metabolism from hyperthyroidism creates a ravenous appetite despite weight loss, muscle wasting, increased thirst and urination, vocalizing, increased heart rate, and an unkempt coat. It can be diagnosed by checking thyroid levels in the blood and can be characterized by checking both TSH and TRH levels. If TSH is high, it may be a primary anterior pituitary problem, while if TRH is high, it may be a primary hypothalamus problem. If both TSH and TRH are low, it is a primary thyroid problem. Hypothyroidism, or too little thyroid hormone production, is more often seen in dogs.

The other hormone produced in the thyroid is calcitonin. Calcitonin is produced in the **parafollicular cells** or **C-cells** found in between the follicles of the thyroid. Calcitonin is one of two major hormones responsible for calcium balance in the body. Calcium is responsible for many crucial body functions like muscle contraction, blood clotting, skeletal maintenance, and milk production. When **hypercalcemia**, or excessive levels of calcium, are sensed in the bloodstream, calcitonin is released from the C-cells. Calcitonin works to drive the excess calcium into storage in the bones, which acts as a calcium bank. Deposits to the calcium bank are made by calcitonin, while withdrawals are made by **parathyroid hormone (PTH)**.

Parathyroid Gland

The **parathyroid gland** is found at the cranial pole of the thyroid gland in the ventral neck. The parathyroid gland produces one hormone: **PTH or parathormone**. PTH is secreted when the body senses **hypocalcemia** or low levels of blood calcium. It works to withdraw calcium from the bones and increase calcium absorption into the body from the kidneys and gastrointestinal tract.

Many reptiles need a high level of calcium in their diet. If they do not get enough calcium and are chronically hypocalcemia, they will overproduce PTH, leeching too much calcium from the skeleton, weakening it considerably, and creating bony deformations. This can also happen to mammals that have chronically low calcium levels from other diseases, particularly kidney disease. This is called **secondary renal hyperparathyroidism**. The kidney is diseased and losing too much calcium via urine which results in hypocalcemia and hyperparathyroidism. Persistent hyperparathyroidism can result in **rubber jaw**, in which the mandible and maxilla become soft or rubbery due to extreme calcium withdrawal from the bone due to PTH.

The Adrenal Gland

The **adrenal gland** plays a major role in three specific areas: the autonomic nervous system, the reproductive system, and general metabolic rate and efficiency. The **adrenal cortex**, or outer layer of the gland, has multiple layers and produces several types of hormones: **glucocorticoids, mineralocorticoids**, and **sex hormones** (Figure 10.3). All of these have a common chemical structure and fall into the category of steroids. The adrenal cortex responds to the hormone ACTH, released from the anterior pituitary gland.

Glucocorticoids are important because they stimulate functions like **gluconeogenesis**, which refers to the process of manufacturing glucose. They also have strong anti-inflammatory properties. As inflammation is caused by the immune system, in response to a disease or injury, glucocorticoids do in effect suppresses the immune system. The glucocorticoids include **cortisol** and **corticosterone**. As suggested earlier, many drugs are based on the action of these molecules and their properties. Glucocorticoids have a hyperglycemic effect (increase blood sugar) and work to catabolize proteins and lipids.

On the other hand, glucocorticoids inhibit the formation of **fibroblasts**, which are important in wound healing. An animal receiving therapeutic glucocorticoid drugs or who has a hyperactive adrenal gland will not heal as quickly or completely as a healthy animal. This is an important issue in wound management in the clinic. Glucocorticoids are also indirectly involved in the "stress response." They can be associated with an increase in systemic blood pressure.

One of the most common metabolic diseases in dogs is **hyperadrenocorticism (Cushing's disease)**, which increases the output of many adrenal hormones dramatically. Patients can present with weight loss, skin and haircoat changes, vomiting and diarrhea, and an increase in drinking and urinating. This last phenomenon is known as **PU/PD**, short for **polyuria** (PU) (urinating large amounts) and **polydipsia** (PD) (drinking large amounts). While PU/PD is associated with dozens of diseases, it is one of the classic symptoms of hyperadrenocorticism. Cushing's disease is seen in horses and cats, but nowhere near as commonly as in dogs. This disease can be caused, again, by any part of the negative feedback loop organs from the hypothalamus to the anterior pituitary or the adrenal cortex itself.

Pituitary-dependent Cushing's disease is a condition whereby there is dysfunction of the pituitary, causing it to send out excessive ACTH. Usually, this dysfunction is related to the presence of a benign tumor, although there are rare instances of malignancy. The high levels of ACTH cause the adrenal gland to produce high levels of steroid hormones. These hormones cause increased levels of protein and glucose in the blood, the former the result of catabolism (breaking down existing proteins) and the latter because of the push to gluconeogenesis (producing glucose). The glucocorticoids, in particular, also suppress the immune system. The combination of these changes is what leads to the clinical signs.

The difficulty lies in the fact that the high levels of steroid hormone production cause the adrenal gland to increase in size, a phenomenon called **adrenal hyperplasia**. The bigger the gland, the more hormones it puts out, exacerbating the problem. Note that there can be hyperplasia of the adrenal gland in the absence of any problem with the pituitary. In fact, this is quite common.

Under ordinary circumstances, the high levels of steroids would trigger the hypothalamus to order the pituitary gland to stop sending out ACTH. Unfortunately, at a high enough steroid level, the pituitary (and perhaps even the hypothalamus) is not able to respond, and the feedback loop ceases to be effective.

In fact, one of the ways we test for the presence of Cushing's disease is to administer a steroid called **dexamethasone**. Its presence in the bloodstream should cause the pituitary to stop pumping out ACTH. Therefore, the blood level of steroid hormones in the system should drop over the next few hours. If no such drop occurs, the feedback loop is not working. In essence, steroid hormones are at such high levels that administering more has no effect.

The most important mineralocorticoid is **aldosterone**. It plays a key role in regulating electrolytes, particularly sodium in the blood. This hormone prompts the kidney to reabsorb sodium. Water follows sodium within the body, and by prompting the body to conserve sodium, it also causes the body to conserve water. It also promotes the excretion of ions like potassium and hydrogen. Hydrogen balance is important in maintaining pH (the relatively acidic or alkaline nature of the blood). Potassium is particularly important in the transmission of nerve impulses and in muscle function. As we have noted, keeping potassium levels in check is a key element of healthy metabolism. Excess potassium can be fatal. In fact, it is a component of many euthanasia solutions.

In Chapter 22, we discuss the **renin–angiotensin–aldosterone (RAA) system**. When the kidney senses low blood pressure, it will release **renin**, which is made in cells near the glomerulus. Renin, in turn, leads to effects on **angiotensin**. Among the other steps, this system triggers the production of aldosterone. By acting on the kidney to keep fluid content within the body, aldosterone helps increase blood volume and thus blood pressure.

The disease resulting from insufficient adrenal gland function is **Addison's disease**, or **hypoadrenocorticism**. This too is most common in dogs but is seen in cats as well. It is more common for the issue to be the decrease in adrenal function, but there can be an insufficiency in the pituitary as well.

Causes of adrenal gland atrophy may include immune-mediated diseases or may be the result of an unknown mechanism. This can also be **iatrogenic** or caused by medicine. In giving steroid medications, used in treating anything from allergy to cancer, we sometimes cause the adrenal gland to stop functioning. Basically, the high level of steroid in the blood occasioned by the drug causes the pituitary to stop producing ACTH, which stops stimulation to the adrenal gland. Without stimulation, the organ can atrophy, just like a muscle would if it were not used. As a result, when the gland is needed, it may not respond.

The symptoms of Addison's disease can be frustrating as a decrease in adrenal cortex hormones like glucocorticoids and mineralocorticoids can have system wide effects. Patients tend to present with intermittent signs that resolve on their own and then recur. These can include gastrointestinal signs like diarrhea and vomiting, lethargy, and weakness. These patients can also experience loss of appetite, weight loss, PU/PD, and dehydration. A simple blood test to check the cortisol levels can be performed on any patient experiencing these waxing and waning signs.

In cases of hypoadrenocorticism, aldosterone production is also compromised. This impairs the kidney's ability to reserve sodium and to excrete potassium, as those functions are mediated by aldosterone. There is a condition called **Addisonian crisis** that results from this electrolyte imbalance. The dog will exhibit signs of weakness, bradycardia (slow heart rate), hypoglycemia (low blood glucose level), and possibly even seizures. It is referred to as a crisis because, if left untreated, even for a short time, it can result in the death of the patient. If only glucocorticoids are affected, the disease is called **"atypical Addison's disease."** Hypoadrenocorticism is overrepresented in certain dog breeds including the Standard Poodle, West Highland White Terrier, Bearded Collie, Great Dane, Labrador Retriever, and Wheaten Terrier, among others.

The adrenal cortex also produces sex hormones. It produces small amounts of estrogens and androgens in both males and females. It is not a significant enough quantity to produce any pronounced effects.

The **adrenal medulla**, or inner portion of the gland, releases **catecholamines:** epinephrine and norepinephrine (or adrenalin and noradrenalin; the names are interchangeable). Epinephrine is the basis for the sympathetic nervous system response to the environment. Anything that is exciting or threatening to the animal will trigger certain pathways within the central nervous system that instruct the adrenal gland to release epinephrine. The hormone is a strong stimulant and increases the activity of the heart, respiratory tract, and muscular systems. In its capacity as a neurotransmitter, it also puts the rest of the body on alert for sudden changes. Refer to Chapter 20 for the relative functions of the sympathetic and parasympathetic nervous systems.

The Pancreas and Insulin

The part of the pancreas that produces digestive enzymes is known as the **exocrine pancreas**. This distinguishes it from the **endocrine pancreas**, the parts of the pancreas that produce hormones. The endocrine pancreas has special clusters of cells, called the **islets of Langerhans** or **pancreatic islets**. These specialized cells produce **insulin, glucagon,** and **somatostatin**. The islets of Langerhans are composed of three types of cells: α **cells**, β **cells**, and δ **cells**.

The α cells produce glucagon which is stimulated by the condition of low levels of glucose in the bloodstream or by the sympathetic nervous system. When glucagon is released by the pancreas and reaches the liver, it stimulates the liver to break down the compound glycogen, which results in the production of more glucose. The δ cells produced somatostatin, which inhibits GH, insulin, and glucagon.

The β cells produce insulin. The production of insulin is triggered by high levels of glucose or amino acids in the blood, digestive activity, and/or parasympathetic nerve stimulation. Insulin serves to escort the glucose within the bloodstream into the cells of the body so that the glucose can be used to create energy. It is the only hormone in the body that works to lower blood sugar levels. When insulin levels are insufficient, or when the insulin is of poor quality, or if the cells of the body become resistant to it, excess glucose remains in the bloodstream. High levels of glucose in the bloodstream, so high that the glucose spills out in the urine, is the disease state known as **diabetes mellitus**. As an aside, it is important to use both words here. There is another kind of diabetes, called **diabetes insipidus or arginine vasopressin deficiency**, which has nothing to do with the pancreas, but rather a lack of ADH or antidiuretic hormone. They are named similarly because, historically, they appeared to have the same symptoms, which are mainly PU/PD. Early testing for these symptoms in the 1600s was to taste the urine. Sweet urine indicated diabetes mellitus, where flavorless urine indicated diabetes insipidus, from the word insipid: lacking flavor.

Other Endocrine Activities

There are other organs that play a role in hormone production. The gonads of both sexes produce hormones which will be discussed in more detail in Chapter 26. The testes produce androgens in response to LH, while the ovaries produce estrogens in a cyclical pattern governed by FSH and LH. The corpus luteum, created from the follicle, also becomes a hormone-producing body, which secretes progesterone.

The kidney produces **erythropoietin** which directs the bone marrow to produce red blood cells. Erythropoietin production increases in response to hypoxia or low oxygen levels in the body. This is because red blood cells primarily function to carry oxygen to tissues, so if oxygen levels are low, a solution may be to increase the number of carriers for oxygen by making more red blood cells. **Renin** is also produced by the kidneys. It is an enzyme and hormone that stimulates the RAA system when blood pressure is low.

The gastrointestinal tract has endocrine capabilities as well. The stomach produces **gastrin** when digesting, which acts as a local hormone to stimulate the production of gastric acid and digestive enzymes. The small intestine secretes **secretin** and **cholecystokinin** with both work to aid in digestion.

Prostaglandins and Pheromones

Prostaglandins and **pheromones** are chemicals somewhat similar to hormones in that they are secreted by the body as some form of chemical messenger. Pheromones are hormones in the sense that they are chemical messengers that stimulate reactions, but they work outside rather than inside the body in terms of their effect. Pheromones are only detected by members of the same species as the one producing them. Felines are able to distinguish feline pheromones, but humans are not sensitive to them. Pheromones are associated with a wide range of behaviors, some related to the reproductive cycle and some to emotional state. Certain pheromones have a calming effect, for example.

Prostaglandins are hormone-like substances that are derived from fatty acids. They tend to act locally and can have profound effects on a number of bodily functions, including reproduction, GI functions, blood clotting, blood pressure, and inflammation. Prostaglandins regulating inflammation is of particular interest to practitioners as we use this medically. **NSAIDs** or **non-steroidal anti-inflammatory drugs** work by blocking the creation of prostaglandins.

Clinical Case Resolution: Cooper

A full physical examination is completed on Cooper. Based on Coopers presentation, the owner is offered to run routine blood work, as well as blood work for certain endocrine function – particularly the adrenal cortex. The doctor discusses concerns for a primary endocrine disease. It is also recommended that Cooper have an abdominal ultrasound.

The owner elects to move forward with blood work but forego the abdominal ultrasound at this time.

Bloodwork results come back the next day and are consistent with hyperadrenocorticism. It is recommended that Cooper be brought back for confirmative testing using a timed test for Cushing's and an abdominal ultrasound. The owner agrees, and once confirmed, Cooper is started on medications to manage his hyperadrenocorticism.

> **Clinical Case Critical Thinking**
>
> 1) *Which of Coopers signs led the veterinary team to consider endocrine testing for him?*
> 2) *If Cooper's adrenal cortex has a benign tumor creating his Cushing's disease, what do you expect ACTH levels to be? Why?*
> 3) *What might the abdominal ultrasound be able to tell us in this case?*
> 4) *Refer back to the hyperthyroidism case, Eloise, presented in Chapter 8. Consider the symptoms Eloise presented with: weight loss despite increased food intake, increased drinking and urination, muscle loss, and poor hair coat. Based on what you have learned in this chapter, explain why these symptoms occur with this disease.*

Review Questions

1 Where do hormones get secreted to?
  A Endocrine glands
  B Exocrine glands
  C The blood stream
  D The nervous system

2 Which is the most common type of feedback loop?
  A Negative feedback
  B Positive feedback
  C Neutral feedback
  D All of the above

3 Which type of hormone has receptors INSIDE the cell wall?
  A Peptide hormones
  B Catecholamines
  C Steroid hormones
  D Neurotransmitters

4 Which thyroid hormone is considered the more potent/active hormone?
  A Tetraiodothyronine
  B Ionized calcium
  C Calcitonin
  D Triiodothyronine

5 Which hormone from the hypothalamus directs the anterior pituitary to produce LH?
  A Testosterone
  B Gonadotropic-releasing hormone
  C Follicle-stimulating hormone
  D Somatropin

6 Which of the following hormones is responsible for decreasing blood calcium by driving excess calcium into bones?
  A PTH
  B Thyroxine
  C Calcitonin
  D Aldosterone

7 Which hormone is directly under the control of the sympathetic nervous system?
  A Prolactin
  B T4
  C T3
  D Norepinephrine

8 What hormone helps to control sodium?
  A Cortisol
  B Glucocorticoid
  C Aldosterone
  D Testosterone

9 Which cells in the pancreas are responsible for the production of insulin?
  A δ cells
  B α cells
  C β cells
  D Exocrine cells

10 Which chemicals are primarily targeted by drugs like NSAIDs?
  A Neurotransmitters
  B Prostaglandins
  C Insulin
  D Pheromones

22

Renal Physiology

Clinical Case: Gigi, a 13-Year-Old Female Spayed DSH

Gigi is brought into the clinic because the owner is concerned about her. The owner says Gigi has always been in great health but lately has had a decreased appetite and isn't grooming as much as normal. They noticed that Gigi has been drinking and urinating much more than normal, but her energy seems slightly decreased.

Introduction

All of the blood in the body, at some point, circulates through the **kidney**. This emphasizes the great importance of the kidney in the maintenance of homeostasis within the organism. When blood enters the kidney, it undergoes a series of changes, which we will discuss here.

The **renal artery** enters the kidney at the **hilus**, bringing oxygen-rich and unfiltered blood into the renal circulation. As it branches, the arteries head toward the **renal cortex**, or the superficial layer of the kidney, eventually landing at the **glomerulus**. The glomerulus is composed of a tuft of capillaries, which acts as a filter. The capillaries of the glomerulus are **fenestrated** or perforated with microscopic holes. The glomerulus acts as a coffee filter or colander in that as blood travels through, anything small enough to fit through the fenestration leaves, and anything big enough stays behind proceeding through. Blood that is not sent along into the systemic circulation continues through to the rest of the **nephron**. The nephron is a series of tubules that dip down into the **renal medulla**, or deeper layer of the kidney, and then back up again toward the cortex, and finally toward the **renal pelvis** at the center of the kidney. The goal of the nephron is to filter blood and get rid of waste products and excess water through the creation of urine.

The Nephron

The nephron works to filter the blood and its products, including low-molecular-weight proteins, water, and electrolytes, and forego large items such as cells and proteins (especially **albumin**), so they are not excreted or lost in urine. Other materials are sent back into the body at other points along the system. What passes from the glomerulus into the tubules of the nephron is known as the **glomerular filtrate**. As its larger molecules have been filtered away, it actually has almost the same specific gravity as blood plasma.

Clinically, this is quite important. If the specific gravity of the urine, which is, after all, the eventual product of all the filtering the nephrons do, is no different from that of plasma, the nephron has not done its job. One indicator of renal disease is **isosthenuria**, which is when the specific gravity or molecular "thickness," relative to water, of urine, is like that of the glomerular filtrate. If the urine is isosthenuric, almost nothing has happened to it from the time it entered the tubules to the time it exited the body – which is to say that the tubules are not functional.

The glomerular capillaries are fenestrated, allowing material to be funneled into the tubules and filtered. The speed and, by extension, efficiency with which this transfer occurs is known as **glomerular filtration rate (GFR)**. There are many factors that determine GFR, which will be discussed below. For the moment, keep in mind that the liters of fluid that pass through the glomerular capillaries will be filtered to a greater or lesser extent. The nature of this filtering is a life-or-death function for mammals. It is important to understand that the size of the fenestrations in the glomerulus is what dictates the items filtered. The fenestrations are very small and only allow molecularly small items to pass through. If the glomerulus is damaged by disease, larger molecules, like proteins, will pass through the now larger fenestrations, resulting in proteinuria.

The glomerular capillaries sit in an epithelial nest called Bowman's capsule. The space the fluid crosses in going from the glomerulus into the first of the tubules is known as **Bowman's space** or the **capsular space**. The filtrate crosses that space into the **proximal convoluted tubule (PCT)**, the first part of the tubular section of the nephron. Once this fluid enters the PCT, it is called **tubular filtrate**. The majority of fluid and components that are reabsorbed from the kidney and sent back into the body comes out of the PCT. There are a few mechanisms that encourage the movement of fluids and amino acids back into the body. Among those, mechanisms are **passive transport** and **co-transport**. Passive transport occurs when material is drawn from one area to another, in this case, from the tubule to the surrounding space called the **interstitial space**. This is done by **osmosis** and **diffusion**, in which differences in local fluid and tissue pressure cause water and particles to passively move. Co-transport occurs when sodium uses a carrier protein to get back into the body from the nephron. When it attaches to the protein, two other molecules hitch a ride: glucose and amino acids. Note that all the glucose, which is so crucial for energy production, is sent back to the body. It is only when glucose levels in the bloodstream are very high that glucose overcomes the ability of the glomerulus and tubule to reject it, and it is passed on out of the body in the urine. The combination of **hyperglycemia** (high blood level of glucose) and **glucosuria** (glucose in the urine) is the major indicator of **diabetes mellitus**, a common metabolic disease in dogs and cats (and in humans, for that matter). When we speak of the "**renal threshold**" for glucose, we refer to the level at which blood glucose levels are so high that not all of it can be resorbed by the kidney. In this case, it will move out of the body in urine (Figure 22.1).

Active transport also plays a role in moving needed material out of the proximal tubule. Much of this type of transport is accomplished via the **Na-K-ATPase pump**. As sodium and potassium exchange places, powered by the "energy molecule" ATP, other electrolytes are dragged along as well (e.g., calcium and chloride). It is important to understand that in the process of reabsorption, anything leaving the tubules of the nephron will enter the interstitial space and then get picked up by the small capillaries surrounding the nephron called the **peritubular capillaries**. The peritubular capillaries take things back into the bloodstream. The opposite can also be true, where the peritubular capillaries push something out into the interstitial space with the intent to have the tubules of the nephron pick it up to deposit in the urine as waste. This process is called **tubular secretion**.

The proximal tubule leads into the **loop of Henle**, which has descending and ascending limbs. First is the **descending limb** in which water continues to be reabsorbed into the body from the nephron. In the **ascending limb** of the loop of Henle and into the **distal convoluted tubule (DCT)**, aldosterone helps to reabsorb sodium in exchange for waste items like hydrogen ions, potassium ions, and ammonium. Calcium will also be reabsorbed in the ascending loop under the control of calcitonin, vitamin D, and parathyroid hormone. Chloride ions are there to help balance the charges inside and outside of the nephron. While the nephron is giving molecules back to the body, the body is using tubular secretion to continue dumping wastes like ammonium and urea back into the nephron to be urinated out. The swapping of these chemicals continues until the final product of urine leaves the kidney. The goal is to dispose of a perfectly balanced waste product in which everything the body needs to get rid of is gone, while everything the body needs to keep remains behind. One of the waste products, **blood urea nitrogen (BUN)** will diffuse back into circulation, despite being waste, as the particle concentrations in the tubular filtrate must be balanced. As such, it is expected that there are some measurable levels of BUN in the blood even though it is a waste product.

Tubular secretion plays an important role in medications like antibiotics. Knowing how antibiotics are processed is particularly important. For example, if a particular antibiotic undergoes tubular secretion, it will be pushed out of the blood at the peritubular capillaries and picked up by the nephron to be put into urine. This is particularly helpful when trying to treat a urinary tract infection. We want to be sure that we can reach the area of infection, in this case, the bladder, with antibiotics through the urine. Further, other drugs that are mostly filtered out of the body through the kidney may not be appropriate for a patient with severe kidney malfunction. In this case, it is possible that too much of the drug will remain within the system due to the kidney's inability to filter it appropriately. Knowing an animal's general health is thus particularly important in prescribing medications.

Figure 22.1 The nephron. Note that this schematic also appears in Chapter 9. Cats have fewer nephrons than most other animals, predisposing them to kidney disease.

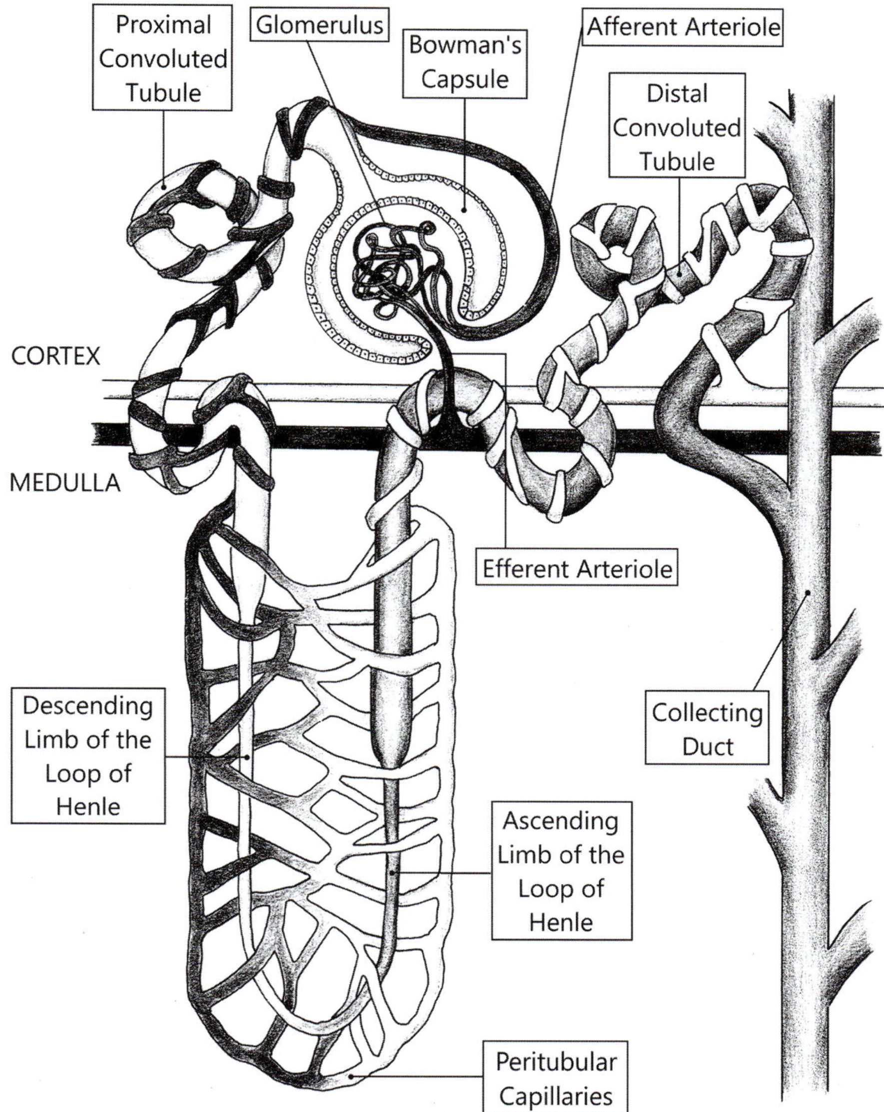

Renal Excretion and Reabsorption of Water

Water tends to follow sodium, so reabsorption of sodium means that water is also being resorbed. Excreting large amounts of sodium means that more water will exit the body. Clearly, loss of too much water is dangerous to most body systems. As a result, not all of the nephron allows water to leave the system. For example, the thick ascending loop of Henle and the DCT are impermeable to water. Even if sodium is resorbed, water won't follow it.

Permeability to water is not a static thing. Certain hormones affect the nephron's permeability to water. Aldosterone, produced by the adrenal gland, and vasopressin, produced in the pituitary gland, alter how water is exchanged in the nephron and can cause the system to retain more water than it would otherwise.

The excretion of urea is another key element in pulling water out of the body or keeping it within the body. Urea is produced in the liver and excreted mostly by the kidneys in mammals. Like sodium, it "pulls" water along with it. High levels of urea, which do not generally get resorbed, are kept within the nephron. This favors the excretion of water as it follows urea and sodium out of the body. When urine contains a great deal of water content, it is said to be **dilute**. It will be a pale color and will be of low specific gravity. If, on the other hand, the nephron resorbs most of the fluid, the remaining urine will be **concentrated**. Concentrated urine has a dark color and a high specific gravity. It has less water and more materials like proteins and sediment. If there is at least some concentration or dilution of urine, this is an indication of at least some degree of renal function, whether normal or not.

Another factor in the nature of filtrate traveling through the nephron is the **countercurrent mechanism**. The descending and ascending limbs of the loop of Henle run right next to each other. The descending limb has a tendency to pick up solutes that need to be excreted, and the ascending limb picks up more water. The relative amount of material surrounding the loop varies because of this. That variation creates more or less oncotic pressure and allows the nephron to reabsorb more water into the body while concentrating urine.

Having traveled to the DCT and undergone its fluid and solute exchanges, the filtrate moves on to the collecting duct. Each collecting duct accepts tubular filtrate from multiple nephrons. The collecting ducts are one of the primary sites of action for antidiuretic hormone (ADH), resulting in the reabsorption of water at the last part of the nephron if necessary. From the collecting duct, the tubular filtrate moves toward the renal pelvis where it is finally referred to as urine.

Ninety-nine percent of the glomerular filtrate is taken back into the body as it journeys through the nephron. The corollary is that there is always a certain amount of water that is excreted, regardless of how much (or even if) the animal drinks. This is of clinical significance. Even an animal that is not eating or drinking much should still be urinating at least a little, albeit very concentrated urine. An animal in the hospital that is not urinating at all is suffering renal shutdown and needs to be treated as an emergency.

It is also important to note that kidney disease can cause many parts of the nephron to fail. It generally creates urine that has excess losses like water and proteins, while waste products remain inside the body like ammonium and BUN due to the kidney being unable to balance needs versus wastes.

Acid–Base Balance

The kidney's activities contribute to acid/base balance in the body. One of the characteristics of blood and urine is its pH. A low (**acidic**) pH, associated with high levels of hydrogen ions, can be damaging to body tissues. On the other hand, high levels of bicarbonate are associated with a high pH (**alkaline**) state. This is not desirable either. The mammalian blood should remain at a pH of 7.4, which is slightly alkaline. Any deviation from this number by more than a few tenths of a point can have clinically appreciable effects.

Several systems help regulate the body's acid/base balance, including the respiratory system. The latter contributes by removing more or less CO_2 from the body as CO_2 is an acid. Removing large amounts of CO_2 helps raise blood pH. It is for this reason (among others) that hypoxemic animals often pant; the body is trying to raise the pH of the blood as it brings in more oxygen.

The kidney plays a role in this as well. Particularly in the proximal tubule and collecting duct, the nephron can either retain hydrogen ions or excrete them. Part of the series of exchanges of molecules involves bicarbonate (an alkaline molecule) and ammonium ion. The latter is actually produced within the proximal tubule. The eventual outcome of these functions is that in cases of acidosis (pH levels that are too low), bicarbonate is resorbed and hydrogen ion is excreted. This helps raise blood pH and return it to a normalized state. It does not matter if the cause of an altered pH is respiratory or metabolic in nature, the body will use any functioning systems to compensate and bring the pH back to 7.4.

Blood Pressure and the Renal System

The control of systemic blood pressure is also in part a function of the kidney. First, in order for the glomerulus to function appropriately, the blood pressure within the glomerulus must be high. In fact, in a normal animal, the blood pressure in the **afferent arteriole** entering the glomerulus is about 80% of that of the aorta. This is very high considering how far from the heart it is and how small the vessels are. This pressure is maintained in the glomerulus by an anatomical feature. The arteriole entering the glomerulus, the afferent arteriole, is a wider diameter than the arteriole exiting the glomerulus, the **efferent arteriole**. This means that more blood can come into the glomerulus than can exit, essentially causing an intentional traffic jam to keep the pressure adequately high.

Further, the kidney has the ability to help control systemic blood pressure. The **renin–angiotensin–aldosterone (RAA) system** helps control blood pressure, GFR, and water resorption. When systemic blood pressure is low, the release of the hormone **renin** is triggered. Renin comes from cells located near the glomerular capillaries called **juxtaglomerular cells**. Juxtaglomerular cells have the ability to sense blood pressure at the level of the afferent arterioles. Another special set of cells called the **macula densa** is able to sense NaCl concentrations in the same location. Low blood pressure, or a low flow rate as detected by the amount of passing NaCl, will trigger the release of renin. Renin, in turn, stimulates the conversion of a compound called **angiotensin I** from **angiotensin**. Angiotensin is a naturally circulating protein. Angiotensin I gets converted to angiotensin II by **angiotensin-converting enzyme (ACE)**. Angiotensin II causes the arteries to constrict, which helps to increase blood pressure. At the same time, angiotensin II also causes the release of aldosterone. Aldosterone triggers the reabsorption of sodium from the kidney, and because water follows sodium, the increased water volume in vessels increases the blood volume, which increases the blood pressure. The use of many medications that control systemic blood pressure is based on this series of reactions, particularly blocking ACE by using **ACE inhibitors**.

Further, the level of angiotensin II in the bloodstream is a signal to the pituitary gland to release vasopressin, also known as ADH. This increases water resorption in the nephron, among other things, and helps to increase blood volume thereby raising blood pressure.

Of course, if these cycles continued indefinitely, systemic blood pressure would rise too high. To avoid this, a negative feedback loop is built into the system. When plasma levels of angiotensin II reach a certain level, the production of renin is suppressed. This brings the cycle of hormones and enzymes to a halt.

Uremia

Uremia is the increase of kidney waste products, BUN and creatinine, in the blood. Uremia can occur in three different ways: **pre-renal uremia, renal uremia**, and **post-renal uremia**. When there is a buildup of kidney wastes in the blood, it is not always the direct responsibility of the kidney. In pre-renal uremia, the kidney works fine, but blood is not getting to the kidney in sufficient enough amounts. This is in situations like dehydration or decreased blood pressure, where the blood volume to the kidney is decreased and not being filtered appropriately. This can also happen in heart disease, where circulation and thus filtration is disturbed.

Renal uremia is when blood is getting to the kidneys appropriately, but something is wrong with the kidney function. This can be from toxins or infections damaging the kidney, or it can be from inflammation or kidney disease damaging the kidney.

Post-renal uremia is where blood can get to the kidneys appropriately, and the kidneys are working fine, but for some reason, the waste can't exit the body, creating a build-up of toxins. This can be caused by a urinary obstruction from tumors, urinary stones, or blood and mucous clots.

Finding the primary cause of uremia or increased renal values is critical to treating the patient. Pre-renal, renal, and post-renal causes have different approaches to treatment and different prognoses. Simple dehydration can have a much more positive prognosis than damaged kidneys, depending on the reason for dehydration (Figure 22.2).

Anemia and the Kidney

Another renal hormone is **erythropoietin** (EPO). This hormone is released in response to a low level of erythrocytes in blood entering the glomerulus. EPO travels to the bone marrow and stimulates red blood cell production. This is of clinical importance. In animals with severe

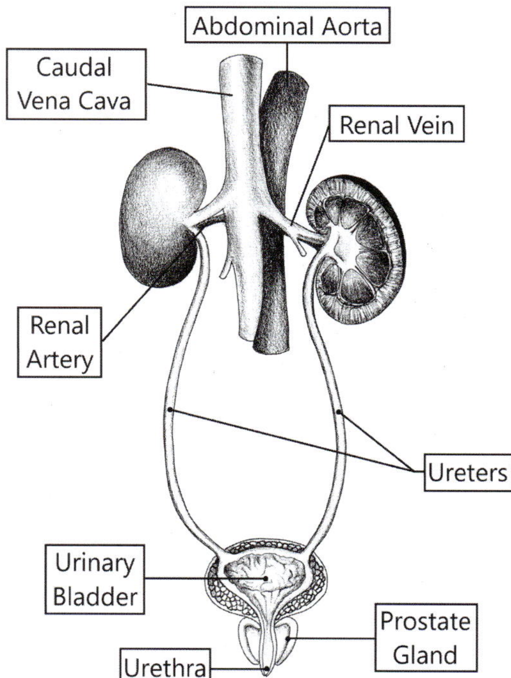

Figure 22.2 The urinary system of a male as noted by the presence of the prostate gland. Blood supply to the kidneys comes directly from the abdominal aorta to the renal artery. After filtration in the kidneys, the waste product, urine, exists in the ureters toward the bladder and then out of the body through the urethra.

kidney disease, EPO production is affected, and the patient can become anemic. The anemia can be quite severe, in which case, we can offer a synthetic EPO in injectable form. It has both advantages and disadvantages, like any drug, and its use is an issue that should be discussed with any client whose pet is suffering from renal malfunction.

A note about **bilirubin** should be made. Bilirubin is a constituent of red blood cells. In the liver, it is converted to **urobilinogen**, which is partly excreted in the feces. Some of it undergoes conversion in the bloodstream and is excreted in urine. In fact, it contributes to the yellow color of urine. There should not be intact bilirubin in urine. If there is, renal and/or circulatory and/or hepatic disease should be investigated.

Species Differences

Avians have three renal arteries. They also have no loop of Henle in the nephron. Most of the salt resorption in their system is achieved in the gastrointestinal (GI) tract. The GI and urinary excreta are channeled to the same exit point, the cloaca. Note that avians excrete urea crystals, and there is little or no liquid urine eliminated by a healthy animal.

Clinical Case Resolution: Gigi

On physical examination, Gigi appears dehydrated with a dull haircoat, a decreased body condition score (BCS), and evidence of muscle wasting. When the client hears this, they are confused as Gigi seems to be drinking regularly. Gigi also seems to have slightly pale mucous membranes indicating possible anemia.

Routine blood work and urine is run on Gigi and reveals a mild anemia, increased kidney values (BUN and Creatinine), and a low specific gravity of urine. All of these are indicators of chronic kidney disease.

Gigi is placed on a lower protein, lower sodium diet as well as an oral drug to help with high blood pressure. Her anemia will be monitored as it is not yet severe enough for intervention, and she does not have clinical symptoms of anemia.

Review Questions

1   Which part of the nephron performs filtration?
    A The glomerulus
    B The PCT
    C The loop of Henle
    D The DCT

2   What is the interconnected network of vessels around the nephron that allows for reabsorption and secretion?
    A The afferent arteriole
    B The efferent arteriole
    C The peritubular capillaries
    D The glomerulus

3   What is the liquid called when in the PCT?
    A Glomerular filtrate
    B Tubular filtrate
    C Urine
    D All of the above

4   What is the process of pulling necessary molecules from the glomerular filtrate back into the blood?
    A Filtration
    B Secretion
    C Reabsorption
    D Osmosis

5 True or False: Specific antibiotics must be selected to treat urinary tract infections.

   A True

   B False

6 What renal waste product is normally found in low levels in the blood?

   A BUN

   B Bilirubin

   C White blood cells

   D Red blood cells

7 Which of the following is the superficial layer of tissue inside the kidney where the glomeruli are?

   A Renal medulla

   B Renal pelvis

   C Renal cortex

   D Renal hilus

8 Which of the following particles move out of the PCT with sodium by co-transport?

   A Amino acids

   B Calcium

   C Bicarbonate

   D Magnesium

9 Which vessel allows blood to flow out of the glomerulus?

   A The afferent arteriole

   B The renal artery

   C The aorta

   D The efferent arteriole

10 What is the role of renin in the RAA system?

   A Splitting angiotensin to angiotensin I

   B Converting angiotensin to angiotensin II

   C Encouraging the reabsorption of sodium

   D Direct stimulation of arterial constriction

23

Cardiovascular Physiology

> **Clinical Case: Turbo, a 6-Year-Old Male Neutered Boxer**
>
> *Turbo is brought in to be assessed after seemingly passing out at the dog park. The owner is concerned that Turbo seemed fine and was playing and then suddenly fell down and was unresponsive. By the time the owner had run across the dog park to get to Turbo, he was beginning to stir and seemingly normalized completely shortly thereafter. This occurred yesterday, and the owner felt comfortable waiting until this morning to have Turbo assessed since he bounced back so quickly. At a glance, Turbo appears to be normal and alert with an excited demeanor.*

Introduction

Conventionally, discussion of the circulatory system begins with the **heart**. As the primary muscle controlling the movement of blood throughout the body, it is the key player in distributing blood and its contents throughout the system. The continued pumping of the heart is associated with the living animal; indeed, the methods of euthanasia we commonly employ indirectly or directly involve the circulatory system.

Cardiac Muscle

The cardiac muscle, also known as **involuntary striated muscle**, is uniquely designed. It is only found in one place in the body, the heart. The cardiac muscle cells have branches that connect end to end to the next cardiac muscle cells. The connection point between the cells is made of special tissue called **intercalated discs**. These hold the cells together and serve as a path of electrical communication between the cells. This is extremely important, as cardiac muscle must always act in a synchronized manner in order to sustain life.

Cardiac muscle makes up the bulk of heart tissue and has a specialized feature that must be discussed. There are sets of cells within the heart that are **autorhythmic**, meaning they can generate their own electrical impulse without needing external nervous system input. This means some cardiac muscle cells are capable of triggering their own contractions. This special group of cardiac muscle cells make up the cardiac conduction system within the heart, responsible for orchestrating timed and synchronized beats. The initiation of this electrical impulse begins in the right atrium, just as the vena cava enters the chamber, in the group of specialized cells called the **sinoatrial node (SA node)** (Figure 23.1).

It is important to understand that, at rest, the cardiac muscle cells are **polarized**, in that they have an electrical difference between the inside of the cell compared to the outside of the cell. In the cardiac muscle cells, the inside of the cell contains potassium ions and is more negatively charged, while the outside of the cell has sodium and calcium ions and is more positively charged. These ions and electrical charges play an important role in contraction and cardiac conduction.

Anatomy and Physiology for Veterinary Technicians and Nurses: A Clinical Approach, Second Edition. Lori Asprea.
© 2026 John Wiley & Sons, Inc. Published 2026 by John Wiley & Sons, Inc.
Companion website www.wiley.com/go/asprea/anatomy_vettech2e

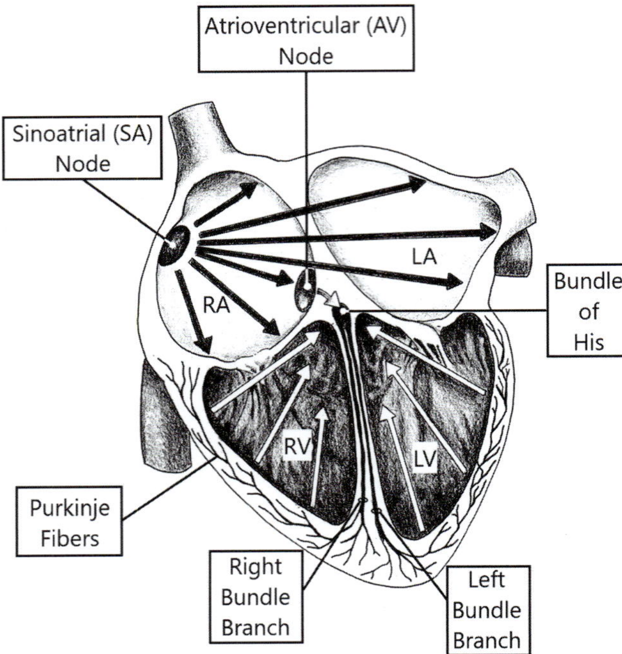

Figure 23.1 The direct control of the heartbeat arises from the sinoatrial node. The signal travels from there to the atrioventricular node and onward along the ventricular septum toward each side of the heart.

The Heartbeat

As previously discussed, the heart generates its own electrical stimulus, called an **action potential**, allowing it to maintain direct control over its function to a large degree. The SA node is the pacemaker that initiates the impulse.

De- and Repolarization

The cardiac muscle cells are polarized at rest, and the **depolarization** of the SA node generates an electrical impulse that flows to the left and right atria, inciting a change in the muscle fibers that ultimately causes them to contract. When depolarization occurs, it happens in two different steps.

In the first stage of depolarization, sodium and calcium ions flood into the cell. This shift in positive ions reverses the polarity, or charges, in the cell. We began with a resting cell in which the outside was more positively charged. Now that the sodium and calcium have entered the cell, the inside is more positive than the outside. Immediately after this, in the second step of depolarization, potassium will leave the cell and restore the charges. Although the cell charges have returned to the normal resting state, the ions are in the wrong locations, leaving sodium and calcium in the interior of the cell and potassium outside. This depolarization allows the cardiac muscle cell to contract.

In order to get the cell ready to depolarize, or contract, again, it must now undergo **repolarization**. During repolarization, specialized channel pumps push sodium, potassium, and calcium back into their original locations. When the cell repolarizes, it relaxes. The cell must complete this cycle in order to be ready for the next wave of stimuli that allow for the next contraction or initiation of the heartbeat.

Cardiac Conduction System

As a result of the branching structure of the muscle fibers and the intercalated discs between them, the muscle fibers are able to fire in concert. This lends strength to the muscle movement.

In the normal animal, the stimulus for contraction begins at the SA node, which sends the signal over both atria. The signal then lands at its next stop at an area near the atrial septum, where the atrium and the ventricles meet. This area is called the **atrioventricular (AV) node**. From the AV node, the wave of electrical energy continues through a "cable" of cells called the **bundle of His**, located in between the atria and ventricles.

From the bundle of His, the wave of energy then separates into two sections. They are called the **left bundle branch** and the **right bundle branch**. These cells transmit the signal down along the **ventricular septum**. When they reach the apex of the heart, they split off and go along the myocardial wall of each ventricle, climbing up the wall of the left and right ventricle back toward the base of the heart by way of the **Purkinje fibers**.

It is important to note that this transmission is carried by cells, not nerve fibers. In other words, the internal changes in the electrical charge within the cells of the heart that lead to muscle contraction are spread by cells and soft tissue, not by nerves. As noted in the chapter regarding muscle function (Chapter 19), the autonomic nervous system does have some input to the heartbeat, but the heart itself generates direct control over its movements.

The impulse actually slows down as it crosses the AV node. This plays a crucial role in the generation of the heartbeat. Slowing the energy wave down allows it to gather itself together and generate a strong, organized "push" so that the ventricles contract as a whole.

Rhythm

Each part of the electrical energy in the heart is able to be read on the surface of the skin via an **electrocardiogram (EKG or ECG)**. The ECG has a series of electrical spikes or waves that represent the internal workings of the heart. Each wave is named and correlates to a specific electrical event in each heartbeat. Please refer to Figure 23.2.

The **P-wave** represents atrial depolarization and, presumably, the contraction of the atria. The **QRS complex** represents ventricular depolarization, and presumably, the contraction of the ventricles. It can be broken down further, where the **Q-wave** represents depolarization of the interventricular septum, the R-wave represents depolarization of the main mass of the ventricles, and the **S-wave** represents the depolarization of the final parts of the ventricle toward the heart base. Finally, the T-wave represents the repolarization and presumably relaxation of the ventricles. We do not see the repolarization of the atria represented on the ECG, as it occurs during the time of ventricular depolarization, which has a much larger electric stimulus and essentially overwrites the atrial repolarization.

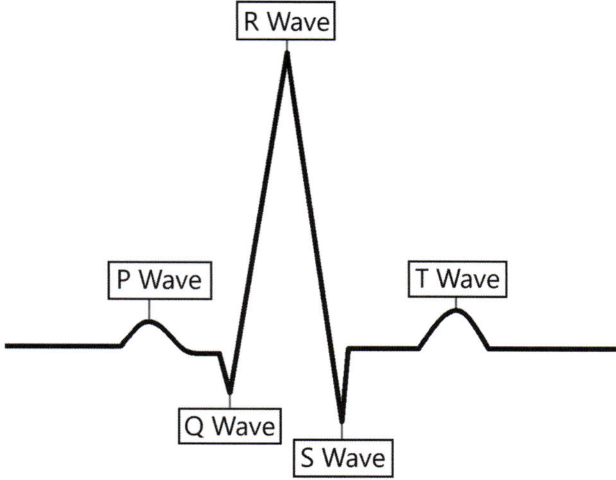

Figure 23.2 The anatomy of the EKG wave.

One of the unique features of this system is that cells anywhere along the route of the depolarization wave can initiate the electrical energy change; that is, the SA node is not the only place where the heartbeat can be triggered. By the same token, if the electrical stimulus is generated further down the system, it will not necessarily be transmitted in an organized fashion. This has significant importance for diagnosing heart disease. If the pacemaker cells are not firing in a synchronous manner, the heartbeat will be irregular. It may "skip" a beat or beat less efficiently. An irregular heartbeat can be a direct result of irregular/disorganized transmission of the electrical wave that stimulates the heart muscle. This abnormal order of events in contraction is referred to as an **arrhythmia**.

Arrhythmias can be caused by a number of factors including electrolyte disturbances, genetic issues, primary cardiac disease, or secondary to systemic disease like anemia. Because any area within the system can generate a beat, if the system malfunctions, we can have serious consequences. **Premature atrial contractions (PACs)** or **atrial premature complexes (APCs)** are interchangeable terms for when the atria depolarize and contract prematurely, or too early, resulting in an irregular beat. If PACs happen one after the other in succession for long periods of time, we call it **atrial tachycardia**. While a single PAC can feel like a "skipped" heartbeat, atrial tachycardia can lead to fainting and decreased blood pressure among other symptoms that need medical intervention. **Premature ventricular contractions (PVCs)** or **ventricular premature complexes (VPCs)** are interchangeable terms for when the ventricles originate a signal for the beat and result in the atria contracting prematurely. VPCs alone, like PACs, can feel like a skipped beat or flutter, but when VPCs persist consistently, we call that **ventricular tachycardia**. Ventricular tachycardia can also cause fainting and decreased blood pressure among other symptoms and also generally requires medical interventions.

As is true in the neurological system, the transmission of energy within the pacemaker cells and from them to the muscle fibers relies in large measure on the electrolytes sodium, calcium, and potassium. Abnormalities in any one of these can have serious consequences for the function of the heart. In fact, when we mentioned euthanasia earlier, we are referring to the drugs used for euthanizing our patients, which act to disrupt the sodium channels in cardiac tissue, causing it to stop functioning. Without the ability to contract and pump blood (and thus oxygen) to the cells, death of the animal results. Euthanasia drugs used today are also anesthetic so that the animal does not feel any of the intended effects.

One other note concerns the metabolism of the muscle fibers within the heart. We mentioned several ways that skeletal muscle fibers generate energy. In contrast, the heart specifically uses cellular respiration to generate ATP. It makes very little use of carbohydrate derivatives. Therefore, oxygen is particularly crucial to heart function, more so than to skeletal muscle.

Cardiac Output

A number of factors are involved in the heartbeat. The electrical energy that sparks the initial muscle contraction is only a part of the picture. For example, part of what determines how much blood is pumped out of the heart is related to the rate at which the heart beats. The amount of blood pumped out of the heart in one single beat is called **stroke volume (SV)**. Multiplying that number by the speed of the heartbeats, or heart rate (HR), yields a number that is referred to as **cardiac output (CO)**. CO is the reflection of the amount of blood sent out to the body over a period of time. Any change in SV or HR will affect CO. This results in a simple formula to calculate cardiac output: $\textbf{CO} = \textbf{HR} \times \textbf{SV}$. As each of these values change, so too will the result and efficacy of the heart.

SV can be affected by a number of factors. These include level of exercise, general health of the animal's heart, systemic blood pressure, and the autonomic nervous system. If systemic blood pressure is high, for example, the heart has to beat harder. Eventually, the abnormal strain on the heart will damage it, and SV will actually decrease, leading to a decrease in CO. SV is also impacted by **preload** and **afterload**.

The volume of blood the ventricle receives from the atrium is called preload. The ventricles eventually reach a point where they are filled. At that point, the ventricles will expel the blood out of the heart by contracting, called **systole**. If the preload is lessened for any reason, the ventricle will push out less blood, meaning the CO will be reduced. The ventricle can only push out what it contains when contraction occurs.

Afterload is the amount of resistance in the space the blood from the ventricles is pushed into. If pressure in the **aorta**, where the left ventricle pushes blood to, is very high, it will impede the attempt of the ventricle to empty completely, thus reducing SV and CO. Small increases in afterload generally can be overcome by a healthy heart, but in cases of heart disease, it can become a significant impairment.

Enlargement of the heart muscle causes abnormalities in the HR. As is true for any muscle, the harder it works, the larger it will grow, and the more rapid the HR needed to keep up the pace. If the heart is too big, it will no longer beat in an organized fashion.

There are genetic factors in some animals that affect CO. Certain breeds of dogs are prone to something called **dilated cardiomyopathy (DCM)**, where the heart muscle becomes weakened and does not effectively pump blood. Some cat breeds have a very high incidence of genetically based **hypertrophic cardiomyopathy (HCM)**, where the cardiac muscles thicken, which reduces its filling capacity and therefore efficiency. In either case, the enlargement causes a number of other problems, including the inability of the heart to sustain normal CO. In dogs, breeds affected include Doberman pinschers and German Shepherds. In cats, Maine coons and Norwegian Forest cats suffer from heart disease much more commonly than domestic shorthair cats.

As might be expected, the greater the pressure/blood content in the ventricles, the stronger the force of the blood that is pushed out of them (e.g., into the aorta). The relationship between the preload and the SV is described by Starling's law. As a result of this relationship, the more blood in the ventricle when it is filled, the greater the SV will be.

This does not seem to be a remarkable statement, but it has tremendous importance for the circulatory system. For example, if SV increases on one side of the heart, by Starling's law, the other side will try to match it so that the amount of blood remains constant. As a clinical example, the presence of **heartworms**, a parasite infection spread by mosquitoes, in the pulmonary artery will cause an increase in pressure in the right atrium (the chamber from which blood comes into the pulmonary artery). Unfortunately, the pulmonary artery is where uncontrolled heartworm infestation often settles. This increase in pressure will be reflected in increased preload and thus increased CO.

Another factor affecting CO is the **contractility** of the heart muscle. The stronger the heart muscle's contraction, the more blood can be expelled. Both the sympathetic nervous system and certain medications can increase contractility. If the heart muscle cannot contract enough to produce a strong burst of energy, not all of the blood can be expelled from the ventricle. In other words, SV decreases.

One of the ways that systemic blood pressure is kept at a normal level is by maintaining normal CO. Less blood entering the peripheral circulation means less fluid pressure, which means that the flow of blood throughout the body will be less efficient, and oxygenation of body tissues will be compromised. The types of heart enlargement mentioned above also affect contractility.

The circulatory system can be thought of as two circuits. One goes from the heart to the lungs and back to the heart and can be referred to as the **pulmonary circuit**. The other goes from the heart to the rest of the body and then back again. The circulation throughout the body is referred to as **peripheral** or **systemic circulation**. Please refer to the chapter on circulatory anatomy to recall the vessels involved in the flow of blood through the body. For the moment, think of the circulation of blood from the heart as traveling through the arteries, narrowing as they approach the capillaries, and then from the capillaries through veins that widen as they approach the cranial and caudal vena cava, which return the blood to the heart.

Flow Through the Heart and Back

Blood flowing back from the body after dropping off oxygen to tissues will travel toward the heart through venules and veins until it reaches either the cranial or caudal vena cava. They merge and enter the heart at the right atrium. Therefore, all systemic circulation leads back to the right atrium of the heart. As the atrium fills, the **right AV valve**, or **tricuspid valve**, will open when the atria contract. At this point, the blood is forced through the opening into the right ventricle. When the right ventricle has filled sufficiently, the right AV valve snaps shut, and the **semilunar valve** of the pulmonary trunk, called the **pulmonary valve**, will open. The pulmonary trunk is an artery in which blood is flowing away from the heart. It does not carry oxygenated blood, unlike other arteries. In fact, the destination of blood from the pulmonary trunk is the lungs, where oxygen and carbon dioxide will be exchanged.

Once the blood travels to the lungs to collect oxygen and drops of carbon dioxide, the newly oxygenated blood is carried toward the heart in the pulmonary veins which lead directly into the left atrium. As it fills and then contracts, the **left AV valve**, or **mitral valve**, will open, and blood will enter the left ventricle. When the ventricle is full, the mitral valve closes, and the contraction of the heart pushes the blood through the semilunar valve that guards the entrance to the aorta called the **aortic valve**.

Please note that both left and right atria contract simultaneously, which means both the left and right AV valve open and close simultaneously. Immediately after this, both the left and right ventricle contract simultaneously, while both the pulmonary and aortic valves open simultaneously. The right and left side of the heart are always working in tandem to ensure appropriate circulation.

When blood fills the ventricles, a signal is triggered by the increase in fluid pressure that causes the AV valves to snap shut. At this point, the semilunar valves of the aorta and pulmonary artery open and the ventricles contract. This strong contraction is called **systole**. Systole exerts the maximum pressure from the heart on the arteries. Once most of the blood has been expelled from the ventricles, the AV valves open and the semilunar valves close, and the cycle repeats. Opposite to systole, when the ventricles relax and refill, it is called **diastole**.

Clinical measurement of the strength of the diastolic and systolic contraction is usually done indirectly, using the measure of **systemic blood pressure** as an indicator. We refer to **diastolic** and **systolic pressure**. As the atria are smaller and send blood a relatively short distance to the ventricles, the resting pressure during atrial contraction is much lower than during ventricular contraction. Therefore, the diastolic number should also be smaller than the systolic number when measuring the strength of the contraction. When an animal's blood pressure is reported as, say, 110/80 mmHg (one hundred and ten over eighty with a measurement unit of millimeters of mercury), we are reporting that the systolic pressure is 110 mmHg and the diastolic pressure is 80 mmHg.

As might be imagined, the transmission of force as the blood circulates will diminish as the blood goes further away from the heart. The aorta is the largest in diameter of all the arteries and is composed mainly of elastic tissue. This reflects the fact that the full force of the systolic pressure is accepted by this vessel. In fact, one of the reasons that many arteries, particularly those nearest the heart, follow a circuitous route relates to an attempt to dampen some of this great force as the blood enters the narrower blood vessels.

One may also use this to their advantage when doing physical examinations. The heartbeat and the pulse of blood through the arteries should be simultaneous. The doctor or the technician will often auscultate the heart while feeling for the rhythm of the pulse of the femoral artery. We mentioned in an earlier chapter that the heartbeat and the femoral pulse should be simultaneous. If there is an audible lag between the two, there is some disruption of the circulatory system. This phenomenon is referred to as **pulse deficit**.

On the subject of auscultating the heart, it is worthwhile to remember that dogs and cats (as is true in the primate) should have two distinct heart sounds. Each sound is associated with the closing of the AV valves or the semilunar valves; that is, diastole and systole have a sound associated with each. This is not true across all species. For example, the heart of the dog has two sounds, but that of the horse has four sounds, when it beats.

A **heart murmur** reflects turbulence in the flow of blood. Instead of flowing in a single, smooth course from the atrium to the ventricle to the body through the valve, the blood may reach a structural abnormality that causes a whirlpool or some other swirling effect. Sometimes, the valves are abnormal and do not close completely. This allows blood to stream backward instead of forward. It is common in older, small-breed dogs to find abnormalities in the mitral valve. The valve is often thickened or deformed and does not close all the way. Thus, blood travels backward through the small opening from the ventricle, back into the atrium. This produces a swishing sound.

There are causes of heart murmurs that are not from primary heart disease. For example, anemia can be associated with **turbulent blood flow** as the lack of red cells reduces blood viscosity. Hyperthyroidism can also cause heart murmurs; the high level of activity of the gland forces the blood to swirl as it travels through the heart.

Vasculature

As blood is expelled into the aorta, there are a series of vessels called **coronary arteries** that branch off the aorta to bring fresh blood to supply the heart tissue itself with oxygen. It is crucial to the rest of the body that the heart be in good working order. Thus, it is no surprise that the most highly oxygenated blood goes to the heart muscle first. The **coronary veins** return the deoxygenated blood directly back to the right atrium.

Recall that there is a greater or lesser degree of smooth muscle tissue in the lining of the arteries. Making the arteries narrower by constriction increases the pressure of the blood flowing through it. While this is efficient in speeding the blood along to where it is needed, it also means that the force involved can, over the long term, damage the vessels themselves. The constriction and **dilation**, or widening, of blood vessels is accomplished by the smooth muscle in the lining of the vessels, mediated by the autonomic nervous system. The greatest control is actually in the arterioles. Some of them actually have sphincter muscles that can narrow these vessels tremendously, allowing pressure to build up. In contrast, the venules have no muscle tissue as their acceptance of blood returning to the heart is passive.

As arteries reach the outskirts of their travels, they have not only narrowed in diameter but have also undergone physical changes. There is less elastic tissue and more muscle tissue in arterioles than in the aorta and in some of the other major vessels. This will come into play as we discuss the control of blood pressure.

Eventually, the arterioles reach the **capillaries**, which are the smallest blood vessels. Their diameter is usually less than $10\,\mu m$. This fact, in addition to the presence of small pores in the walls of the capillaries, allows material to be exchanged with the tissue surrounding the vessels.

A combination of **diffusion** and **hydrostatic pressure** helps determine what materials are absorbed by the surrounding tissue and what materials are resorbed by the capillaries to continue through the venous system back to the heart.

Since there is less oxygen in the surrounding tissue than in the artery, the oxygen will flow into the local tissues. The reverse is true for carbon dioxide. Some hormones and lipids can also pass through the pores. All of these materials are conveyed to the cells so that they can use the energy contained therein to produce protein or whatever else the cell is designed to manufacture.

Hydrostatic pressure has to do with fluid exchange. As the relative water pressure is higher within the capillaries than in the surrounding area, water tends to flow out of the capillaries to hydrate the tissues. Changes in the normal balance of these pressures, as might be the case in dehydration, will lead to an inefficient exchange, exacerbating the water deprivation of the surrounding area by encouraging water to go into the capillaries instead.

As noted in previous chapters, the capillaries in certain areas, such as the liver and the kidney, are **fenestrated** or have microscopic openings on them. Some have large pores that allow bigger molecules (like proteins) to flow into and out of the capillaries. In the liver, where toxins are processed, it is desirable to have a way to "flush" them directly into the liver from the circulatory system.

Blood Pressure

The mere act of flowing through the blood vessels means that the blood will be affected by the stiffness or natural pressure within the vessel itself. The resistance of the circulatory system is analogous to a person walking into the wind. Under normal circumstances, the resistance is the equivalent of a light breeze; in disease states, or under "deliberate" increases in resistance caused by the hormonal and/or neurological system, it is more like walking into a storm.

The combination of the CO and the resistance of the peripheral vasculature determines arterial pressure. Note that there is also resistance in the veins. The greatest resistance to blood flow is actually in the arterioles. The fierce pumping of the blood provided by the heart propels the blood through the arteries. This, combined with the structure of the arterial wall, means that the blood should flow under a certain amount of pressure as it travels toward the organs and other tissues. As it reaches the smaller-diameter vessels such as the arterioles, the blood is flowing under higher pressure.

This is clearly advantageous. Any disease states that lower CO, or weaken the stiffness of the arteries, will have a negative effect on the ability of blood to circulate. Arterial stiffness in animals, unlike in humans, is relatively rare. Changes in CO, however, do occur. Note that certain drugs lower CO; when using these drugs or anesthetics, it is important to measure systemic blood pressure carefully.

When the animal is exercising, the arterioles in the skeletal muscles dilate. This means that they can accept a much greater volume of blood. This explains, in part, how the animal can cope with the greater activity required during exercise. It also explains why the animal suffers from exercise intolerance with significant cardiac disease.

Note also that the blood vessels within the lung are quite sensitive to the amount of oxygen within the blood. In cases of oxygen deprivation, their diameter will be adjusted, lowering their resistance and allowing more blood to flow, and exchange more carbon dioxide for oxygen.

CO is affected by contractility and HR. Other factors also control the resistance of the arterioles, increasing or decreasing blood pressure. Factors such as neurological input, hormones, and/or the condition of the destination tissues also have an effect.

Autonomic Nervous System Involvement

The **autonomic nervous system** controls both the function of the heart itself and the degree of constriction of the arteries and veins. The **sympathetic nervous system** uses epinephrine and norepinephrine as transmitters to increase the rate of impulses through the pacemaker cells and to increase the strength of the cardiac muscle contraction. The **parasympathetic system**, by way of acetylcholine, has the opposite effect.

The sympathetic nerve fibers control the peripheral arterioles and veins by two methods. One is the constriction of the arterioles and veins. There is one class of sympathetic nerve receptor cells that actually causes vasodilation. These receptors are present in the coronary arteries and in skeletal muscles. Dilation of these vessels allows more oxygen-carrying blood to reach these tissues.

The parasympathetic fibers in the heart stimulate muscarinic **cholinergic receptors** that slow its rate and thus CO. **Muscarinic receptors** are also present in the arterioles, and their stimulation causes vasodilation.

Hormonal influence is a subset of neurological input, as the release of hormones such as epinephrine and norepinephrine are mediated by the sympathetic nervous system. However, the increase in production of these hormones (used as neurotransmitters) is not possible without the function of the adrenal gland, so the endocrine system is crucial to the control of blood pressure.

Specialized cells within the local organs and tissues also contribute to influence blood flow. **Baroreceptors** are pressure-sensitive nerve fibers. When arterial pressure goes above or below its desired amount, the change in pressure within the vessel is sensed by these cells. It is the stretching of the walls of the surrounding tissue that triggers the response. What is engendered is an increase in the number of action potentials over time. The neural impulse is directed to the hypothalamus. This message will result in the autonomic nervous system adjusting CO and vascular resistance to counteract the undesired changes. Baroreceptor cells are located in the aortic arch, the right atrium of the heart, and the carotid arteries. Note that these adjustments do not necessarily bring the systemic blood pressure all the way back to normal. In addition, they do not address the source of the disturbance; they merely alert the brain to the problem.

There are also stretch receptors within the atria. These respond to the volume of blood present. They work in concert with the baroreceptor cells to speed up or decrease the frequency of the action potentials sent to the central nervous system.

There are other mechanisms related to the outside world that mediate vascular circulation. For example, the "fight or flight" response is triggered by the perception of stimuli perceived as threatening. The central nervous system's interpretation of any menacing event (including everything from a loud noise to a leaping tiger) will set off the release of hormones such as **vasopressin** and **angiotensin II** in response to the sympathetic nervous system's engagement. Certainly, the cardiovascular system will respond with increased CO and systemic blood pressure. Anyone who has auscultated the chest of a timid cat in the clinic is well aware of this phenomenon.

The mechanism works in the opposite way as well. As the animal's activity slows, the parasympathetic system becomes more active (and the sympathetic system less so). This allows for the "rest and digest" state, in which case the CO and systemic blood pressure will return to its resting level. Sleep, of course, is a strong expression of this change.

If blood pressure becomes low enough and the CO and vascular system do not compensate, the animal can undergo **syncope** (fainting). This is rare in animals, although not uncommon in humans. Again, animals receiving treatment or medication that lowers blood pressure must be monitored carefully. Syncope or decreased consciousness may be a sign that there has been an overdose of the medication or an underlying cardiac condition.

Measurement of systemic blood pressure is usually accomplished indirectly, by way of monitoring the strength of the pulse through a systemic artery. As with measuring core temperature by way of a thermometer placed away from the major organs, the measurement of blood pressure using a distal artery yields a slightly different result from that which would be found measuring these levels closer to the heart.

The Lymphatic System

Blood and other molecules along for the ride travel from the capillaries through the venous system. The majority of the veins actually have a larger diameter than that of the arteries (the aorta being a notable exception). Thus, the venous system can actually carry a large percentage of blood volume.

Along the way, **lymphatic vessels** exit from the organs and other structures. These vessels have the ability to draw off larger molecules, like plasma proteins and fragments of dead cells. These vessels travel throughout the body, just as blood vessels, although they are lesser in number.

The lymph nodes perform a valuable filtering service. The white blood cells they contain have the ability to destroy pathogens such as bacteria. Cells called **macrophages** can scavenge unwanted material and "digest" it so that it ceases to be a threat to the system.

The lymph nodes assist in the storage of white blood cells as well, which can then be sent out into the system to respond to inflammation. Materials that have been processed in the lymph node are then funneled into the efferent vessels toward the veins, usually the vena cava. Thus, the venous system not only carries blood cells back to the heart for diversion to the lungs to pick up oxygen. It also provides a way for the disposal of filtered lymphatic fluid.

Clinical Case Resolution: Turbo

Turbo is examined thoroughly, and his exam is mostly within normal limits. An intermittent arrhythmia is auscultated, but otherwise Turbo appears to be in good body condition with normal energy levels. A blood pressure is obtained, which is normal.

It is recommended that Turbo have routine screening bloodwork, an EKG performed, and that echocardiogram be considered. The owner agrees to all diagnostic tests.

The EKG reveals intermittent VPCs, and the echocardiogram is normal. It is recommended that Turbo be fitted with a Holter monitor, which is a device that will measure the EKG from home 24 hours a day. This will help capture any abnormalities that Turbo might have.

Blood work results returned and they are normal. The Holter monitor continues to catch frequent intermittent VPCs. The owner notes normal behavior and activity throughout the time that Turbo wore the monitor.

Based on Turbo's breed, presenting history, and EKG findings, he is diagnosed with arrhythmogenic right ventricular cardiomyopathy. This is a genetic condition in Boxer's that causes the heart muscle to be replaced with fibrous and fatty tissue. This in turn causes an electrical instability in the heart which results in arrhythmias, particularly VPCs. Occasionally, these VPCs will occur in "runs" or consistently, replacing each beat called ventricular tachycardia. When this happens, the heart is not pumping blood correctly and CO falls, which makes blood pressure fall, and the patient experiences syncope or collapse.

Turbo is prescribed an antiarrhythmic drug to help stabilize his heart. He will need frequent regular follow up with the cardiologist to ensure his disease is managed appropriately.

Review Questions

1 Where does the left atrium pump blood into?
  A The right atrium
  B The left ventricle
  C The right ventricle
  D The aorta

2 Cardiac muscle has special cells that are ______________________ which means they can create their own impulses.
  A Sympathetic
  B Parasympathetic
  C Autorhythmic
  D Voluntary

3 Which vessel brings deoxygenated blood back to the right atrium?
  A The aorta
  B The pulmonary artery
  C The coronary artery
  D The vena cava

4 Where does the impulse for each heartbeat begin?
  A The SA node
  B The AV node
  C The bundle of His
  D The Purkinje fibers

5 When measuring blood pressure, diastolic pressure represents which of the following?
  A The pressure when the ventricles are contracting
  B The pressure within the pulmonary vessel
  C The pressure when the atria are contracting
  D The pressure within the glomerulus

6 Which wave on the EKG represents the repolarization of the ventricles?
  A The P wave
  B The Q wave
  C The R wave
  D The S wave
  E The T wave

7 A heart murmur is
  A Turbulent blood flow in the heart that can be auscultated
  B A misfire of the heart's electrical system
  C The flow of blood during diastole
  D The lymphatic system returning lymph fluid

8 If HR and SV decrease, what will happen to CO?
  A It will increase
  B It will decrease
  C It will not be affected

9 What ions move into the cardiac cell during the first stage of depolarization?
  A Sodium and potassium
  B Sodium and chloride
  C Potassium and calcium
  D Sodium and calcium

10 What is preload?
  A The amount of blood delivered to the right atrium
  B The amount of blood delivered to the left atrium
  C The amount of blood delivered to the right ventricle
  D The amount of blood delivered to the left ventricle

24

Respiratory Physiology

Clinical Case: Tictac, a 3-Year-Old Male Intact Pomeranian Mix
Tictac is presented to the emergency room after being hit by a car. He got out of the yard unexpectedly and ran into the street. The owner saw this happen and can confirm that he was hit by a car. He is presenting with dyspnea, or difficulty breathing, and seems to be orthopneic. Orthopneic breathing is when an animal stretches its neck, spreads its front legs, and sits or stands upright, all in an effort to increase airflow into the chest. The orthopneic breathing position is seen in moderate to severe respiratory distress and constitutes an emergency.

Introduction

The main goal of the respiratory system is to pull air into the animal so that oxygen can be extracted and spread to the tissues and to provide a pathway for carbon dioxide to be expelled. In mammals, it does serve some other purposes as well, including warming and humidifying the air that enters, as well as filtering what is inhaled. The respiratory system is comprised of two parts: the **upper respiratory tract** and the **lower respiratory tract**. The upper respiratory tract contains the nose and nasal passages, the pharynx and larynx, and finally the trachea, while the lower contains the bronchi, bronchioles, and alveoli.

The Basics

The entrance to the nasal passages is the nares or nostrils. Air moves into the nasal passages, which are ciliated mucous membranes with an extensive amount of blood vessels. These cilia and the mucous help to filter the air that enters and traps any particulate matter. This includes dust and dirt but also microscopic items like allergens and pathogens. The mucous membrane also helps to humidify the air, while the large volume of blood vessels helps to warm the air.

The air then moves to the pharynx, where the oropharynx and nasopharynx meet. The area immediately caudal is the larynx, which serves to protect the airways from any contents entering them during eating or drinking. The larynx is also where the "voice box" allows the animal to make sounds like meowing or barking.

The trachea helps to bring air into the lungs and splits into the two main bronchi, which continue to branch through the lower respiratory tract. The branches, or **bronchioles**, continue to branch, and the smallest tubes—the **alveolar ducts**—take air to the alveoli, which are responsible for gas exchange. This will be discussed in more detail later in this chapter.

The bronchial tree has smooth muscle in it that can constrict or dilate the airways, a process called **bronchoconstriction** or **bronchodilation**. This is in response to instructions from the autonomic nervous system.

A few definitions are in order. **Ventilation** refers to the movement of air/gases into and out of the respiratory tract. It is not a specific quantitative measure but a description of a general action.

Tidal volume actually refers to measurement. Tidal volume is the amount of air that is moved with each breath. **Minute ventilation** is an even more specific number; it is the total amount of air that is breathed in and out in 1 minute. Minute volume is calculated by multiplying tidal volume by breaths per minute (BPM). In effect, if either the total amount of air being moved or the rate at which it is moving varies, minute ventilation will be affected. The clinical significance of this lies in disease states or medication effects that change the depth or shallowness of breathing and/or change the respiration rate or BPM. For example, **hyperthermia** (fever) will often cause panting, as the body attempts to decrease its core temperature. As a result, the minute ventilation will be adversely affected, in that abnormally rapid rates of air intake do not allow for large amounts to be inhaled.

Another important term is "**dead space**." Dead space refers to areas of the respiratory tract in which there is no active gas exchange. There are two kinds: **anatomical dead space** and **physiological dead space**.

The term "anatomical dead space" refers to the area from the entrance to the respiratory system at the nares through the major bronchi. This area serves to conduct air into the lungs. It does not move oxygen or other gases on a cellular level, as is the case in the alveoli of the lungs. While respiration is dependent upon the channeling of air to the alveoli, this space is considered dead, in that there is no exchange of oxygen and carbon dioxide at this level. Were it not for the anatomical dead space, air would have to be conducted to the lungs through the skin, as is the case in some amphibians, or by some artificial means such as a **tracheostomy tube**, which is a tube inserted directly into the trachea and can be used for mechanical ventilation.

Physiological dead space is related to the alveoli themselves, where the actual exchange of gases occurs. Not all alveoli are perfused to the same degree; that is, some of them are inactive at any given time, and there is no gas exchange taking place. If only as a result of the effects of gravity and movement, the capillary blood supply to each alveolus is different. The ones that are not perfused sufficiently (do not have much blood passing by) do not actively engage in gas exchange. The term physiological dead space encompasses the dead space in the alveoli as well as the anatomical dead space.

The more physiological dead space, the less surface area there is for the animal to exchange carbon dioxide and oxygen to a sufficient degree for normal function. A particular concern arises during surgery when the animal is **intubated**. The **endotracheal tube**, or breathing tube, itself is dead space. Using a tube that is too long or too wide interferes with the motion needed for respiration and may provoke decreased gas exchange, even though the animal is receiving oxygen directly into the airway. It is for this reason, among others, that we monitor oxygen and carbon dioxide levels in the blood during surgery.

One other point needs to be made in reference to ventilation. Once gases reach the alveoli, they are processed so that some elements are absorbed into the bloodstream and others passed into the alveolus so that they can be exhaled. This exchange, as noted above, happens by way of local blood vessels. If the minute ventilation of the animal is too high or too low relative to the rate and amount of blood flowing past the alveolus, the gas exchange will be inefficient. Put another way, if the amount of air exchanged does not match the ability of blood to pick up oxygen and discharge carbon dioxide, the "hand-off" of gases does not go smoothly. This is referred to as **ventilation/perfusion (V/Q) mismatch**. A slight amount of mismatch is normal in a healthy animal, as BPM and rate of blood flow are variable enough in the normal animal that they do not match up at all times. However, an abnormal amount of V/Q mismatch makes it harder to get oxygen into the body.

Ventilation and Temperature

A major factor in the changeable nature of minute ventilation is the interplay of **ambient** (outside the body) and **core temperature**. An animal suffering from heat stress, like the febrile animal we discussed earlier, will decrease activity in an effort to avoid building up more heat. In contrast, a **hypothermic**, or cold, animal will have a slower respiratory rate but an increase in tidal volume. This increases the efficiency of the gas exchange and allows the animal to increase metabolic energy production—in short, to warm up.

Considering the animal under anesthesia again, it should now be evident that another corollary of increasing dead space is that the animal will shed heat. An animal under anesthesia is already experiencing a decrease in core temperature as metabolic activity is slowed by the drug. Add to that more heat loss through an inappropriately placed endotracheal tube, and the problem of surgical hypothermia will be even worse. Warming blankets or other devices are often used during or after surgery to counteract this problem.

Residual Capacity

Functional residual capacity is a phrase that refers to the fact that there is a small amount of air that remains in the lungs after exhalation. This amount of air helps maintain the slightly negative air pressure in the chest cavity, relative to air pressure outside the body. The consistency of the level of air in the cavity is enough to ensure that ventilation will be relatively consistent with the animal at rest. As is true for all body systems, regular rhythms contribute to consistency (see Figure 24.1).

Thoracic Pressure

It is important to remember that in the normal animal, the thoracic pressure is slightly more negative than the environment. If the chest cavity is punctured, say, by traumatic injury, the balance between the air pressure inside and outside of the body is now changed as more air enters the cavity. This increased pressure will cause the lung to collapse down in size. The collapse of a lung is called **atelectasis**. It is actually more likely to occur in thoracic injuries to a young animal than an older animal. Adult tissue is stiffer and less likely to collapse. There are other causes of atelectasis, but this one is germane to our discussion.

As the thoracic cavity expands and contracts during mammalian respiration, the diaphragm moves. The muscles of inhalation include the external intercostals and the scalenus muscle. The diaphragm is active during inhalation and recoils (passively returns) during exhalation. It is a **musculotendinous** tissue, having both strength and flexibility from muscles and tendons. As muscles contract to allow the animal to inhale, the diaphragm is drawn caudally and flattens. This helps increase the size of the thoracic cavity. The expansion causes the relative air pressure in the thorax to be even lower than that of the ambient air. The condition of negative air pressure in the thorax is an enticement for air from the outside to come in.

Once the muscles have reached their furthest expansion, they will stop. The elastic properties of the lungs and the thoracic cavity will cause these tissues to rebound to their normal position. The diaphragm will also recoil to its relaxed position and take on a curved appearance. This will cause air to be expelled from the animal.

The process of exhalation in dogs and cats is, for the most part, passive. It is not so much the force of muscle contracting as it is the return to a resting state that causes air to flow out of the respiratory system. There is some minor contribution, however, to exhalation by muscles such as the internal intercostals.

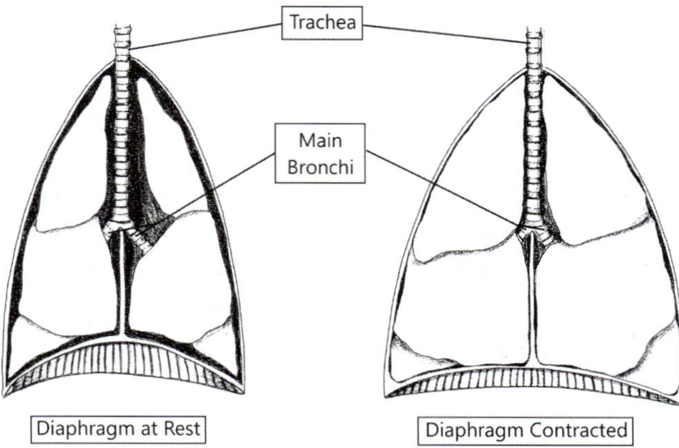

Figure 24.1 The expansion of the thorax allows the diaphragm to expand, and the pressure change brings air into the lungs. Exhalation in dogs and cats is passive, and so the diaphragm returns to its resting position without an external force.

The Nervous System and Respiration

In an animal that is having difficulty breathing, the central nervous system will attempt to apply more muscular force to inhalation. For example, additional abdominal muscles will be recruited. Large excursions of the chest and abdomen denote increased respiratory effort and are a clear marker for respiratory disease/distress in a patient who presents with this symptom called **abdominal breathing**.

Another factor assisting the movement of the lungs during respiration is the presence of a scant amount of viscous serous fluid between the parietal and visceral pleura. This provides lubrication for the movement of the tissues.

There is another relevant point regarding the movement of air through the respiratory apparatus. As the flow of air approaches the alveoli, it is going through narrower airways. This causes airflow to slow down considerably and make less noise as it is moving. As a result, when auscultating the thorax in a normal animal, what is being heard, in terms of respiratory sounds, is mostly the upper respiratory tract noise rather than the bronchioles. This is why thoracic radiographs are so important in diagnosing respiratory disease. While auscultation may not yield anything remarkable, clear abnormalities may be identified on diagnostic imaging.

The Rhythmicity of Breathing

The rate and volume of air inhaled and exhaled during respiration is mediated by many factors, some of which have already been noted. There are other features that also participate.

Within the **lung parenchyma** (the specific cells associated with the organ and their supporting connective tissue), there are stretch receptors. These receptors are also present in the airways and even the surrounding musculature. For example, as the lungs fill with air, the stretch receptors sense the expansion and signal the nervous system regarding the degree of movement.

The autonomic nervous system plays a large role in the function of the respiratory system. There is smooth muscle from the trachea all the way down to the alveoli. The smooth muscle within the bronchi and bronchioles responds to parasympathetic stimulation from the **vagus nerve (cranial nerve X)**. Acetylcholine is released, which causes the muscle to contract and thus constrict the airway. This, in turn, will cause changes in air intake, which may have been triggered by the central nervous system perceiving hypoxia. In contrast, there is also sympathetic innervation to the smooth muscle. Triggering these neurotransmitters will cause dilation of the airways.

Gas Exchange

Just as the pressure within the chest leads to inhalation or exhalation, gas exchange itself is based on pressure differentials. Gas exchange includes a number of molecules. For our purposes, the term "gas exchange" refers to the delivery of oxygen to the bloodstream and the infiltration of carbon dioxide into the alveolus so that it can be exhaled (see Figure 24.2). We generally talk about **partial pressure**, which refers to the pressure of a particular gas relative to the overall gas/air pressure of the surrounding area. The abbreviation "**Pa**" is used to indicate partial pressure. Thus, **PaO$_2$** is the partial pressure of oxygen in an area, and **PaCO$_2$** is the partial pressure of carbon dioxide.

Note that neither PaO$_2$ nor PaCO$_2$ is a static number. PaO$_2$ will necessarily fluctuate with inhalation and exhalation. The amount of oxygen, and thus its pressure, will vary based on how much air is entering or leaving the system. In fact, the exchange of oxygen and carbon dioxide that occurs between the alveolus and the capillary is the source of fluctuation of oxygen pressure in the alveolus itself.

Despite the fluctuation, the alveolus will normally have a higher PaO$_2$ than the capillaries flowing past it. The blood flowing from the heart to the lung carries a very low PaO$_2$, the oxygen having already been depleted by the body as the blood passes through the animal. The oxygen will diffuse from where its pressure is the highest (the alveolus) to the capillaries, where PaO$_2$ is lower. The reverse occurs with PaCO$_2$, which is higher in the capillaries than in the alveoli.

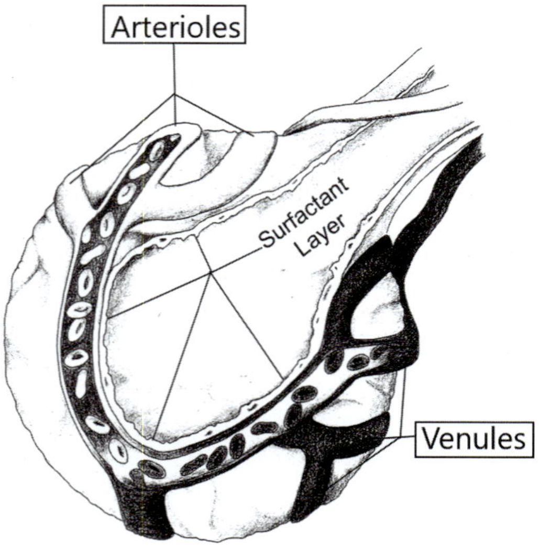

One of the things that make the surface of the alveolus more efficient in gas exchange is a material on its luminal surface called **surfactant**. Surfactant is a liquid containing proteins and fats that serves to decrease the surface tension within the alveoli. Remember that alveoli are made of very thin walls and that air in the respiratory system is moist. This moisture is necessary to help with gas exchange but can cause an issue without surfactant. Surfactant reduces the surface tension within the alveoli or, in other words, helps the alveoli remain open and avoid collapsing in and sticking to themselves. Puppies or kittens (or humans, for that matter) that are born prematurely have not developed a sufficient layer of surfactant and thus have significant neonatal respiratory distress, as their alveoli cannot open as efficiently and perform adequate gas exchange.

Certain diseases and toxins can alter the permeability of the alveoli. In inflammatory conditions, gas exchange is less efficient as a result of the increased thickness of the swollen tissues. One of the basic principles underlying the administration of pure oxygen to an animal with respiratory distress is the increase of PaO$_2$ that results within the

Figure 24.2 The alveolus. The venules and arterioles pass around the alveolus, and gases are exchanged across the surface of the interior.

alveolus. This strengthens the ability of the oxygen to cross the alveolar border and to enter the capillary. The increased movement of oxygen into the bloodstream will allow more CO_2 to diffuse out of the bloodstream.

Having discussed pressure ratios in a little more detail, it is time to return to the subject of the V/Q mismatch. If the normal function of the respiratory system depends on the gas pressure and the speed of the bloodstream being ideally synchronized, anything that interferes with that match may make gas transfer less efficient. Potential interferences with V/Q matching include increased cardiac output. It is akin to trying to catch a taxi while it is still moving by; the greater speed and volume of blood passing by the alveolus hinder the efficiency of gas exchange.

The other side of this problem is that of an insufficient respiratory rate. If the PaO_2 is not high enough in the alveolus, it will not cross over to the capillaries. Animals that have been exercising will often pant; this increases oxygen intake by way of increasing the respiratory rate, in an effort to balance out the increased cardiac output that accompanies exercise. Note that panting without sufficient tidal volume will create a significant deficit in the alveolar PaO_2.

Hemoglobin

Once the blood is oxygenated, it returns to the heart so that it can be pumped out into the body. However, oxygen is poorly soluble in water. Very little of it will enter the plasma, and thus it would be difficult for it to get into the cells of the body. The solution to this is a molecule called **hemoglobin**. Refer to Figure 14.2 to review the structure of hemoglobin.

Hemoglobin is a pigmented molecule that has four substructures called **hemes**. Each heme is associated with a particular protein. These proteins are the same within a given species of animal but usually differ among species. The hemoglobin is a constituent of the red blood cell. Its pigment is what gives the cell its characteristic color; the oxidation of the iron within the pigment leads to the color change.

Since there are four hemes for each molecule of hemoglobin, and each heme holds a molecule of oxygen, each red blood cell carries four oxygen molecules. Multiplying the number of red blood cells (erythrocytes) by four will yield the amount of oxygen molecules the bloodstream is carrying. Given that there are millions of red blood cells in a typical dog or cat, the number is impressive.

Another constituent of hemoglobin is **iron molecules**. **Anemia**, the condition of having insufficient red blood cells, can be associated with iron deficiency. Animals with severe anemia are often given iron supplements in recognition of this concept.

Hemoglobin acquires oxygen by way of the binding of oxygen to the ferrous (iron) components of the hemoglobin molecule. The more oxygen that is acquired, the more readily the hemoglobin will take more oxygen on. This phenomenon is called **affinity**. It is analogous to opening a door a little wider each time a person comes in, until all four people have come in (i.e., all four hemes have attached to oxygen, making it **oxyhemoglobin**).

Thus, oxygen is carried through the bloodstream by hemoglobin. At some point, it needs to dissociate itself from the blood so that it can be taken up by the tissues. The **oxyhemoglobin dissociation curve** is a mathematical representation of what it takes for the oxygen molecules to "free themselves" from the hemoglobin.

Hemoglobin does have a limit to how much oxygen it can carry. When the hemoglobin is at 100% of its carrying capacity, it is said to be saturated. As the blood leaves the lungs, the hemoglobin is close to its saturation point. Traveling through the body, the oxygen will be drawn off whenever the surrounding tissue has a relatively low amount of oxygen (low oxygen pressure). This is known as the **dissociation point**.

The exact amount of oxygen that reaches the dissociation point is not a fixed number. Several factors have an effect on how many oxygen molecules have to build up before they "jump off" the hemoglobin. For one thing, the dissociation point varies depending on the relative oxygenation of the tissue that surrounds it. If the local cells are full of oxygen, there is not enough of a pressure difference to encourage the oxygen to leave the hemoglobin.

In anemia, the overall carrying capacity of oxygen in the blood is diminished. Because not much oxygen is getting to the tissues, it does not take much for there to be a big difference between the oxygen pressure in the hemoglobin and that in the tissues. Once there is enough of a difference, the oxygen will dissociate. Since the oxygen dissociates sooner than it ordinarily would (say, by the time it gets to the abdominal organs), the hemoglobin that gets around to the later parts of the system has already depleted its reserves.

When an animal is hyperthermic, the increased temperature of the blood will make it easier for oxygen to dissociate. The point at which the ratio of hemoglobin oxygen concentration and body tissue oxygen concentration will be more favorable occurs at a lower level of oxygen when there are higher local temperatures. In essence, it is easier to off-load the oxygen at a higher blood temperature.

The reverse is true when the animal is hypothermic. The oxygen pressure in the tissues of the body must be lower than normal in order for oxygen to dissociate from the hemoglobin. Warming the animal gradually will allow the normal gradient (relative amount of difference between one thing and another) of oxygen pressure to reassert itself so the dissociation point returns to normal.

Unfortunately, oxygen is not the only thing that binds to hemoglobin. **Carbon monoxide** has 200 times the binding capacity to heme that oxygen does. Animals exposed to high levels of carbon monoxide will have so much of it bound to their heme that there will be no room for oxygen to bind with it. Nitrites and other toxins can bind to the iron in the heme and also prevent the binding of oxygen to the hemoglobin. Nitrites are a particular problem in ruminant feeds in that they are found to be a contaminant in food that has been poorly processed or stored.

Methemoglobin is a type of hemoglobin molecule in which the typical ferrous iron molecule of hemoglobin has been changed to ferric iron through oxidation. Ferric iron cannot bind to oxygen, and the remaining ferrous iron in the molecule then has a strong affinity to bind oxygen. This process means that methemoglobin cannot effectively deposit oxygen to tissues. Small amounts of methemoglobin typically do not have systemic effects and can even be converted back to regular hemoglobin; however, if there is a condition of high levels of methemoglobin, **methemoglobinemia**, the patient will be symptomatic. Methemoglobinemia can be caused by genetic disorders or by toxicities from ibuprofen and acetaminophen.

Carbon Dioxide

Just as the blood that enters systemic circulation from the left ventricle is heavily oxygenated, the blood that enters the venous system has dropped off most of its oxygen and is now carrying the metabolic by-product, carbon dioxide. Carbon dioxide can be carried in solution in the blood. It can also be carried in the cytoplasm of the red blood cell in the form of its metabolites: **bicarbonate** and oxygen. In fact, when blood is analyzed chemically in standard clinical practice, the measurement of bicarbonate levels is used to infer levels of carbon dioxide in the blood. The measurement of carbon dioxide is much more difficult than the measurement of bicarbonate.

As the venous blood circulates and arrives at the alveoli, the CO_2 pressure is much higher in the bloodstream than in the alveoli. It will thus be drawn into the alveolus, where the $PaCO_2$ is normally low and will be exhaled.

Carbon dioxide can cause significant illness if not expelled from the body. High levels of carbon dioxide in the bloodstream result in **acidemia**, or **low blood pH**. Remember that the normal pH of the mammalian blood is about 7.4, and anything that changes the pH greater than ±0.5 points (7.3 and below or 7.5 and above) can cause clinical signs.

Anything that impedes the exchange of gases across the alveolar boundary, such as pulmonary disease, can result in acidemia. Increased respiratory rate is a method of literally blowing out more carbon dioxide in an attempt to raise blood pH back to normal. The term **respiratory acidosis** refers to the increase in blood levels of carbon dioxide associated with the inability of the lung to absorb and eliminate this gas.

Respiratory alkalosis is associated with hyperventilation, or too high of a respiratory rate. In cases of hypoxia or pulmonary disease, respiratory rate will increase. In this case, carbon dioxide leaves the body at a greater-than-normal rate, and the body is not able to keep up with its production. Having less than a normal amount of carbon dioxide in the lung is actually problematic in that it raises blood pH beyond the norm. Some normal metabolic functions are only possible with pH at an optimal level. Therefore, either respiratory alkalosis or acidosis is a problem. Testing of blood pH is easily done with conventional blood testing equipment.

Chemoreceptors

There are chemoreceptors in various locations. They monitor the relative amounts of oxygen and carbon dioxide in the bloodstream, as well as blood pH. Chemoreceptors are located in the carotid and aortic bodies, and in the medulla oblongata.

The **carotid body** is a collection of receptors near the branching of the external and internal carotid arteries. The **aortic body** is, not surprisingly, seated in connective tissue around the aortic arch. They are particularly responsive to hypoxia (low levels of oxygen), hypercapnia (high levels of carbon dioxide), and acidemia (low pH). The central chemoreceptors are present on the ventrolateral surface of the medulla oblongata. This area is even more sensitive to carbon dioxide levels. Anything, respiratory or metabolic, that causes changes in pH or gas levels will be sensed by these chemoreceptors.

The carotid body is more active in juveniles, and the aortic body in older animals. The medulla of the brain is very sensitive to pH throughout the animal's life. Together, these chemoreceptors monitor blood gases and pH and help determine the respiratory rate and tidal volume. The information from these areas is also used by the renal system. When pH is sensed as being too high (alkaline), the renal tubules will excrete more bicarbonate, which is alkaline. When the pH is sensed as being too low (acidic), the renal tubules will excrete more H+ ions, which are acidic. The body will use anything it can to compensate, so if the animal has respiratory acidosis, the kidneys will try to correct that by excreting acids. Similarly, if the animal has respiratory acidosis, the body will increase the respiratory rate in order to expel more acids in the form of CO_2.

Mechanisms to Increase Oxygenation

If a lack of oxygen is sensed by the chemoreceptors, there are a number of resources with which to work. As noted earlier, increasing core temperature will encourage oxygen dissociation from hemoglobin, making more of it available. Increasing cardiac output will also help. The increased amount of blood in circulation allows for the availability of more oxygen.

Two minor ways are also available for increasing oxygen supplies. One is **splenic contraction**. The spleen has a large number of erythrocytes in it, which, in turn, carry oxygen as they normally do. The organ can contract and add to the total blood volume. This is only a minor contribution.

As noted in Chapter 19, one of the materials in skeletal muscle is called **myoglobin**. Myoglobin does have a small store of oxygen in it. If the oxygen level of the blood brought to the muscle is not enough, the myoglobin can contribute at least a little so that muscle function may continue.

Species Differences

Fish, amphibians, and lizards all have somewhat different respiratory systems, and all differ from those of mammals. Avians, however, are unique.

The body of the bird contains air sacs, extending from the neck to the caudal abdomen. It is the air sacs that do the contraction and expansion that draws air in and pushes it out of the body. While the actual gas exchange is done in the lung, just as in a mammal, the lung is relatively quite small and does not undergo any rhythmic change in size or shape. Refer to Figure 11.6 in the respiratory anatomy chapter for a diagram.

As the main bronchus travels cranially to caudally, it runs through the entire horizontal axis of the lung. It gives off airways of diminishing diameter, fed by the air sacs, which are eventually the size of capillaries. These air capillaries are paired with blood capillaries in the lung, and gas exchange occurs across their surfaces.

The air sacs are large enough, and the lung parenchyma is dense enough, that rupture of one area of the air sac is not enough to cause atelectasis. On the other hand, the tissue of the air sacs, which have the appearance of Bubble Wrap, is rather delicate. This fact, coupled with the necessity of strong muscle contraction so that the entire system of air sacs can move as one, has great clinical significance. When restraining a bird for examination, it is important not to hold the body of the bird too tightly, particularly in the mid-thorax. Excess pressure on the muscles of inhalation will strangle the bird, as the lung has no way to draw air in for itself.

Clinical Case Resolution: Tictac

It is evident from a brief physical examination that Tictac is in critical condition. He is given 100% oxygen through a mask and an intravenous catheter is placed. At the time of intravenous catheter placement, blood gases are checked, which reveal that Tictac is experiencing respiratory acidosis. Auscultation reveals reduced breath sounds and cardiac arrythmia.

In order to better understand what is happening to Tictac after being hit by a car, radiographs of the chest and abdomen are recommended along with other emergency stabilization steps. The owner agrees to this plan.

Tictac's thoracic and abdominal radiographs show that there is intestine inside the thoracic cavity. This is called a diaphragmatic hernia, where the diaphragm is torn, allowing abdominal organs to enter the thoracic cavity.

Steps are taken to stabilize Tictac with oxygen supplementation, supportive care, and pain management. Once Tictac is stabilized, he will have to undergo surgical correction of his diaphragmatic hernia to resolve his inability to appropriately ventilate. Patients with trauma-induced diaphragmatic hernias always carry a guarded prognosis and require extensive hospitalization and care.

Clinical Case Critical Thinking

1) *Consider the patient history. What likely caused the diaphragm to have a tear in it? Do you think the patient's size had any effect on this injury?*
2) *Why does a diaphragmatic hernia cause dyspnea? What happens to the lungs and the pressure in the thoracic cavity?*
3) *Why would supplementing oxygen for Tictac be helpful?*
4) *Why was Tictac given pain medications along with his stabilization?*
5) *What other complications might arise from having abdominal organs enter the thoracic space?*

Review Questions

1 What is physiological dead space?
- **A** The anatomic spaces in the respiratory tract that do not participate in gas exchange
- **B** The alveoli that are not participating in the same level of gas exchange
- **C** The small amount of air that remains in the lungs after exhalation
- **D** Both A and B
- **E** Both B and C

2 What is the term for the amount of air moved in one single breath?
- **A** Tidal volume
- **B** Minute volume
- **C** Stroke volume
- **D** Cardiac output

3 What temperature increases oxygenation of tissues?
- **A** Lower body temperatures
- **B** Higher body temperatures
- **C** Temperature does not affect oxygenation

4 What is the term for a lung collapse?

5 True or False: PaO_2 is a static number that will be the same at all times.
- **A** True
- **B** False

6 What is the dissociation point?
- **A** The point at which all hemoglobin molecules are saturated with oxygen
- **B** The point at which CO_2 is too high
- **C** The point at which O_2 is released to the tissue based on low oxygen pressure
- **D** The point at which ferrous iron changes to ferric iron

7 When might we expect to see respiratory alkalosis?
- **A** Tachypnea
- **B** Bradypnea
- **C** Hyperthermia
- **D** None of the above

8 Which part of the autonomic nervous system causes bronchodilation?
 A The parasympathetic nervous system
 B The sympathetic nervous system
 C The somatic nervous system
 D The rest and digest system

9 What is surfactant?

10 True or False: Methemoglobinemia is the condition where hemoglobin molecules cannot fit into the alveoli to pick up oxygen.
 A True
 B False

25

Digestive Physiology

> **Clinical Case: Laney a 5-Year-Old Female Spayed Miniature Schnauzer**
>
> *Laney is brought into the clinic with watery diarrhea and a very painful abdomen. As per the owners, she was mildly lethargic yesterday and a little bit less interested in food. They joked that she must have been spoiled because, over the weekend, a houseguest fed her bacon and eggs with cheese for breakfast, but now she won't eat anything at all and is presenting with the signs above. Laney yelps when she is lifted from the ground, supporting her owners concern about pain.*

Introduction

In Chapter 12, it was noted that the system is extraordinarily complex, both within and among species. In discussing physiology, the complexity increases. This chapter will concentrate on cats and dogs, with a nod toward other species. The basic function of the digestive tract is to receive, mechanically reduce, and chemically process materials such that nutrients are absorbed, and unnecessary materials are excreted. Nutrients are absorbed so that they can be directed to the rest of the body by way of the bloodstream. **Feces** are the materials excreted from the digestive tract. While the renal system also excretes material, it has a completely different biochemical function and so is treated as a separate entity.

The Entryway

Any material the animal ingests that preserves life is considered a **nutrient**. This includes things that may not be considered as food by the layperson.

In critical nursing, one of the first considerations is **hydration status**. Water is not only a nutrient, but it is also one of the most important ones. Animals can live longer without food than without water. As noted earlier, much of the composition of the cells of the body is water. The accessibility of potable water is crucial, and the ability to drink it is essential.

In dogs and cats, most food is accessed by a combination of the lips, tongue, and teeth. Food can be brought in by lips, tongue, and teeth to varying degrees, depending on the nature of the food and the species. In horses, the lips are **prehensile**; they are very mobile and can actually wrap around grass and other food material in order to bring them into the mouth, almost like an elephant's trunk.

Once inside the mouth, a number of activities begin. **Mechanical digestion**, which is to say the physical grinding down of the food, is accomplished by grinding of the teeth and movement of the **bolus**, or ball, of food by the tongue and **buccinator** (cheek) **muscles** so that the material is shifted from one side of the mouth to the other. This would be difficult if the material were dry. The **salivary glands** are stimulated by the smell and/or feel of food in the mouth. They produce **saliva**, which, in addition to moisture, has small amounts of enzymes that aid in digestion. For example, canine saliva contains some **amylase**, which helps digest starches. There is little, if any, amylase in feline saliva. This is not surprising, considering that felines are true carnivores, while canines are omnivores. Felines thus have much less starch in their diet (at least, they should).

Note that the mouth has functions other than those of digestion. The mouth has a role in amplifying sound. It also serves a respiratory function, allowing air to pass in and out when the nasal passages are not able to conduct enough air during breathing. The mucous membranes of the mouth help in thermoregulation in that their moisture allows for the evaporation that aids in cooling when the mouth is open. Finally, the teeth serve as a method of defense or aggression (or both).

Teeth

In dogs and cats, the "puppy" or "kitten" teeth that grow during the first few months of life are referred to as **deciduous**, meaning temporary, teeth. The adult teeth start to grow underneath them, and eventually, the deciduous teeth are pushed out of the mouth and the adult teeth remain. The adult, or permanent, teeth in dogs and cats stay the same size for the rest of the animals' lives. Dog and cat teeth **brachydont**, meaning they have finite growth or stay the same size.

The term "**hypsodont**" refers to teeth that continue to grow throughout the animals' life. In horses, the teeth continue to increase in length and thickness as the animal ages. Only the acts of chewing and food abrasion keep the teeth from growing too big. In rabbits, the incisor teeth are also hypsodont.

Dental care is important for all animals. Diseases of the teeth and gums can be associated with problems in many organ systems, particularly in the gastrointestinal (GI) tract and heart. Since equine teeth can easily overgrow, particularly if the animal's diet is inappropriate or if there is an abnormal chewing pattern, regular dental care is crucial. The abnormal size and shape of teeth under these conditions can cause pain and even reluctance to eat. Filing the teeth down to a normal size and shape is called **floating** the teeth.

Neglected rabbits can have such severe overgrowth of the maxillary incisors that they are unable to eat; the teeth can curve over the lower teeth and start to curl toward the chin. Most often, a Dremel drill is used to bring the teeth down to a normal size. The same procedure is used to trim the beak of a bird. A rabbit whose teeth are severely overgrown will sometimes have to have part of the crown of the tooth cut off by a clipper-type instrument called a **rongeur**. Any abnormality that causes the upper and lower teeth to not meet properly when biting down is called a **malocclusion**.

The tartar that forms on the teeth of dogs and cats contains bacteria. Left uncleaned, the bacteria can travel throughout the bloodstream and GI tract as they are swallowed. At one time, dental disease was one of the main causes of **endocarditis** or infection of the heart valves or interior of the cardiac chambers, as some of the bacteria would settle into the nooks and crannies of the valve structure.

See Figure 25.1 for a modified **Triadan chart**. The Triadan system is a way of numbering the teeth so that they can be identified easily. It is more efficient to note that tooth 204 is missing than to say that the maxillary left canine is missing. Using a chart like this, which can be printed onto the dental medical record, makes it easy to record which teeth are missing or extracted when dental work is done.

In dogs and cats, the teeth accomplish both biting and tearing functions. This breaks food into manageable pieces so that it can be swallowed. These pieces are shepherded toward the caudal oral cavity by the tongue. As the bolus of food reaches the caudal oral cavity, the swallow reflex is triggered.

Moving Toward the Stomach

Recall that as the **oropharynx** extends caudally, it leads to two different paths. One, **the trachea**, is designed only to transport air. If food or water were to travel down the trachea, it would access the bronchi and significantly interfere with the function of the lungs. One reason we insist that dogs and cats be fasted before undergoing anesthesia is that, if there is food in the upper GI tract and the animal has an **emetic** reaction to anesthesia (i.e., vomits in reaction to the drug), the food may be aspirated, or drawn down the trachea instead of remaining in the esophagus. The epiglottis closes when the animal swallows, and the vocal cords close in order to prevent this occurrence when the animal is eating.

When eating or drinking, the food and water follow the path down into the **esophagus**. A combination of striated and smooth muscles contracts and expands in a rolling wave to push the bolus of food toward the stomach. This wave is referred to as **peristalsis**.

The actions of smelling food, chewing, and swallowing set in motion the production of digestive enzymes in the stomach. As the bolus of food reaches the distal esophagus, its sphincter opens, allowing the food to enter the stomach. If the sphincter were open at all times, food could proceed from the stomach into the esophagus and even exit the body. Some diseases cause reverse peristalsis, such that ingesta exit the body. This is known as **emesis**, better known as vomiting.

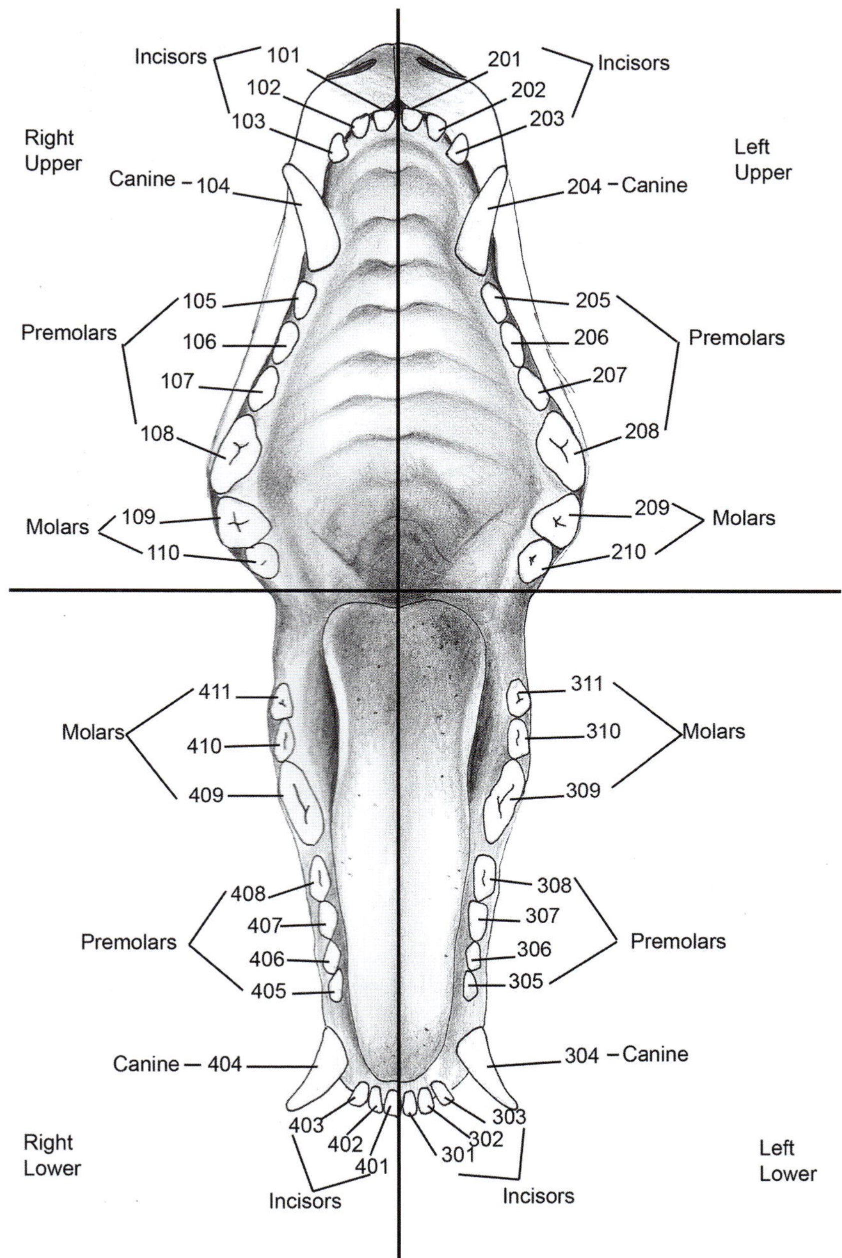

Figure 25.1 The modified Triadan chart is a way of identifying each tooth by a separate number, such that it is clear which teeth are on the left or right and which are maxillary or mandibular. For numbering purposes, the mouth is divided into four quadrants: upper left, upper right, lower left, and lower right. This image also appears in Chapter 12.

While most people use the term GI tract to refer to the entire tube from mouth to anus, GI stands for gastrointestinal. Therefore, properly, GI only refers to the system from the stomach to the exit from the body. It is also important to remember that digestive activity is mostly mediated by the parasympathetic nervous system.

The Stomach

Once food reaches the stomach, a number of changes occur. The **rugae**, or folds, of the stomach are more convoluted and greater in number than the rugae of the dorsal oral cavity. These gastric luminal ridges expand and contract, as do the muscles of the stomach wall, and serve to increase the surface area of the stomach. They also help to some extent in mechanically breaking down food.

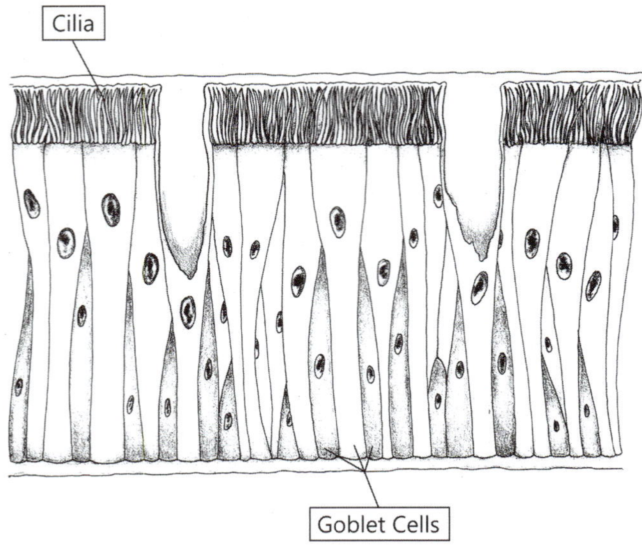

Figure 25.2 Goblet cells.

The luminal surface of the stomach is covered with microscopic **goblet cells**, which produce mucus. Mucus not only helps lubricate the ingesta (which is what the food and water are now called) but also helps buffer the tissue of the stomach against the low pH of its fluids (Figure 25.2).

Deep to the mucus-producing cells, and also on a microscopic level, are a series of peaks and valleys. The peaks resemble a finger being pointed and are referred to as **villi**. Halfway down the villi are **parietal cells**, which produce **hydrochloric acid (HCl)**. At the bottom of the villus, in the "valley," are **chief cells**, which produce an enzyme called **pepsinogen**. Pepsinogen leads to the production of **pepsin**; this transformation is triggered by low pH. Pepsin is particularly important in protein digestion and thus plays a major role in the GI tract of carnivores and omnivores. The goal of antacid medications is to reduce the overproduction of these fluids.

The production of HCl is helpful in breaking down food products by virtue of its acidic nature. The byproduct of HCl production is **bicarbonate (HCO$_3$)** in the bloodstream. HCO$_3$ is quite **alkaline** or **basic** on the pH scale. As it enters the bloodstream, it may raise the pH of the blood. These fluctuations in pH are also of clinical importance in both evaluating the overall acidity of the system and fashioning drugs to treat various disorders.

A material called **gastrin** is produced by **G cells** in the stomach lining (and in the pancreas and duodenum). Gastrin has an effect on parietal cells (and, on a lesser level, chief cells) to produce more HCl and pepsin. As mentioned earlier, HCl production causes an increase in HCO$_3$ in the blood. This is then circulated to the pancreas, which picks the HCO$_3$ up and secretes it into the small intestine via pancreatic secretions. Once pH reaches a certain point, a negative feedback loop is triggered regarding gastrin. In other words, as digestion continues, less gastrin is needed, and so rising pH signals the cells to stop producing gastrin.

Another "side effect" of gastrin production is the release of **histamine** in the stomach, which also contributes to the eventual lowering of stomach pH by promoting HCl production. Thus, antihistamines can also play a role in changing gastric pH.

As the enzymes do their work, a number of chemical changes occur, involving the breakdown of nutrients into their constituents. Proteins are broken down into amino acids. Starches are broken down into short-chain polysaccharides.

The gastric parietal cells of canines produce **intrinsic factor**, which is a glycoprotein that helps the body absorb vitamin B12. B12 is an essential vitamin in mammals that is integral to many body functions like DNA synthesis, red blood cell production, protein synthesis, and more. In cats, intrinsic factor is produced by the small intestine.

Entering the Small Intestine

Once the food bolus reaches the pyloric antrum and enzyme activity increases, the pyloric sphincter will open, allowing the ingesta, now called **chyme** after gastric breakdown, to continue into the duodenum. Chyme is an acidic mix of broken-down food and water with the addition of HCl. When the chyme enters the duodenum, it triggers the release of two important chemicals: **cholecystokinin** and **secretin**. Cholecystokinin helps to slow gastric emptying, so the release of acidic material into the duodenum is slow enough to be processed. It also causes an increase of HCO$_3$ secretion to neutralize some of the acidic chyme, while triggering the gallbladder to release **bile** and the pancreas to secrete digestive enzymes. Secretin helps to lower the production of HCl in the stomach and increase HCO$_3$ and pancreatic secretion.

The digestive enzymes produced by the pancreas are **amylase, lipase**, and **trypsin**. In the pancreas, these are **proenzymes** or inactive enzymes. They will become activated once they enter the duodenum. Amylase is an enzyme that helps digest starches. Lipase, as the root word "lipid" implies, helps digest fats. By the process of elimination, trypsin "digests" proteins.

In discussing the endocrine system, the role of the pancreas as an endocrine organ is noted in that it produces several hormones. Insulin is one of those. Digestive enzymes are not hormones. The production of these enzymes is called **exocrine** rather than endocrine. Thus, the pancreas is both an exocrine and an endocrine organ. It is the exocrine function that we discuss in connection with digestion.

In addition to providing a place for preliminary digestion of starches, fats, and proteins, the duodenum has a role in **enterohepatic circulation**. As is implied by its name, there is a loop between the small intestine (root word "entero-") and liver (hepatic is the adjectival form for the liver) that involves the circulation of substances like **bile acids**. These help the system regulate itself.

As discussed, when chyme reaches the duodenum, a signal is sent to the gallbladder, telling it to release bile by way of cholecystokinin. The bile enters the duodenum through the biliary duct into the duodenum. Bile acids are vital for fat digestion. As the acids continue to work, they eventually reach the ileum. At this point, they are broken down enough to circulate back to the liver to suppress bile production. This, too, is a negative feedback loop and another example of the way in which the system is self-sustaining without the animal's conscious control.

Throughout the small intestine, digestive molecules produced in the enterocytes (cells of the small intestine) percolate through the lining of the intestine and are directed out into the lumen of the intestine. This is known as the **membranous phase** of digestion. There are specific enzymes for the various **polysaccharides** and **peptides** (protein products) allowing them to be processed.

Cranially in the GI system, carbohydrates are broken down into **lactose, starch**, and **sucrose**. In the membranous phase of digestion, these items are further broken down into various sugars.

Of all of the materials the organism ingests, some are not needed. However, many of them are needed. It is mostly within the small intestine that material is absorbed to be channeled into systemic circulation. This absorption is accomplished in a number of ways. Some material passively moves from within the lumen of the intestine to the surrounding tissue and circulation. For example, water is able to "slip out" between cells of the intestinal wall. Passive transport usually is most efficient when the balance of molecular weight favors osmotic movement.

Another method of exchange is called **cotransport**. The most common example of this involves sodium. An electrolyte crucial to the production of many types of energy, its exit from the intestine can "drag along" other molecules such as glucose. Water is another molecule that tends to follow sodium, described in detail when looking at the function of the nephron in the kidney.

Active transport involves the production of energy that pushes or pulls material into or out of a cell. In the case of the GI tract, it is ATP that, when hydrolyzed, forces sodium out between the cells of the intestinal wall (and allowing potassium in). Recall that **hydrolysis** is the action of breaking chemical bonds by inserting a water molecule. Hydrolysis is a major player in digestion and is another reason that hydration status is a key part of normal function. It should also be noted that a by-product of hydrolysis is HCO_3.

The absorption of nutrients is not the only function of digestion. Some materials do need to be excreted; these do not normally transport out of the intestine. In fact, one of the hallmarks of GI disease is that materials are not absorbed or excreted properly. For example, if the ingesta has a high salt content, it will draw water into the intestine from the surrounding tissue, and thus too much water will be excreted.

The microscopic structure of the jejunum and ileum includes the presence of villi. They are tallest in the jejunum and get shorter and broader as the system continues toward the anus. The enzymes produced in the villi differ from place to place.

The small and large intestines also maintain a wave of peristalsis. Different sections of the bowel are active at any given time, which is why the intestine appears to change shape as the animal is digesting. The term **motility** refers to the movement of the walls of the digestive tract. We generally refer to intestinal motility in describing some digestive diseases.

Under normal circumstances, motility of the intestinal tract is different when food is present and when it is not present. When food is present, the small intestine engages in **propulsion**, moving food along from stomach to colon. **Segmentation** results when small areas of the intestine form a series of expanded areas and very narrow areas, forming what appear to be sausage links. Segmentation allows for mixing and breaking up material but does not actually push the ingesta very far along the tract. When food is not present, there is some very slow wave motion, most likely designed to get rid of any amounts of undigested material. As the ingesta moves forward, it will approach the **ileocecocolic** junction, where the end of the ileum ("ileo-") becomes a blind-ended pouch called the **cecum** ("-ceco-") and connects to the colon ("-colic"). The cecum is a blind-ended pouch that plays a role in digestion of some species.

Transit time refers to the speed and nature of the motility of the intestines. If transit time is too fast, material will not have a chance to be digested and will come out as more liquid than solid. This is the case in diseases that cause diarrhea. If transit time is slow, material can come to obstruct the intestine. If transit time is slow through the colon, in particular, the animal will be constipated.

The Colon

The major function of the colon, in addition to funneling the material out of the body, is to resorb water. This is the body's last chance to reserve fluid from the GI tract before it is expelled from the body. When faced with the continuing presence of material in the distal colon, it will continue to withdraw more and more fluid. This is why feces from a constipated animal are small and hard; the water content has been almost totally removed. Unfortunately, the drier the feces, the harder it is to expel them, and the more time there is for water to be withdrawn. This condition is called **constipation**. This condition is treated with drugs called **laxatives**. Most laxatives have an osmotic effect that increases the colonic water content to rehydrate the fecal material. They may also work as a stimulant to generate colonic contractions to expel fecal material.

Recall that the anal sphincter has both smooth muscle and striated muscle sections. What this means is that the animal does have some voluntary control over defecation. By the same token, though, if the pressure to defecate is strong enough, it will overcome that control, and the smooth muscle section will open enough to cause feces to emerge. Inflammatory conditions put the control of these muscles under great stress. It is also of great importance if any surgery is done in the area of the anus. Interruption of the nerve controlling the anal sphincter can cause incontinence.

The Liver

The liver is a highly vascularized organ that is involved in the majority of the bodily systems, including the digestive tract. The gallbladder produces bile, which is conducted through the liver by way of a series of small ducts until it reaches the duodenum. Bile enters the intestines and gets converted into **stercobilinogen** and then into **stercobilin**. Stercobilin is dark brown/red and gives feces its color. The liver also participates directly in digestion in its role in filtering out material that has been resorbed from the intestines.

The enterohepatic circulation is also known as **portal circulation**. Some dogs are born with an abnormality in the vessels of the liver that affect the portal circulation. Instead of blood and waste products flowing back from the liver to the intestines, the material escapes through an abnormal blood vessel that **shunts** (diverts) the unwanted material into the systemic circulation. Known as a **portosystemic shunt**, it is characteristically associated with what appear to be neurological signs. This is because among the liver's roles is that of assisting with the breakdown of proteins. One of these breakdown products, **ammonia**, can be transported directly to the brain when a shunt of this type is present. Ammonia causes damage to the brain tissue, and neurological signs emerge. The condition is surgically remediable and medically manageable in the short term.

Another role of the liver is the storage of **glycogen**. In times of stress, the liver can use this to assist in regulating blood glucose. A condition called **diabetic ketoacidosis** occurs when prolonged states of very low blood glucose occur. This happens in a diabetic animal when insulin is not regulated well and/or given properly, as insulin allows the cells to use the glucose. The liver will engage in the production of glucose to replenish the body's supply, in a process called **gluconeogenesis**. Unfortunately, if this continues over a long period of time, the liver can start to produce a by-product of this process known as a **ketone**. Ketones are damaging to any tissues that surround them and also cause the pH of the blood to drop.

As alluded to earlier, the liver plays a role in filtering toxins. It is also able to break down many medications. This can make them easier for the body to use or to eliminate. The liver also participates in the production of some of the elements that allow blood to clot. All of this is in addition to its role in assembling materials that are used to form feces.

In the dog, heart disease can affect the liver directly. This is because enlargement or inefficiency of the heart can cause a pressure "backup" in the vena cava, which passes near the liver on its way to the heart. This, in turn, causes pressure within the liver to increase dramatically. Fluid from within the soft tissue of the liver can actually be forced out of the liver and into the surrounding space of the abdomen. **Ascites**, excess fluid in the abdomen, can thus be caused by effusion of fluid from the liver, in response to cardiac disease or other inflammatory processes.

Species Differentiation

There are a few issues regarding other species that contrast to the system in dogs and cats. For example, equines and lago-morphs do most of their digestion in the cecum. The cecum is relatively large in comparison to the cecum of dogs and cats, and it is crucial to their ability to metabolize food. Animals that are cecal digesters actually ferment their food rather than utilize the enzymes we discussed earlier. One of the reasons that horses and rabbits do not vomit is that the digested food is so far along in the system that it cannot work its way back to the surface.

The reader will have noticed that horses and rabbits have much in common from a metabolic standpoint.

The ruminant digestive system, as the reader will recall, has a four-chambered stomach, not four stomachs. It does not help that mammals like dogs and cats are referred to as monogastric, implying that other species have more stomachs. The construction of the ruminant GI tract is designed to accommodate its diet in an extraordinary manner.

The cow subsists on a diet consisting mainly of **cellulose**, the major constituent of grass/hay. Cellulose, like fats, is hard to digest. From the outset, the bovine uses aggressive methods to break down food. The amount of amylase in cow saliva is multiplied many times compared to that in dogs. As amylase is designed to digest starch, it is clear that some aspects of digestion occur before the food reaches the stomach.

Material travels through the esophagus into the cranial-most part of the bovine stomach, known as the **reticulum**. The reticulum is positioned near the heart. The reticulum and the next chamber, the **rumen**, work together to process food. The rumen is the largest of the chambers. Food processed in these areas is returned to the oral cavity to be broken down further. A cow "chewing her cud" is regrinding her food and adding more amylase so that the pieces are small enough to be pro-cessed further.

The reticulum, rumen, and third chamber, **the omasum** are known as the **forestomach**. They contain a normal popula-tion of bacteria and fungi that help the enzymes present to process cellulose. The cellulose is broken down to various saccharides, which, in turn, are used for energy.

The purpose of the forestomach is to process food by way of **fermentation**. This means that the process is **anaerobic** or does not require oxygen. In fact, the use of bacteria, protozoa, and fungi to break down sugars into carbon dioxide and fatty acids provides the main source of energy for the animal. Proteins and other materials can also be utilized, but they form a small part of the diet.

Fermentation is the main method of breaking down food in ruminants, equines, and lagomorphs. There is a "true stomach" in the ruminant, called the abomasum. This is a small section of the four-chambered stomach that performs some enzymatic functions similar to those of the dog and cat.

The pH balance in large animals is a more complex subject than in dogs and cats. Suffice it to say that rumen acidosis is a major problem in cattle, leading to illness and even death. In equines, it is believed that nutrition-related acidosis is a factor in laminitis, a hoof problem that is one of the leading reasons horses are euthanized due to the severity of its symptoms.

Clinical Case: Laney a 5-Year-Old FS Miniature Schnauzer

Laney has a physical examination which reveals an increased heart rate and respiratory rate. She has a fever and appears to be mildly hypersalivating. Her abdomen is tense and painful.

Given her history, the team is concerned that Laney has a primary GI issue and would like to pursue a few different tests—namely blood work, abdominal radiographs, and an abdominal ultrasound.

Abdominal radiographs show some gas-filled intestines but no obvious signs of a foreign body or something stuck in the intestines.

*Full blood work is pending, but a rapid test in the hospital is available to check for elevated pancreatic lipase. This value increases in the blood whenever the pancreas is inflamed. This rapid test reveals a positive result, indicating pancreatic inflammation or **pancreatitis**. Abdominal ultrasound reveals some abdominal effusion and a mildly enlarged pancreas.*

Pancreatitis is a condition in which the pancreatic enzymes are activated too early and start to digest the pancreas itself, causing inflammation. The enzymes can also spill out into the abdominal cavity and cause inflammation of other organs. This is a very painful process and can be a progressive disease resulting in serious complications.

It is thought that dietary indiscretion, particularly of high-fat foods, can be a trigger for pancreatitis; however, it can be idiopathic or possibly genetic. Miniature Schnauzers are overrepresented in cases of acute pancreatitis.

Laney is admitted to the hospital and given IV fluids, antiemetics, and pain medication. As she recovers, a low-fat prescrip-tion diet is introduced, and when her appetite returns and her pain is absent, she is sent home to remain on the low-fat diet for some time before transitioning back to her regular diet while monitoring at home for any changes or concerns.

Clinical Case Critical Thinking

1) *Why might Laney have an elevated heart rate and respiratory rate?*
2) *Why is Laney hypersalivating?*
3) *Why might pancreatic enzymes cause inflammation of other organs?*
4) *Why might Laney have abdominal effusion?*
5) *What part of Laney's history might be related to her diagnosis?*
6) *What advice might you give Laney's owners for the future?*

Review Questions

1 Where is intrinsic factor produced in dogs, and what does it do?
  A Within the small intestine, aids in the digestion of starches
  B Within the stomach, aids in the digestion of fats
  C Within the small intestine, aids in the absorption of B12
  D Within the stomach, aids in the absorption of B12

2 Which cells are responsible for producing pepsinogen?
  A Mucous neck cells
  B Parietal cells
  C Chief cells
  D G cells

3 What is the purpose of microorganism fermentation in the ruminant stomach?
  A To breakdown complex proteins like polypeptides
  B To breakdown complex fats like triglycerides
  C To breakdown complex carbohydrates like cellulose
  D None of the above

4 Which of the following inhibits or slows gastric emptying?
  A Cholecystokinin
  B Pepsinogen
  C Gastrin
  D Hydrogen chloride

5 Which organ is responsible for concentrating and storing bile?
  A The gallbladder
  B The liver
  C The pancreas
  D The stomach
  E The duodenum

6 Which group of pancreatic enzymes are responsible for breaking down starches?
  A Lipases
  B Amylases
  C Proteases
  D Proenzymes

7 Where do equines perform fermentation?
  A The ascending colon
  B The reticulum
  C The cecum
  D The rumen

8 True or False: Depending on the species, the labia oris and the tongue can be used for prehension.
  A True
  B False

9 Which species has hypsodont teeth?
  A Humans
  B Canines
  C Felines
  D Equines

10 If an animal is significantly dehydrated, what do we expect from the stool?
  A Very firm formed stool
  B Very soft stool
  C Diarrhea
  D Normal stool

26

Reproductive Physiology

<table><tr><td>Clinical Case: Diamond, a 6-Year-Old Female Intact Pitbull Terrier</td></tr><tr><td>Diamond is brought into the clinic because she seems lethargic and has a decreased appetite. She also appears to be drinking and urinating much more. She has never been bred before and had a heat cycle approximately 3 weeks ago. She is not up to date on vaccines and has not been to the vet since she was a puppy.</td></tr></table>

Introduction

There is a strong connection between the survivability of a species and its ability to bear viable young on a consistent basis. The combination of physical and chemical changes that occur in order for fertilization, pregnancy, and birth to occur in mammals has some things in common across species. There is much more variety in lizards and avians, for example. However, the clinician in small animal practice will be well served by investigation of mammalian reproduction.

The Female

The series of events preceding and following **ovulation** are known as the **estrous cycle**. **Estrus** (note that the spelling of the noun is different from the spelling of the adjective) is the part of the cycle that denotes the time of female sexual receptivity to the male. It is also known as "**heat**." The only species that has a cycle that occurs every month, year-round, is the primate. That cycle is referred to as **menstrual** rather than estrous. The word "menstrual" comes from the root word for month, while the word "estrous" refers to one of the major reproductive hormones, **estrogen**.

The combination of the **ovum** (egg) produced by the female and the **sperm** (fertilizing agent) produced by the male forms the basis of the developing **embryo**. There are some mammals that are born with sets of both male and female reproductive organs. These animals are **sterile**, or unable to reproduce. This is not true for all species; however, a single clownfish can produce both ova and sperm that are viable and lead to a newborn.

The **ovary** is the cranial-most part of the female reproductive system in dogs and cats. When a puppy or kitten is born, she has all the ova (egg cells) she will ever have. Whether she mates or not, there will be a steady decrease in the number of ova available throughout life. As a result, fertility decreases over time.

The ovarian or estrous cycle refers to the series of physical and hormonal changes that occur from one estrus to the next. The cycle has four parts. **Proestrus** is the series of chemical and structural changes that prepare the animal for ovulation. It includes the growth of the follicle under the influence of rising levels of estrogen (Figure 26.1). The follicle is the round "cushion" within which the ovum sits. Follicles might be seen as a protrusion from the ovary, like a blister, during **ovariohysterectomy** (spay surgery) if the surgery takes place during this part of the cycle. Proestrus is the time during which there may be bloody discharge from the vagina.

Estrus, as mentioned above, is the part of the cycle that is literally dominated by the female's receptivity to the male. From a hormonal standpoint, a cascade of events takes place. A peak level of estrogen leads to a surge of **luteinizing hormone (LH)**, which, in turn, stimulates a sharp increase in progesterone levels. The level of LH declines so rapidly that

Anatomy and Physiology for Veterinary Technicians and Nurses: A Clinical Approach, Second Edition. Lori Asprea.
© 2026 John Wiley & Sons, Inc. Published 2026 by John Wiley & Sons, Inc.
Companion website: www.wiley.com/go/asprea/anatomy_vettech2e

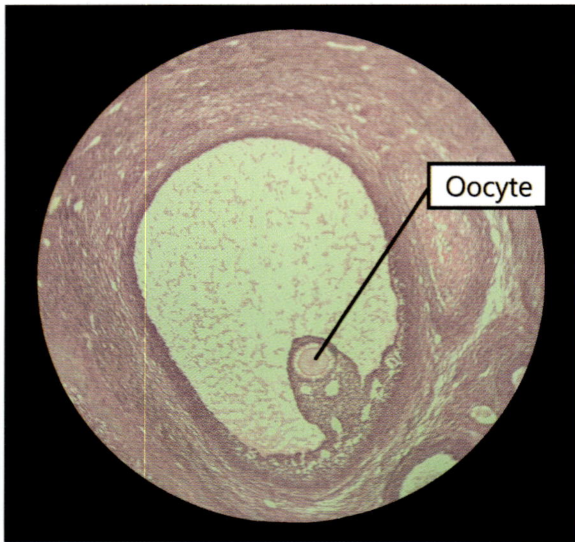

Figure 26.1 The developing oocyte and surrounding follicle in the ovary as seen under the microscope.

it is actually back down to its resting level before the estrus phase is over. Estrus is associated with ovulation.

Progesterone, which is produced in the adrenal gland and by the placenta in the pregnant animal, continues to rise through **diestrus**, the next phase in the cycle. Estrogen, manufactured in the adrenal gland and the ovary, continues to decrease. If the animal were to become pregnant, the presence of progesterone would help maintain the pregnancy. If the animal does not become pregnant, the cycle enters **anestrus**. Anestrus is basically a time of reproductive system inactivity.

Hormonal Control

A closer look at the hormones involved in the reproductive cycle will be helpful. Most of the hormones controlling the progression of steps through the ovarian cycle come from the pituitary. In particular, the **anterior pituitary** produces **follicle-stimulating hormone (FSH)**, **LH**, and **prolactin**. The latter is associated with the production of milk. The **posterior pituitary** produces **oxytocin**. We have discussed oxytocin in its connection to milk letdown. It is also produced as the time of parturition nears. Its effect is to increase the contraction of the muscles of the uterine wall so that the puppy or kitten can be propelled out into the world.

Some of the hormones involved come from the tissues of the reproductive tract itself. Specifically, the ovary produces estrogen and testosterone, steroid compounds that provide an internal signal for the hypothalamus to monitor. If the animal does become pregnant, the membrane that grows around the infant will also produce these hormones. This membrane is known as the **placenta**.

As the ovum begins to grow, it is important that the **follicle** around it continue to develop. FSH is released from the pituitary in response to the appearance and early growth of the follicle. In addition to this stimulus, the cells of the follicle itself can take androgens such as testosterone and convert them to estrogen. As both are steroids, their chemical structure is not dissimilar, and the conversion is thus possible.

Estrogen helps the follicle to grow, providing a good environment for the ovum. In addition, the early follicle adds receptors for FSH, furthering its stimulation to grow. However, as estrogen levels in the follicle continue to rise, the presence of receptors to LH increases. With more LH receptors, the follicle is more sensitive to this hormone, which eventually causes the follicle to open and release the ovum into the reproductive tract, called ovulation.

Once the follicle collapses, it is referred to as a **corpus luteum**. The corpus luteum is still viable for a time and in fact has an important role to play in the reproductive cycle. Under the continued influence of LH and other hormones, the corpus luteum is maintained and produces progesterone, which prepares the uterus for pregnancy. This is called the **luteal phase** of the estrous cycle. In the absence of pregnancy, **prostaglandin F2 alpha (PGF2a)** causes disruption of the corpus luteum, and the remnant of the follicle becomes fibrous tissue. New follicles will start to form, and the process repeats.

Diestrus is, as noted above, the stage after estrus. The production of progesterone is a part of the luteal phase of the cycle. If the animal has mated successfully, endocrine signals from the developing embryo will cause the corpus luteum to persist and continue pumping out progesterone. If there has been no mating (or mating has been unsuccessful, perhaps related to fertility issues), the corpus luteum will regress upon itself. This occurs during diestrus.

The canine estrous cycle lasts approximately 21 days, with the actual period of estrus from a matter of few days to a week (approximately; there are individual variations). Canines go through cycles twice a year.

During anestrus, the reproductive system undergoes little, if any, activity. Progesterone levels are very low, and other hormones, while present, do not undergo fluctuations.

A notable feature of the feline reproductive cycle is that the cat is a **stimulated (or induced) ovulator**; that is, the stimulation for the release of the oocyte from the follicle is, in large part, the act of copulation itself. While most mammals "automatically" ovulate, at which point they are in estrus, felines do not ovulate until they mate. There is still a follicle, and estrogen levels have to be at a certain point for the ovulation to occur. However, the corpus luteum does not form, in response to LH, until after copulation.

Felines produce a number of follicles at a time. In the absence of mating, these follicles will involute. What occurs is a series of follicular growth and collapse that persists over a number of days. Given that a number of follicles are available, and that the act of mating provokes ovulation, it is quite possible to have a litter of kittens in which some have different sires.

Briefly, then, a series of hormonal changes leads to the growth of the follicle (FSH) and its discharge of the egg (LH). Estrogen stimulates the onset of estrus and rises again when birth is imminent. Progesterone prepares the uterus for pregnancy.

Prolactin, one of the pituitary hormones, is associated with maintaining the corpus luteum. In other words, it continues the ovary's production of progesterone, which maintains the pregnancy. If prolactin is released in the absence of fertilization, the result is something called **pseudopregnancy**. In this condition, the animal will exhibit the behavioral signs of pregnancy but will not actually be carrying an embryo.

Many domestic animals are **seasonally polyestrous**. This means that they have more than one estrous cycle, but only at certain times of the year. Felines are a good example of this.

Other Factors Affecting the Estrous Cycle

Puberty is defined as the time the female begins to ovulate or the time a male can produce enough sperm to impregnate a female. The first ovulation does not generally result in pregnancy even if mating occurs. The onset of puberty is about 6 months for dogs and cats, although it can occur many months later in larger-breed dogs. Poor nutrition and certain disease states can delay the onset of puberty.

Photoperiod also has an effect on the estrous cycle. Longer hours of daylight in a 24-hour period are one of the triggers of the development of the follicle and the growth of the oocyte. Interestingly, sheep actually are more prone to be in estrus during times when daylight hours are fewer.

Ovarian activity can be affected by lactation. In some species, such as swine, lactation actually suppresses activity in the ovary, and successful mating cannot take place until after piglets are weaned.

Pheromones play a role in the estrous cycle. In a kennel or cattery, male pheromones will often cause the estrous cycles of the animals to become synchronous. In return, female pheromones will increase the male's desire to mate.

During feline estrus, the widely fluctuating hormones can be a cause of unusual behaviors. Arching of the back and increased vocalizations are some of them. These behaviors also serve to "advertise" the female's receptivity to any males in the area.

The Male

The production of sperm is the province of the testicles. As the sperm continues along the **deferent duct**, various fluids are added, and the resulting solution is called **semen**. Many of the same hormones discussed in conjunction with the female will be discussed in conjunction with the male.

Spermatogenesis is the process of producing sperm. It must occur at a specific temperature in mammals. However, that temperature does vary by species. The testicles are extra-abdominal (on the outside of the body) in dogs and cats, intra-abdominal or retractable in other species. All of these structural differences exist to ensure that the production of viable sperm is possible. The more favorable the temperature, the better the quality of the sperm.

The production of sperm begins in the **seminiferous tubules**, microscopic channels within the testicle. The process of producing sperm cells is under the direction of LH. FSH also plays a role here. FSH stimulates some of the cells that assist in building the spermatozoa (sperm cells) to produce a small amount of estrogen (Figure 26.2).

As the spermatozoa continue to develop, they begin to move through another series of tubules until they reach the **epididymis**. As they move along the epididymis, they have extra time in which to mature. Eventually, they reach the **ductus deferens**, which bring the sperm cells along through the penis. The sperm are actually discharged from the urethra as the deferent duct meets up with the urethra proximal to leaving the body (Figure 26.3).

The process of **erection** is related to the presence of cavernous tissue. This tissue has many hollows that allow it to stiffen when filled with blood. **Ejaculation** is the process of expelling semen from the body. These actions are under parasympathetic and sympathetic nervous system control, respectively. There are other factors as well, including psychobehavioral ones, although these are less common than in humans. Hormonal imbalances can affect the ability of the male to produce and/or discharge semen. The proper word for the introduction of the penis into a female reproductive tract is **intromission**.

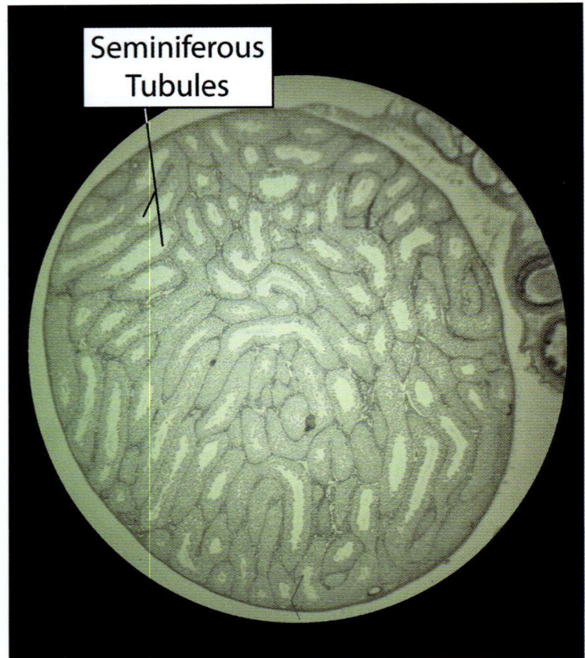

Figure 26.2 The seminiferous tubules of the testicle under the microscope. Each of these channels is lined with cells producing spermatozoa.

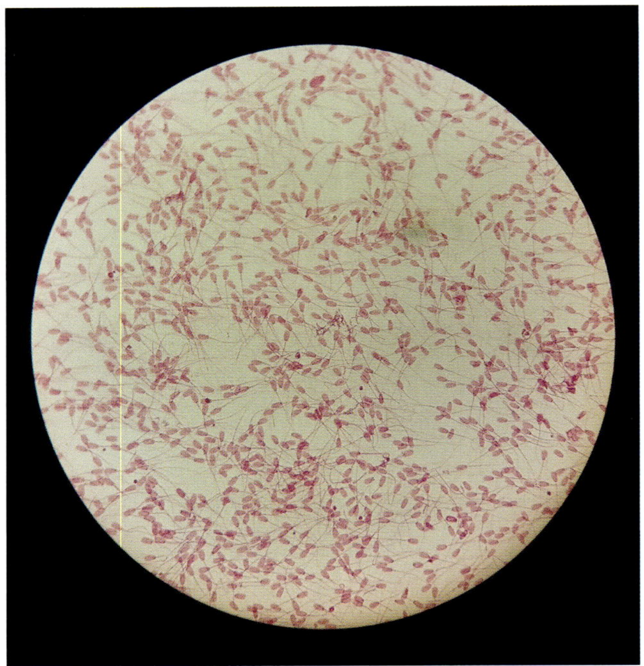

Figure 26.3 Spermatozoa.

Oxytocin is released in males in response to copulation. The muscle contraction in the reproductive tract caused by this helps move the sperm along into the more cranial parts of the tract.

While in the reproductive tract of the female, the sperm begins to undergo a process called **capacitation**. This involves the release of enzymes that allow the sperm to penetrate the ovum. Spermatozoa will try to implant in a number of places on the ovum. Once one has penetrated the ovum, the membrane will not allow other sperm to enter. As there are multiple ova, the number of spermatozoa that find an ovum in which to achieve entry is greater than in primates, who generally only produce one or two ova.

Fertilization and Pregnancy

Once the ovum is fertilized, it is called a **zygote**. Each sperm cell or ovum has only half the normal number of chromosomes an adult cell has. It is only when the zygote is formed that the chromosomes join together.

A significant difference between dogs and cats has to do with the location of fertilization and pregnancy. Ovum and sperm actually come together in the **oviduct**. As they begin to work together, they move slightly caudally to rest in the **uterine horns**. The growth of the embryo and fetus occurs in the uterine horns, not in the body of the uterus.

The newly fertilized ovum will begin to divide itself to make new cells, using the genetic material of the sperm as well as its own. At this point, it does not increase in size. Until the time it implants itself in the walls of the uterus, it is referred to as a zygote. Once it implants itself, it is called an **embryo**. Once it begins to show differentiated organs, it is referred to as a **fetus**.

The small cluster of cells that will become the fetus implants in the **endometrium**, which is the inner lining of the uterine horn. As the zygote settles into the uterine lining, a membrane begins to develop around it. This membrane is called the placenta. Nutrients and oxygen-rich blood will be provided to the embryo through this membrane. The placenta is connected to the embryo by way of a stalk-like structure called the umbilicus.

Note that the embryo/fetus does not breathe air but receives oxygen through the bloodstream. As a result, there is no need for blood to circulate through the lungs as it journeys around the fetus's body. Blood entering one side of the heart

> **Box 26.1 Approximate gestation period for a variety of species.**
>
> | Species | Approximate gestation period (in days) |
> | --- | --- |
> | Brown rat | 22 |
> | Rabbit | 31 |
> | Canine | 63 |
> | Feline | 65 |
> | Pig | 115 (3 mo, 3 wk, 3 d) |
> | Sheep | 150 |
> | Equine | 337 |
> | Donkey | 365 |
> | Elephant | 660 |

is immediately shunted to the other side of the heart, bypassing the lungs altogether. The reader will recall structures like the **ductus arteriosus** and **foramen ovale** that help blood pass through the fetal heart without circling through the lungs.

There is tremendous variation in the location and complexity of the attachment of the placenta to the uterus. The structure is actually more complicated in large animals than it is in dogs and cats, and even less complicated in primates. The attachment of the placenta to the uterus in cattle is so firm that the placenta occasionally will not be expelled after the calf is born. This condition is called **retained placenta**.

Under normal circumstances, the pregnancy of the dog or cat is approximately 63 days. This contrasts favorably with the gestation period (length of pregnancy) of the elephant, which is approximately 21 months. See Box 26.1 for approximate gestation periods of a sample of animals.

The dog or cat generally has four to six newborns in a litter. However, this number varies, particularly in the case of larger dogs. It is of great concern if only one or two animals are born, and the mother should be checked carefully for any signs of retained fetuses or other problems.

Parturition

As mentioned earlier, progesterone helps keep pregnancy viable. As the size of the fetus and the weight of the uterus reach a certain point, a number of changes occur. The amount of **cortisol** in the fetus rises and triggers secretion of estrogen. The rise in estrogen level, in turn, causes the release of oxytocin from the maternal pituitary gland.

Oxytocin causes contraction of the uterine muscles, leading each fetus to gradually move toward the body of the uterus. From there, the fetus is pushed toward the exit of the body. At this point, the cervix has relaxed enough that the puppy or kitten can slip through. Note that the muscle contraction will continue past the point that the last fetus is delivered. This will make sure that all placental material has been expelled as well.

Release of prostaglandin from the uterus eventually leads to regression of the corpus luteum and decline in progesterone levels. The placenta produces a hormone called **relaxin**. Relaxin, as the name implies, decreases the stiffness in the muscles and ligaments surrounding the pelvis, easing the passage of the newborn through the birth canal (vagina).

Although not directly related to the birth process itself, another hormonal event at this time is the release of prolactin from the pituitary gland. The rise in prolactin levels that accompanies pregnancy stimulates the production of **colostrum**, which is rich in maternal antibodies. As mentioned in an earlier chapter, prolactin continues to stimulate the production of milk once the colostrum has been used up. It is joined in this effort by growth hormone. Milk production does not occur during pregnancy, in part because of the levels of progesterone and estrogen, which have an inhibitory effect on lactation.

Clinical Case Resolution: Diamond

A physical examination is performed on Diamond which reveals tachycardia, a slightly painful and tense abdomen, prolonged skin turgor, tacky mucous membranes, and hyperthermia.

*The top concern for Diamond, given the history, is for **pyometra**, or an infected uterus. Pyometra occurs within the first month or two after the heat cycle. It is generally caused by both hormones and bacteria creating the perfect storm. The hormones during heat allow the cervix to open slightly, giving access for bacteria to enter the uterus. This is usually by way of an ascending infection, which is when bacteria make their way up to the target, in this case up the vagina and into the uterus. Recall that progesterone also causes the uterus to thicken, and after repeated heat cycles, the uterine lining can become cystic or contain fluid-filled sacs. This thickened lignin with fluid leads to an ideal growing environment for bacteria. The uterus then fills with pus and bacteria begin producing toxins that can enter the bloodstream.*

Pyometra can either be "open" or "closed". In an open pyometra, the purulent material is able to exit the uterus and is often seen as vaginal discharge on examination. In a closed pyometra, pus is unable to exit the uterus and remains trapped. Closed pyometra cases often get sicker more quickly than open, but both require immediate medical attention.

Diamond has abdominal X-rays and an AFAST (abdominal-focused assessment with sonography for trauma/triage/tracking), which both confirm suspicion for a closed pyometra. The only option for Diamond is to have an emergency ovariohysterectomy.

Diamond recovers from surgery in the hospital and is discharged 3 days later.

Clinical Case Critical Thinking: Diamond

1) *What part(s) of Diamond's history led the veterinary care team to place pyometra so high on their list of concerns?*
2) *Is Diamond's ovariohysterectomy any different than a normal routine spay? Why or why not?*
3) *Is there any way Diamond's condition could have been prevented?*

Review Questions

1 What is the term for when the female is sexually receptive to the male?
   A Estrous
   B Estrus
   C Anestrus
   D Diestrus

2 At which stage of the female cycle might there be bloody vaginal discharge?
   A Anestrus
   B Estrous
   C Diestrus
   D Proestrus

3 Which hormone from the anterior pituitary helps with milk production?
   A LH
   B FSH
   C Prolactin
   D Oxytocin

4 After ovulation, the follicle is further developed into:
   A The corpus luteum
   B The zygote
   C The embryo
   D The placenta

5 True or False: Spermatozoa are fully developed within the seminiferous tubules.
   A True
   B False

6 What is the term for semen exiting the male reproductive organ?
   A Erection
   B Intromission
   C Ejaculation
   D Capitulation

7 At what point are the developing cells called an embryo?
   A When the sperm and ova meet in the oviduct
   B When the sperm and ova start to create cells
   C When the cells are implanted into the uterine wall
   D When the cells begin to produce organs

8 What is spermatogenesis?

9 What is the role of relaxin?
   A To relax the pregnant female during pregnancy
   B To relax the tissues around the birth canal for parturition
   C To relax the fetus immediately after birth
   D To reduce the heart rate of the newborn

10 What is capacitation?

Appendix 1

Dissection Notes

The use of clean instruments is essential. Follow instructor directions regarding handling sharps and be sure they are disposed of appropriately. Scalpel blades can be reused in laboratory dissection, as there is no fear of contaminating the animal, but a new blade should be put in place when the first one becomes dull. Please visit the online video library for a visual guide on handling sharps, as well as placement and removal onto your scalpel handle.

Scalpel blades are used to incise (make cuts) quite easily, with minimal pressure, when the blade is new. Preserved specimens tend to have tougher tissue than fresh samples. For thicker tissue, like skin, the scalpel blade should be used, but be careful not to press down hard or use a sawing motion. It is easy to cut down through tissue one wishes to examine later if too much force is applied.

For more delicate materials like smaller muscles and internal organs, a scissor and blunt dissector is usually sufficient. This avoids cutting through too many layers at once. In separating layers of muscle, or organs from fascia, it is best to use the blunt dissector rather than a sharp instrument. The goal is to avoid destruction of the organs or tissue surrounding the area on which one is working.

When looking at layers of musculature, work from the superficial layer to the deeper layer. Once a superficial muscle has been excavated, use a scissor to cut across the midline of the muscle, rather than separating it from the bone or joint. This will allow you to reflect (fold back) the superficial muscle and to see what lies underneath. The superficial muscle can be folded back into place for later study.

Hollow organs such as intestines, stomach, and urinary bladder, may still contain digested material or urine, respectively. Use caution when incising these organs and be sure to use appropriate personal protective equipment. The accompanying online media for this text has many videos and images to support your dissection.

Most preserved specimens contain formalin, a solution that is 10% formaldehyde. Formaldehyde can cause injury or illness, and handling any fluid materials within the animal should be done with utmost care. The use of goggles is highly recommended. The use of examination gloves is essential. Nitrile gloves are preferred for working with formalin as they are less permeable to formaldehyde than latex. As is true in any laboratory, the use of protective clothing and closed-toe shoes is required.

Muscle Dissection

When dissecting out muscle, it is useful to remove the white, spiderweb-like material that surrounds it. It is a type of superficial fascia – connective tissue, which should be removed in order to see the muscle clearly. It can be brushed away fairly easily. The very tough, flat, white, or silver connective tissue that encases some muscles or muscle connections is known as muscle fascia. It is generally stuck to the muscle tissue closely; if it is necessary to remove it to see beneath it, use blunt dissection to avoid cutting into the muscle below. A large area of fascia covers the muscles on the dorsum in the area of the lumbar spinal column. This is known as the thoracolumbar fascia.

Once the superficial muscles of each area are identified, transect these muscles through their middle to reveal the layer underneath (i.e., cut them in half at the center so that they can be opened like the leaves of a book). In this manner, one can fold back and reestablish each layer for later study. In preserved organic materials, muscle will usually appear pink or gray. In the living animal, they are a red or brick color.

Anatomy and Physiology for Veterinary Technicians and Nurses: A Clinical Approach, Second Edition. Lori Asprea.
© 2026 John Wiley & Sons, Inc. Published 2026 by John Wiley & Sons, Inc.
Companion website: www.wiley.com/go/asprea/anatomy_vettech2e

Accessing the Internal Organs

Abdominal Cavity

To view the viscera, a midline incision can be made through the linea alba on the abdomen. This should be just large enough to insert a set of dissection scissors with the blunt end in the cavity. This will prevent any unwanted damage to the delicate tissues underneath. Use the scissors to cut along the midline in both directions, reaching the diaphragm at the cranial boundary and the pelvic region at the caudal boundary. It may be helpful to also cut across the abdominal tissues to the left and right at the cranial and caudal incision boundaries. This will yield an overall incision that is "I" shaped. Once you are inside the cavity, note that the greater omentum is a covering of fat over the organs that is generally friable. It is anchored to the greater curvature of the stomach and should be gently lifted and moved out of the way to observe the underlying organs.

Thoracic Cavity

To enter the thoracic cavity, gently dissect the diaphragm away from the body wall. Following this, use your large dissection scissors, with the blunt end in the cavity, to cut along the right or left side of the sternum. When dissecting a cat or small dog, the scissors should be sufficient to cut through the ribs alongside the sternum. Continue this incision cranially until you reach the cervical region. Be cautious to not cut or damage the large vessels in the neck.

Retroperitoneal Cavity

The best manner in which to view the kidney is to leave the abdominal viscera attached to the body and to shift them toward the midline to reveal the kidney. The artery and vein are easily visualized. The ureter will have an off-white appearance and resembles a flat strand of spaghetti. Sever the left kidney from these vessels at the hilus, leaving the right kidney in position. The kidney can be most easily transected and its deeper structure is viewed in this manner. Once the kidney is extracted from the body, remove the renal capsule and make a longitudinal incision to reveal the interior of each half of the kidney.

   Note that craniomedially to the kidney within the abdominal cavity is a small, flat, pink/gray organ with a somewhat rounded shape. This is the adrenal gland. Do not remove it at this time.

   If the bladder is large enough, it too can be dissected to reveal the trigone. You can accomplish this by making a small incision at the cranial pole and then cutting along the ventral plane.

Appendix 2

The Cranial Nerves

Number	Name	Related to	Function
I	Olfactory	Sense of smell	Sensory
II	Optic	Visual images	Sensory
III	Oculomotor	Eye movement, focus of the lens and Pupil size	Motor
IV	Trochlear	Eye movement	Motor
V	Trigeminal	Facial sensation, movement of many muscles of the head	Both sensory and motor
VI	Abducent	Eye movement	Motor
VII	Facial	Movement of facial muscles, sense of taste, tear, and saliva production	Both sensory and motor
VIII	Vestibulocochlear	Balance and sound reception	Sensory
IX	Glossopharyngeal	Movement in tongue and throat, salivation, sense of taste	Both sensory and motor
X	Vagus	Sensation from respiratory and GI tract, laryngeal and pharyngeal movement, functions as part of the autonomic nervous system	Both sensory and motor
XI	Accessory	Movement of muscles in the neck	Motor
XII	Hypoglossal	Movement of the tongue	Motor

Most students use a mnemonic device to remember the names of the nerves. One that uses the first letter of the name of each nerve as the first letter of a word in a sentence is:

On **O**ld **O**lympus the **T**ruth **T**ouches (a) **F**ew **V**ery **G**ood, **V**ery **A**ccepting **H**earts. (olfactory, optic, etc.)

For function:

Some **S**ay **M**y **M**other **B**uys **M**any **B**ananas **S**o **B**aking **B**read **M**atters **M**ost (Sensory, sensory, motor, etc.)

A search of the Internet will yield many other choices, or the reader can construct a new one.

Most of the cranial nerves arise from the brain stem or the medulla oblongata. The accessory nerve has some fibers that arise from the cervical spinal cord. Refer to the chapters on the anatomy of the nervous system and neurophysiology for more information.

Appendix 3

Selected Muscle Origins and Insertions

Masseter: zygomatic arch to mandible
Pectorals: sternum to humerus
Deltoid: scapula to deltoid tuberosity of humerus
Trapezius: neck and cranial thoracic vertebrae to spine of the scapula
Serratus ventralis: cervical vertebrae (and cranial ribs, for thoracic part of muscle) to scapula
Supraspinatus: scapula to humerus
Biceps brachii: scapula to radius
Extensor carpi radialis: lateral epicondyle (area just proximal to the condyle) of humerus to metacarpus
Lateral ulnar: lateral epicondyle of humerus to metacarpal V
Superficial digital flexor: medial condyle of the humerus to the palmar surface of the middle phalanges
Latissimus dorsi thoracolumbar spine to humerus
Internal and external abdominal obliques: ribs to linea alba
Middle gluteal: ilium to greater trochanter of femur
Biceps femoris: ischium to patella, tibia, and calcaneus
Tensor fasciae latae: pelvis to lateral femoral fascia
Quadriceps: actually four different heads in the femoral area that converge at the patellar tendon, which contains the patella itself
Biceps femoris: ischiatic tuberosity to patella, tibia, and calcaneus
Semitendinosus: ischiatic tuberosity to tibial crest and calcaneus
Semimembranosus: ischiatic tuberosity to medial femur and tibia
Sartorius: ilium to medial stifle
Gracilis: pelvic (pubic) symphysis to medial stifle and calcaneus
Cranial tibial: proximal tibia to plantar surface of metatarsals I and II
Gastrocnemius: distocaudal femur to calcaneus
Coccygeus: ischium to tail
Levator ani: pelvis to tail

Appendix 4

Common Abbreviations

Below is a table of common abbreviations used in veterinary medicine. This is by no means an exhaustive list, and many more abbreviations or shorthand terms are used.

Abbreviation	Meaning
AAHA	American Animal Hospital Association
Ab/Abx	Antibiotics
ACE	Angiotensin converting enzyme
ACTH	Adrenocorticotropic hormone
AD	Right Ear
ADH	Antidiuretic hormone
ad lib	Freely, as wanted
ADR	"Aint' doin' right" or Adverse drug reaction
A Fib	Atrial fibrillation
ALB	Albumin
ALK Phos/ALP	Alkaline phosphatase
ALT	Alanine transaminase
ALS	Advanced life support
AMA	Against medical advice
amp	Ampule
APC	Atrial premature contraction
AS	Left ear
ASAP	As soon as possible
AU	Both ears
AV	Atrioventricular
AV Block	Atrioventricular block – 1st, 2nd, 3rd degree AV block
AXR	Abdominal radiographs
BAR	Bright, alert, responsive
bid	Twice daily
BM	Bowel movement
BP	Blood pressure
BSA	Body surface area
BUN	Blood urea nitrogen

Anatomy and Physiology for Veterinary Technicians and Nurses: A Clinical Approach, Second Edition. Lori Asprea.
© 2026 John Wiley & Sons, Inc. Published 2026 by John Wiley & Sons, Inc.
Companion website www.wiley.com/go/asprea/anatomy_vettech2e

Abbreviation	Meaning
BW	Body weight
c	With
C&S	Culture and sensitivity
Ca	Calcium
CBC	Complete blood count
cc	Cubic centimeter
CC	Chief complaint
CHF	Congestive heart failure
CNS	Central nervous system
CPCR	Cardiopulmonary cerebral resuscitation
Creat	Creatinine
CRF	Chronic renal Failure
CRT	Capillary refill time
CSF	Cerebrospinal fluid
CVP	Central venous pressure
CXR	Chest radiographs
D5W	5% dextrose in water
DCM	Dilated cardiomyopathy
Ddx/Dx	Differential diagnosis/Diagnosis
DIC	Disseminated intravascular coagulation
DLH	Domestic long hair
DM	Diabetes mellitus
DOA	Dead on arrival
DSH	Domestic short hair
DV	Dorsal Ventral – position.
ECG/EKG	Electrocardiogram
ECHO	Echocardiogram
EENT	Ears eyes nose throat
ELISA	Enzyme-linked immunosorbent assay
ER	Emergency room
FB	Foreign body
FeLV	Feline leukemia virus
FIP	Feline infectious peritonitis
FIV	Feline Immunodeficiency virus
FPV	Feline panleukopenia virus
FSH	Follicle stimulating hormone
FUO	Fever of unknown origin
Fx	Fracture
g/gm	Gram
gal	Gallon
GDV	Gastric dilatation volvulus
GFR	Glomerular filtration rate
GI	Gastrointestinal
gtt	Drops

Abbreviation	Meaning
GU	Genitourinary
h	Hour
Hb	Hemoglobin
HBC	Hit by car
HCT	Hematocrit
HR	Heart rate
Hx	History
IC	Intracardiac
ICU	Intensive care unit
IM	Intramuscular
IN	Intranasal
IOP	Intraocular pressure
IP	Intraperitoneal
IU	International Unit
IV	Intravenous
IVDD	Intervertebral disc disease
K	Potassium
K-9	Canine
Kcal	Kilocalorie
KCS	Keratoconjunctivitis sicca
kg	Kilogram
LRS	Lactated Ringer's Solution
LSA	Lymphosarcoma
m2	Meter squared
MAC	Minimum alveolar concentration
MAP	Mean arterial pressure
mcg	Microgram
MCT	Mast cell tumor
mEq	Milliequivalent
MER	Maintenance energy requirement
MI	Mitral Insufficiency
ml	Milliliter
MM	Mucous membrane
MRI	Magnetic resonance imaging
Na	Sodium
NPO	Non per os (nothing by mouth)
NRBC	Nucleated red blood cell
NSF	No Significant findings
NSR	Normal sinus rhythm
OA	Osteoarthritis
OD	Right eye
OHE	Ovariohysterectomy
OS	Left eye
OTC	Over the counter

Abbreviation	Meaning
OU	Both eyes
P	Phosphorus
P3	Third phalanx
PCV	Packed cell volume
PDA	Patent ductus arteriosus
PE	Physical exam OR pulmonary edema
PEG	Percutaneous endoscopic gastrotomy
PO	Per os (by mouth)
PRAA	Persistent right aortic arch
Prn	As needed/necessary
PTH	Parathyroid hormone
PTS	Put to sleep
PU	Perineal urethrostomy
q	Every
qXh	Every X hours (q2h = every 2 hours)
qid	Four times daily
R	Right
Rads	Radiographs
RBC	Red blood cell
Retic	Reticulocyte
r/o or R/O	Rule out
RTG	Ready to go
Rx	Prescription
SC or SQ	Subcutaneous
Sig	Prescription label directions
SOAP	Subjective objective assessment plan
sp.	Species
sp. gr.	Specific gravity
SR	Suture removal
STAT	Statum – Immediately
Sx	**Surgery** OR Symptoms
T BILI	Total bilirubin
tab	Tablet
tid	Three times per day
TLC	Tender loving care
TP	Total protein
TPR	Temperature, pulse, respiration
TSH	Thyroid-stimulating hormone
Tx	Treatment
UA	Urinalysis
UG	Urogenital
UO	Urinary obstruction
URI	Upper respiratory infection
USG	Urine specific gravity

Abbreviation	Meaning
UTI	Urinary tract infection
v.	Vein
V Tach	Ventricular tachycardia
VD	Ventral dorsal
V/D or v/d or v+/d+	Vomiting/diarrhea
VECCS	Veterinary emergency and critical care society
VS	Vital signs
WBC	White blood cell
WNL	Within normal limits
XRT or RT	Radiation therapy

Glossary

Abduction Movement away from the midline of the body.

Action potential The wave of electrical energy that is directed toward a target cell or organ.

Acute onset A problem or disease that appears suddenly.

Adduction Movement toward the midline of the body.

Allergen A material that causes a hypersensitivity (allergic) response.

Anastomosis A joining or connecting between two or more tubes in the body, which can be natural or surgical. Examples are within blood vessels and the gastrointestinal tract.

Antebrachium The part of the thoracic limb from the elbow to the carpus.

Antibody A protein made by the immune system that can target and help neutralize harmful pathogens.

Apex The pointed or narrow end of a body part, such as the heart or tongue.

Arrhythmia An abnormal heartbeat or rhythm.

Artery A vessel carrying blood away from the heart.

Articular surface The surface of a bone that is within the joint.

Aspirate To bring anything other than air into the trachea; also, to remove liquid or other soft material from a body structure by way of a needle or catheter.

Atelectasis The collapse of one or more lobes of the lung.

ATP (adenosine triphosphate) A product of chemical reactions that liberate a substantial amount of energy for cells to use.

Atrophy A process in which a body tissue or organ degrades and wastes away.

Auscultate Listen; particularly, to listen to the chest or abdomen in order to assess the status of organs within it.

Autorhythmic The ability of specific cells to generate their own impulse without external stimuli.

Axilla The area ventral to the shoulder joint ("armpit").

Biopsy Surgically taking a sample of tissue so that it can be analyzed.

Brachium The part of the thoracic limb from the shoulder to the elbow.

Cachexia A physical state in which metabolic or cardiac disorders cause extreme muscle and fat loss.

Calculus When referring to medicine, it means a concretion of minerals or other hard materials, informally called a "stone." Calculi (plural) are often found in the urinary bladder and less commonly in the kidneys and gallbladder.

Canthus An angle, particularly one where two structures meet. The lateral canthus of the eye is the spot on the side of the head where the upper and lower eyelids meet; the medial canthus is the equivalent spot toward the midline.

Capillary The smallest blood vessels in the body, which connect venules (the smallest veins) to arterioles (the smallest arteries).

Caudal A directional term meaning toward the tail.

Cavity An opening, usually fairly large, within which are other organs. The major cavities of the body are the thoracic (chest) and peritoneal (abdomen) cavities. Also, a defect in a tooth.

Cellular respiration The way that a cell creates energy to manufacture proteins or other substances needed for normal performance.

Cervid The family of hoofed stock including deer.

Ciliated cell A cell with one or more hair-like structures on its surface.

Circumduction Movement of the appendage in a circular manner from a stationary axis point.

Compact bone Mature bone that has great strength.

Continent/incontinent The ability to urinate or defecate at the appropriate place and time is called continence. An animal that cannot control when or where they urinate or defecate is said to be incontinent.

Cranial A directional term for toward the head.

Chronic A condition or disease that continues over time; it can be intermittent or steady.

Cortex The outer layer of some organs, such as the adrenal gland and the kidney; also, the part of the brain encompassing the areas related to higher/integrative thinking.

Crepitus The crunching, popping, or grinding sound or feeling when bones or cartilage rub against one another.

Cyanosis A blue or purple tint to the mucous membranes resulting from a lack of oxygen in the blood.

Cytoplasm The liquid portion of a somatic cell.

Dermis The layer of the skin deep to, or under, the epidermis.

Diffusion The movement of particles in a concentration gradient, normally from an area of high concentration to an area of low concentration.

Distal Directional term for further away from the trunk of the body or an anatomical landmark.

Distensible Expands and contracts easily, as the urinary bladder.

Diuresis An increased volume of urine produced by the kidney to be excreted.

Dorsal Upward, toward the spine (directional term).

Dyspnea Difficulty breathing.

Ectopic In an abnormal or unusual place, such as thyroid tissue, that appears in the chest instead of in the gland itself.

Electrolyte Molecules such as potassium, calcium, and sodium, which are capable of becoming ions (losing or gaining an electron).

Epidermis The most superficial layer of the skin.

Endocrine organ An organ that produces hormones, chemicals that stimulate the production of hormones, or neurotransmitters. Usually ductless.

Endoplasmic reticulum The energy storage component of a somatic cell.

Endotracheal Within the trachea; often used in the phrase "endotracheal tube," which is a tube inserted through the mouth down into the trachea, used for breathing when an animal is under anesthesia.

Enteric Referring specifically to the small intestine.

Equilibrium A balance of opposing forces, the specialized sense of having balance.

Estrous cycle The series of chemical events that lead to ovulation and either pregnancy or the end of the reproductive cycle.

Estrus The period of time in the estrous cycle in which the female is receptive to breeding.

Fascicle (plural: fasciculi) A collection of muscle fibers into one bundle; also, a collection of nerve fibers into one bundle.

Fasciculation Localized muscle twitching.

Fenestrated Has windows or pores in its walls; often refers to blood vessels.

Gait The way an animal walks or runs; an abnormal gait would imply limping or not being able to coordinate movements of the limbs.

Gestation period The amount of time the animal is normally pregnant.

Gonad The reproductive organs that produce sex hormones and reproductive genetic material.

Gray matter A portion of the central nervous system (CNS) that is primarily comprised of neuron cell bodies and dendrites that appear grey in color.

Hilus An indentation or divot on an organ where blood vessels, lymphatics, and nerves enter and exit.

Homeostasis The level of performance the body needs to maintain in order to continue normal function; applies to many things, but particularly to keeping a normal energy level and pH balance.

Hormone A substance that changes metabolic function or stimulates the neurological system; generally discharged directly into the bloodstream.

Hydrophilic The affinity for water; usually referring to a molecule or chemical that can interact easily with water on a chemical level.

Hydrophobic The "fear" of water; in physiology, this term refers to a molecule or chemical that does not interact easily with water and essentially repels it.

Hypodermis The fatty layer deep to the dermis also called the subcutaneous layer.

Iatrogenic The description of a disease or dysfunction that occurs as an unexpected result of medical treatment; a medical problem caused by the treatment for another disorder.

Ingesta Material that has been taken into the digestive tract at least as far as the esophagus. Note that this material is not necessarily composed of nutrients.

Interstitial space Small spaces or areas of connective tissue within organs or between them, excluding the major body cavities like the thoracic and peritoneal cavities, as well as other spaces like intracellular or intravascular.

Invagination When the surface of something folds in on itself to make a cavity or tube.

Lateral Directional term for away from the midline.

Ligament A connective tissue that attaches bone to bone.

Lipid An organic compound made of fatty acids that are insoluble in water.

Lobe A separate but connected section of a larger organ; for example, both the liver and the lungs are composed of a series of "flaps" called lobes.

Lumen The hollow part of the inside of a tube; the luminal surface is the layer that forms the boundary of the inside of the hole.

Luxate The act of moving out of a normal position, temporarily or permanently; usually refers to bones or joint components.

Manus The paw of the thoracic limb.

Medial Directional term for toward the midline.

Mediastinum The space between the left and right lungs, enclosing the heart as well as sections of the trachea and esophagus, in addition to nerves and blood vessels.

Medulla The inner section of some organs, including the adrenal gland and kidneys.

Metabolism A series of activities that lead to the continuation of basic bodily systems such as digestion, respiration, cardiovascular circulation, and cellular activity, or the rate of speed or strength of response of these functions.

Minute ventilation The amount of air moved in and out of the body in 1 minute; in other words, tidal volume multiplied by breaths per minute or respiratory rate (RR). (MV = TV × RR)

Mnemonic device A way of remembering things by using another (presumably easier-to-recall) word or letter to represent each item.

Nephron The functioning unit of the kidney that filters blood and produces what will eventually be urine.

Neuron The functioning unit of the nervous system, also called a nerve cell or nerve fiber.

Nociception The sense of noxious or painful stimuli from the nervous system.

Olfactory Having to do with the sense of smell.

Oncotic pressure The molecular "attraction" that causes osmotic movement.

Onychectomy A surgical procedure to remove the claws and distal phalanx; declaw.

Orchiectomy Surgical removal of the testicles; neuter.

Orthopneic A posture an animal assumes when it is having trouble breathing, involving the thoracic limbs spread apart, back hunched, and head down.

Osmosis The movement of liquid toward an area of higher concentration of solutes.

Osteon A circular structure containing cells that are the main support for compact bone.

Ovarian cycle The amount of time between estrous cycles.

Ovariohysterectomy Surgical removal of the ovaries and uterus; spay.

Palmar The surface of the pelvic foot that faces the ground.

Papilla Small, raised bumps or elevation in various parts of the body: the tongue, the skin, the intestines, etc. Plural: papillae.

Parenchyma The functional tissue of an organ that is not connective or supportive in its primary role.

Parturition The act of giving birth.

Pathogen Any organism capable of causing disease, i.e., bacteria, virus, fungus, parasite, etc.

Perfusion The movement of blood through the body to tissues.

Peritoneum The membrane lining the peritoneal or abdominal cavity.

Pes The paw of the pelvic limb.

pH A measure of acidity/alkalinity. A low pH means having an acidic quality, and a high pH an alkaline quality. Normal pH in mammals is usually different from that of water, which is 7.0.

Pharynx The throat; separated into the oropharynx and the nasopharynx.

Phlebotomy The removal of blood from a vein or artery by way of a needle.

Pinna The visible, cartilaginous part of the outer ear.

Plantar The surface of the pelvic foot that faces the ground.

Pleura The membrane lining the pleural or thoracic cavity.

Plexus An intricate branching network of nerves or vessels usually interlacing or grouped together.

Polydactyly Having more than the usual number of digits; a polydactyl dog has 21 or more digits, a cat 19 or more.

Prehension The act of grasping something.

Pronate Move a distal limb from palmar/plantar surface up to palmar/plantar surface down; the equivalent of slapping the palm on the ground.

Proprioception A sense that allows an animal (or person) to perceive its own body location relative to the environment.

Proximal Near to; directional term for closer to the trunk of the body or an anatomical landmark.

Pruritic Itchy.

Radiograph The image produced by an X-ray machine.

Reflex A physical reaction by the body in response to a stimulus that does not require the conscious mind.

Rostral Directional term for closer to the nose, replaces cranial, only used on the head.

Rugae The folks or wrinkles in a tissue or organ; the rugae of the stomach or hard palate.

Saline A solution of salt and water.

Sarcolemma The membrane or cell wall of a muscle cell.

Sarcoplasm The liquid portion of a muscle cell.

Sarcoplasmic reticulum The calcium storage container of a muscle cell.

Sebum A waxy, oily substance produced by the sebaceous glands in the integument.

Sesamoid Having the appearance of a sesame seed; usually refers to small bones that appear in association with joints of the limbs and help cushion ligaments or tendons as they move.

Spinal column, divisions of From cranial to caudal, cervical, thoracic, lumbar, sacral, and caudal.

Spinal cord The thick cable of nerve fibers that runs from the brain to the cauda equina.

Stem cell A type of cell made in the embryo during development and in the bone marrow in the adult that can become many different types of cells in the body.

Subcutaneous The fatty layer deep to the dermis, also called the hypodermis.

Supinate On the distal limb, moving the palmar/plantar surface of the limb so that it is facing upward.

Synapse The space between a presynaptic neuron and the postsynaptic membrane, which allows for communication to pass through and from the nervous system.

Tendon A connective tissue that attaches bone to muscle.

Threshold A point of intensity or volume that must be reached or surpassed in order for a certain reaction or result.

Thrombus A blood clot that forms inside the vessels.

Tidal volume The total amount of air moved in one breath.

Trunk of the body The thorax and abdomen taken as one unit; the body of the animal, minus the head, tail, and limbs.

Turgor The rigidity of tissues or cells based on the hydration or level of fluid absorption.

Tympanic membrane The thin layer of tissue that separates the external auditory canal from the middle ear; the eardrum.

Ungulate Mammals that have hooves.

Urticaria Hives.

Valve A set of tissues within a passage that can temporarily close or allow unidirectional movement like the valves within the heart, the vessels, and lymph ducts.

Vascularization How well supplied an area is with blood vessels; neovascularization refers to the formation of new blood vessels in an area.

Vein A vessel carrying blood toward the heart.

Ventral Downward toward the floor (directional term; applies only to the trunk and head).

Vesicle A small structure that can be found in cells or tissues that store, transport, and release substances like neurotransmitters, hormones, or even waste products.

Vibrissae A tactile hair found on the face and head; whiskers.

Viscera The internal organs of the abdomen and thorax.

White matter A portion of the central nervous system (CNS) that is primarily comprised of axons covered in myelin that appear white in color.

Zoonotic disease A condition that humans can develop from contact with an infected animal or animal product.

References

Bibliography

Akers R, Denbow D. *Anatomy and Physiology of Domestic Animals*, 2nd ed. Wiley-Blackwell, Ames, IA, 2013.
Cunningham J (ed.) *Textbook of Veterinary Physiology*, 6th ed. Elsevier Health Sciences, St. Louis, MO, 2019.
Dyce K, Sack W, Wensing C. *Textbook of Veterinary Anatomy*, 5th ed. Elsevier Health Sciences, St. Louis, MO, 2019.
Feldman E, Nelson R. *Canine and Feline Endocrinology and Reproduction*, 3rd ed. Elsevier Health Sciences, St. Louis, MO, 2003.
Pasquini C, Spurgeon T, Pasquini S. *Anatomy of Domestic Animals*, 11th ed. SUDZ Publishing, Pilot Point, TX, 2007.
Reece W. *Functional Anatomy and Physiology of Domestic Animals*, 5th ed. Wiley-Blackwell, Ames, IA, 2017.
Stedman TL. *Stedman's Medical Dictionary*. Wolters Kluwer Health, Inc., Philadelphia, PA, 2023.

Further Reading

Using Anatomy for Clinical Purposes

Ballard B. *Restraint & Handling for Veterinary Technicians and Assistants*, 1st ed. Cengage Learning, Independence, KY, 2009.
Cheville N. *Introduction to Veterinary Pathology*, 3rd ed. Wiley-Blackwell, Ames, IA, 2006.
Colby L, Nowland MH, Kennedy LH, Hrapkiewicz K. *Clinical Laboratory Animal Medicine: An Introduction*. Wiley-Blackwell, Ames, IA, 2019.
DuPont G. *Atlas of Dental Radiography in Dogs and Cats*. Elsevier Health Sciences, St. Louis, MO, 2008.
Fowler M. *Restraint and Handling of Wild and Domestic Animals*, 3rd ed. Wiley-Blackwell, Ames, IA, 2008.
Greene C. *Infectious Diseases of the Dog and Cat*, 5th ed. Elsevier Health Sciences, St. Louis, MO, 2023.
Hyttel P. *Essentials of Domestic Animal Embryology*. Elsevier Health Sciences, St. Louis, MO, 2009.
Lavin L. *Radiography in Veterinary Technology*, 7th ed. Elsevier Health Sciences, St. Louis, MO, 2021.

And What Every Technologist Should Have

Samples OM. *McCurnin's Clinical Textbook for Veterinary Technicians and Nurses*. 11th ed. Elsevier Health Sciences, St. Louis, MO, 2025.
Sirois M. *Principles and Practice of Veterinary Technology*, 4th ed. Elsevier Health Sciences, St. Louis, MO, 2016.
Stedman TL. *Stedman's Medical Dictionary*. Wolters Kluwer Health, Inc., Philadelphia, PA, 2023.

Index

a

A/an- 7
Abdomen vi, 6, 9, 11, 53, 57–58, 60, 64, 79, 83, 86–87, 95, 105, 111–113, 115, 117, 119, 123–124, 213, 217, 221, 226–227, 236, 240, 251, 254
Abdomin/o 9
Abdominal breathing 213
Abdominal-focused assessment with sonography for trauma/triage/tracking (AFAST) 236
Abduction 10, 47, 251
Abomasum 115, 227
Absorption 139, 160–161, 186, 225, 228, 254
Acetabulum 34, 36, 51
Acetylcholine 166–170, 174–175, 177, 207, 214
Acetylcholinesterase 166, 175, 178
Acidemia 216
Acidosis 196, 215–217, 227
Acromion 31
Actin 57, 165–168
Action potential ix, 146, 149–150, 166, 168–169, 172–175, 179, 202, 207, 251
Activated charcoal 178
Acute caudal myopathy (Limber tail, Swimmers tail) 64
Ad 7
Addison's disease 188. *See also* Hypoadrenocorticism
Adduction 47, 251
Aden/o 9
Adenohypophysis 78, 183
Adenosine diphosphate (ADP) 167, 170
Adenosine triphosphate (ATP) ix, 55, 130, 134, 167, 251. *See also* ATP
Adip/o 9
Adipose 9, 15, 50, 133, 137, 139, 142, 161
Adrenergic neuron 177
Adrenergic receptor 177–178
Adrenocorticotropic hormone (ACTH) 183–185, 187–188, 190, 245
Afferent arteriole 196–199

Afferent signal 172, 178
Affinity 215–216, 252
Afterload 204
Agranulocyte 133
Air sac 43, 105, 155, 217
Airflow 23, 105, 211, 213
Alar fold 22–23
Albumin 132, 193, 245
Aldosterone 185, 187–188, 190–191, 194–197
Alimentary tract 107
Alkaline 188, 196, 217, 224, 245, 253
Alkalosis 216, 218
Alopecia 13, 20
Alveolar sac 104
Alveoli:
    mammary alveoli 122, 125, 141
    respiratory alveoli 104–106, 211–214, 216, 218–219
Alveolus 104, 109, 111, 212, 214–216
Amino acid 129–130, 182, 189, 194, 199, 224
Ammonia 226
Ampullae 25–26
Amylase 221, 224, 227–228
Anabolism 130, 183, 186
Anagen 141
Anastomoses 92–93
Anconeal process 32
Anconeus 61
Androgen 79, 188–189, 232
Anemia x, 7, 80, 108, 156, 163, 169, 197–198, 203, 206, 215
Anestrus 232, 236
Angiotensin 188, 196–197, 199, 207, 245
Angiotensin I 197, 199
Angiotensin II 197, 199, 207
Angiotensin-converting enzyme (ACE) 197, 245
Angular process 37
Ante- 7
Antebrachiocarpal joint 51
Antebrachium 6–7, 9, 48, 51, 61, 65, 73, 251

Anterior chamber   27, 146–147
Anti-   7, 27, 64, 184, 187, 189
Antibodies   7, 122, 133, 135, 141, 235
Antibiotics (Ab)   7, 245
Anticlinal   41–42, 45
Antidiuretic hormone (ADH)   184, 189, 196–197, 245
Antler   viii, 19, 137, 142
Anucleate   130
Anus   15, 61, 74, 107, 114, 123, 140, 143, 223, 225–226
Aorta   89–98, 104, 121, 123, 196–197, 199, 204–206, 208–209
  ascending aorta   94
  descending aorta   95
Aortic:
  aortic arch   80, 94, 207, 216, 248
  aortic bulb   94
  aortic hiatus   95, 104
Aortic valve   91–92, 99, 205
Apex:
  bladder   86
  heart   90, 202
  tongue   108, 116
Apocrine   15, 138, 140, 144
Aponeurosis   57, 60
Appendicular skeleton   v, 31, 33–35
Aqueous compartment   27
Aqueous humor   27, 146–147
Arachnoid membrane   68
Arbor vitae   70
Arcade:
  mandibular   108–109
  maxillary   108
Arginine vasopressin deficiency   189. *See also* Diabetes
    insipidus
Arrector pili   14, 17, 138, 144
Arrhythmia   169, 203, 208, 251
Arter/o   9
Arterioles   92–93, 197, 206–207, 214, 251
Artery   vii, 9, 57, 71, 79, 83, 86, 88–96, 99, 112–114, 121, 123,
    193, 197–199, 204–209, 216, 240, 251, 253
Arthrology   47
Articular:
  cartilage   48–50, 155, 160–161, 163
  disc   50, 161
  fat pad   50, 160–161
  fovea   32
  process   40–41
  surface   153, 251
Ascites   111, 226
Aseptic   19, 143
Atelectasis   213, 217, 251
Atherosclerosis   93
Atlas   40–41, 45, 69, 255

ATP   55, 130–131, 166–167, 170, 173, 179, 194, 203, 225, 251.
    See also Adenosine triphosphate (ATP)
Atrial tachycardia   203
Atrioventricular:
  node   202
  septum   92
  valve   91. *See also* Left atrioventricular (AV) valve; Right
    atrioventricular (AV) valve
Atrium   89–92, 94, 96–99, 201–207, 209–210
Atrophy   58, 60, 141, 165, 167–168, 188, 251
Atropine   178–179
Auditory   ix, 23–24, 27, 37–38, 145–146, 148–149, 151,
    175, 254
Auditory nerve   148, 175
Auditory receptor   145
Auditory sense   23
Aural   27–28
Auricle   90
Auriculopalpebral nerve   73
Auscultation   89, 105, 213, 217
Auto-   7
Autonomic nerve   138, 161, 176
Autorhythmic   201, 209, 251
AV node   202, 209
AV valve   91, 205
Avascular   25
Avian   vii, ix, 18, 43–45, 59, 69, 87, 105, 112, 115, 132, 155,
    168, 198, 217, 231
Axial skeleton   vi, 31, 36
Axillary artery   94
Axis   40–41, 45, 47, 50, 91, 112, 123, 217, 251
Axon   67–68, 74, 171–175, 177, 254
Axon terminal   68, 172–173
Azygous vein   95, 97, 99

b

B12   155, 157, 224, 228
Bacteria   7, 14, 122, 129, 133, 137, 208, 222, 227, 236, 253
Baroreceptor   145, 150, 152, 207
Barrow   120
Basal   14
Basement membrane   14
Beak   viii, 4, 18, 115, 142–143, 222
Bi-   7, 133
Bicarbonate   185, 196, 199, 216–217, 224. *See also* HCO$_3$
Biceps brachii   61, 243
Biceps femoris   62, 65, 73, 243
Bicuspid valve   91. *See also* AV valve; Left atrioventricular
    (AV) valve
Bilateral   7, 123
Bile acid   225
Bilirubin   139, 198–199, 248

Billy   120

Bisected   23, 38, 71, 80, 85, 102

Bitch   120, 129

Bladder:
   gallbladder   10, 86, 92, 95, 107, 112, 114, 139, 185, 224–226, 228, 251
   urinary bladder   8, 10, 63, 83–88, 95–96, 120–124, 177, 194, 197, 239–240

Blood–brain barrier (BBB)   69–71

Blood pressure   x, 9, 80, 93, 150, 152, 169, 184–185, 187–189, 203–209, 245
   diastolic   205, 209
   systemic   175, 187, 196–197, 204–205, 207–208

Blood urea nitrogen (BUN)   169, 194, 196–197, 199, 245

Boar   120

Body
   ciliary   25–27, 146–147
   condition score (BCS)   105, 167–169, 198
   dense   57, 168, 170
   penis   124
   stomach   112
   uterus   120–121, 234–235
   vertebrae   41
   vitreous   146–147

Bolus   221–222, 224

Bone marrow   ix, 31, 34, 80–81, 93, 132–133, 153–157, 185, 189, 197, 254
   aspirate   156
   yellow   154

Bowman's space   194

Brachialis   61

Brachii   61, 243

Brachiocephalic trunk artery   94–95

Brachiocephalicus   58, 61, 64

Brachiocephalic vein   96

Brachioradialis   51, 64

Brachium   6–7, 9, 51, 61, 94, 138, 251

Brachy   9

Brachycephalic   9, 38–39, 105, 109, 151

Brachydont   222

Brady-   7

Brain   vi, ix, 9–10, 13, 17, 19, 21–25, 36, 67–74, 77–78, 81, 94, 104, 129–130, 134, 138–139, 146–149, 151, 159, 171, 175–176, 178–179, 183, 207, 217, 226, 241, 252, 254

Brainstem   vi, 38–39, 69–71, 176
   medulla oblongata   69–72, 74, 104, 216, 241
   midbrain   74, 176
   pons   69–71, 74

Bronch/o   9

Bronchial sound   105

Bronchioles   104, 211, 213–214

Bronchoconstriction   211

Bronchodilation   177, 211, 219

Bronchovesicular sound   105

Buccinator muscle   107

Bucco-   7

Buck   120

Bull   120, 123–124

Bundle of His   202, 209

Bursae   50, 54, 160–162

C

Cachexia   168, 251

Calcaneus   34, 63, 156, 243

Calcitonin   154, 184–186, 190, 194

Calcium   55, 78, 139, 154, 165–166, 170, 175, 179, 184–187, 190, 194, 199, 201–203, 210, 246, 252, 254

Callus   154

Calorigenic   186

Calyx   86, 88
   major   88
   minor   88

Canal of Schlemm   27

Cancellous bone   153–154, 156

Cancer   9–10, 18, 87–88, 93, 124, 140, 150, 168, 188

Cannon bone   42, 45

Canthus:
   lateral   146, 251
   medial   15, 25, 146, 251

Capacitation   234, 237

Capillaries   92–93, 104, 193–194, 197–198, 205–206, 208, 214–215, 217

Capsule:
   Bowman's   86, 88, 194
   joint   49, 54, 160–161, 163
   lymph node   93–94
   renal   83–84, 88, 240
   testicle   123

Carbon dioxide (CO_2)   10–11, 22, 106, 130, 132, 150, 170, 196, 205–207, 211–218

Carbon monoxide (CO)   108, 216

Carcin/o   9

Cardi/o   9

Cardiac:
   contractility   177
   muscle   ix–x, 55–57, 64, 91, 165, 167, 170, 201–202, 204, 207, 209
   output   x, 204, 215, 217–218
   sphincter   111. *See also* Lower esophageal

Cardiomyopathy:
   dilated cardiomyopathy (DCM)   204, 246
   hypertrophic cardiomyopathy (HCM)   204

Carotid artery   94, 207, 216

Carp/o   9

Carpal   15, 32–33, 50–51, 140, 142
Carpometacarpal joint   51
Carpometacarpus   43
Carpus   4, 6–7, 15–16, 30–32, 34, 42, 50–51, 142, 251
Cartilage   ix, 29, 37–39, 101–103, 137, 153, 252
  articular   48–50, 155, 160–161, 163
  arytenoid   102, 106
  costal   38
  cricoid   102, 106
  elastic   48–49, 155–157
  fibrocartilage   48–50, 53, 154–157, 160–161
  hyaline   48–49, 155–157, 160–161
  thyroid   102
Cartilaginous joint   vi, 48–49, 53, 160, 163
  primary cartilaginous joint   49. *See also* Synchondrosis
  secondary cartilaginous joint   49. *See also* Symphysis
Cartilaginous rings   79, 103, 106
Caruncle   121
Catabolism   130, 186–187
Catagen   141
Catecholamine   183, 185, 188, 190
Cauda equina   73, 75, 254
Caudal gluteal artery   96
Caudal rectal nerve   74
Cavity:
  abdominal   6–7, 9, 40, 80–81, 83, 106, 111, 121, 123, 227, 240, 253
  medullary   31, 154, 156–157
  nasal   22, 36, 44, 71, 108, 149–150
  oral   viii, 38–39, 44, 58, 102, 107–108, 110, 115, 139, 160, 222–223, 227
  peritoneal   6, 112, 116, 253
  pleural   6
  retroperitoneal   83, 86, 88, 116
  synovial   49, 160–161
  thoracic   6, 8, 10–11, 40, 80–81, 89, 104, 106, 116, 213, 217–218, 240, 254
Cecum   10, 113–114, 116–117, 225, 227, 229
Celiac artery   95–96, 112, 114
C-cell   186
Cell membrane   129, 131, 165, 174, 182–183
Cellulose   227–228
Central canal   72, 154
Cephal/o   9
Cephalic vein   73, 95–97
Cerebell/o   9
Cerebellar hypoplasia   9, 70, 74, 176
Cerebellum   vi, 9, 69–70, 176, 179
Cerebr/o   9
Cerebral cortex   69–70
  frontal lobe   69
  occipital lobe   69
  parietal lobe   69
  temporal lobe   69, 148, 699
Cerebrospinal fluid (CSF)   9, 68–69, 72, 246
Cerebrum   vi, 9, 69–71, 75, 150, 176, 179
Cerumen   27
Ceruminous   27
Cervid   19, 251
Cervix   121, 235–236
Channel   24, 29, 72, 79, 129, 166, 173–175, 202–203, 233–234
  ligand-gated   175
  voltage-gated   175
Chemical receptor   145
Chemoreceptor   xi, 145, 150, 216–217
Chestnut   16
Chief cells   224, 228
Choanae   38
Cholecystokinin   80, 185, 189, 224–225, 228
Cholinergic:
  neuron   177
  receptor   207. *See also* Muscarinic; Nicotinic
Chordae tendineae   91
Choroid   25, 146–147
Chyme   224–225
Cilia   148–149, 211
Circum-   7
Circumduction   47, 251
Cisterna magna   69
Clavicle   43
Claw   v, viii, 10, 13, 18, 33, 137, 142, 253
Clitoris   121
Cloaca   87, 115, 198
Coat   16, 74, 92, 105, 137, 140–141, 178, 186
Coccygeal artery   95, 99
Coccygeus   61, 64, 243
Cochlea   24, 28, 50, 148–149, 151–152
Coffin bone   42
Col/o   9
Collagen   14, 25, 48, 57, 142, 154–155, 159
Colloid   78
Colon   xi, 9–10, 95, 113, 170, 225–226, 229. *See also* Large intestine
  ascending   114, 117, 229
  descending   114–115, 117
  transverse   114, 117
Colostrum   115, 122, 141, 235
Common carotid artery   94
Common digital extensor   61
Compact bone   153–154, 156, 160, 163, 252–253
Compound follicles   17
Conduction   x, 107, 139, 167, 174, 178, 201–202
Condyle   30, 32–34, 38, 69, 243

Condyloid process of the mandible   37
Conjunctiva   25
Constipation   225
Convection   138
Coracoid   43
Cornea   25, 28, 146–148, 151
Cornification   137
Cornified   14, 142
Cornual process   143–144
Coronary artery   90, 94, 206–207, 209
Coronary vein   90, 206
Coronoid process   32
Corpus callosum   69
Corpus luteum   184–185, 189, 232–233, 235–236
Cortex:
   adrenal   79–80, 185, 187–190
   auditory   148
   cerebellar   70
   cerebral lobe   69–70
   hair   17
   renal   83–88, 193, 199
   visual   147
Corticomedullary boundary   83
Corticosterone   187
Cortisol   185, 187–188, 191, 235
Costochondral joint   39, 51
Co-transport   194, 199
Countercurrent mechanism   196
Cowlick   16
Coxofemoral joint (hip)   33–34, 51
Crackles   105
Cranial epigastric artery   94
Cranial nerve   vi, xi, 10, 26, 67, 70–73, 75, 107, 147–149, 173, 176, 214, 241
   I: olfactory   71–72, 241
   II: optic   25–26, 71–72, 75, 147, 176, 241. *See also*
      Optic nerve
   III: oculomotor   71–72, 241
   IV: trochlear   71–72, 241
   V: trigeminal   71–73, 173, 176, 241
   VI: abducens   71–72, 241
   VII facial   71–73, 241
   VIII: vestibulocochlear   71–72, 148, 241
   IX: glossopharyngeal   10, 71–72, 241
   X: vagus   71–72, 176, 214, 241
   XI: spinal accessory   71–72, 241
   XII: hypoglossal   71–72, 241
Creatine kinase   167, 170
Creatine phosphate   131, 167, 170
Cremaster   60, 123, 125
Crepitus   161, 163, 252
Crest   29, 33–36, 243

Crista ampullaris   25–26, 148, 151
Crop   115, 177
Cross bridge   166, 168
Crus   6, 63, 96
Crypto-   7
Cryptorchidism   7, 123
Cupula   25–26, 148–149
Cushing's disease   187, 189–190. *See also*
      Hyperadrenocorticism
Cutaneous   43, 140, 143
Cuticle (hair)   17, 141
Cyan-   7
Cyanosis   7, 108, 139, 252
Cyst   10
Cystocentesis   86
Cyt-   7
Cyt/o   10
Cytoplasm   129, 132–133, 165, 174, 182, 216, 252
Cytoskeleton   129
Cytosol   129–130, 134

d

Dactyl   10
Dam   120
Dead space   212, 218
Debris   27, 89, 133, 143, 148
Dehorn   143
Deltoid   32, 59, 61, 243
Demodectic   20
Dendrite   67–68, 74, 169, 171, 173, 178, 252
Dens   41, 51, 109
   atlas   41, 51
   tooth   109
Dental formula   109, 116
Dental pad   114
Depolarization   166, 173–174, 178–179, 202–203, 210
Derm/a/o   10
Dermis   13–15, 58, 139, 252, 254
Detrusor muscle   87–88
Dewclaw   18, 32–34
Dexamethasone   187
Dextr/o   10
Diabetes:
   insipidus   189
   mellitus   79, 113, 189, 194, 246
Diabetic ketoacidosis   226
Diaphragm   25, 73, 95, 104, 110–111, 116, 213, 217–218, 240
Diaphysis   31, 153, 156
Diastole   205, 209
Diencephalon   vi, 69–70, 77
Diestrus   232, 236
Diffusion   131, 134, 155, 194, 206, 252

Digastricus   58

Digestion   80, 114, 117, 189, 221–222, 224–228, 253

  chemical   80

  mechanical   221

Digit   7–8, 10, 15, 18, 32–34, 42–43, 45, 52, 61, 142, 254

  numbering   33

Digital   15, 18, 20, 61, 63, 142, 243

Digitigrade   142

Dilute   195

Directional terms   4

Dis-   7

Dissociation point   215–216, 218

Distal convoluted tubule (DCT)   86, 194–196, 198

Diverticulum   86, 104

Dolich/o   10

Dolichocephalic   10, 38

Dorsal (direction)   4, 6, 11

Dorsal horn   173

Dorsal root   172

Dorsum   vi, 4, 6, 16, 59–60, 239

Duct   77, 90, 138, 141, 143, 148, 211, 225–226, 233, 254

  alveolar   104, 106, 211

  bile   113

  collecting   86, 88, 196

  efferent   123–125

  pancreatic   113

  tear   101, 146

  thoracic   95, 114

Duct/o   10

Ductus arteriosus   90–92, 98, 235, 248

  patent ductus arteriosus (PDA)   91, 248

Ductus deferens   86, 123–125, 233

Dys-   7

Dyspnea   9, 211, 218, 252

e

Ear   4, 10–11, 21, 23–25, 27–28, 37–38, 50, 90, 148–149, 152, 155, 245–246, 253–254

Eardrum   24, 149, 254

Eccrine   15, 138, 140, 144

Echocardiogram   98, 208, 246

Ectropion   148

Efferent arteriole   196, 198–199

Efferent signal   172, 178

Ejaculation   124, 233, 237

EKG (ECG) wave   203

Elbow   4–6, 32, 51, 53, 61, 94, 161, 251

Electrical charge   130–131, 173–174, 201–202

Electrocardiogram   8, 203, 246. *See also* EKG (ECG) wave

Embryo   7, 121, 231–234, 236–237, 254

Emetic   222

Eminence   29, 34

Encephala/o   10

Encephalitis   19

Endo-   7

Endocarditis   222

Endocrine system   77–81, 181–191

Endocytosis   131

Endolymph   148–149

Endometrium   121, 234

Endoskeleton   29

Endothelium   92–93

Endotracheal tube   102, 108, 212, 252

Enter/o   10

Enterohepatic circulation   225–226

Entropion   148

Epaxial   60, 63

  iliocostal   60

  longissimus   60

  transversospinalis   60

Epi-   7

Epicardium   89, 98

Epidermis   13–14, 18–20, 137–143, 252

Epididymis   123–125, 233

Epidural space   72

Epiglottis   7, 102, 106, 155, 222

Epimysium   57

Epinephrine   170, 177, 179, 182, 185, 188, 207

Epiphyseal plate   31, 153, 160. *See also* Growth plate

Epiphysis   31, 78, 153–154, 161

Episioplasty   9. *See also* Vulvoplasty

Epithelial   9, 13, 22, 71, 86, 93, 113, 194

Epithelial cell   9, 13, 71, 86, 93

Equilibrium   v, ix, 21, 24–25, 28, 148, 252

Erectile tissue   87, 121, 124

Erection   124–125, 233, 237

Ergot   16

Erythema   13, 20, 27

Erythr/o-   7

Erythrocyte   7, 132, 135, 197, 215, 217

Erythropoiesis   10, 132

Erythropoietin   80, 155–157, 185, 189, 197

Esophagus   viii, 8, 80, 97, 102, 104, 107, 112, 115, 222, 227, 253

  abdominal   111, 116

  cervical   110, 116

  thoracic   110, 115–116

Esophagus serosa   111

Esthes/o   10

Estrogen   80, 141, 181, 184, 188–189, 231–233, 235

Estrous   xi, 119, 121, 231–233, 236, 252–253

Estrus   231–233, 236, 252

Ethmoid   22, 36, 101–102

Ethmoturbinate   22

Eu-   7
Eustachian tube   24, 28, 149
Euthyroid   186
Ewe   120
Ex/exo-   7
Excitatory potential   174
Excoriation   27
Exocrine   81, 113, 188, 190–191, 225
Exocytosis   131
Exoskeleton   7, 29
Extension   47, 50, 53–54, 61, 64, 67, 69, 93, 159, 161, 171, 193
Extensor carpi radialis   61, 243
Extensor carpi ulnaris   61
External abdominal oblique   60, 243
External auditory canal   23–24, 27, 149, 151, 254
External auditory meatus   37–38
External carotid artery   94
External ear   23, 27, 149
External intercostal muscle   104
Extra-   7, 233
Eyelash   8, 25
Eyelid   11, 15, 20, 25, 94, 146, 148, 152, 251

f
Facial artery   94
Facilitated diffusion   131
Fascia   57, 62, 65, 108, 162, 239, 243
Fascicle   57–58, 68, 252
Fasciculi   57, 68, 165, 252
Feather   13, 141, 184
   contour   17–18
   down   17–18
Feces   9, 74, 198, 221, 226
Feedback loop   150, 184, 190
   negative   177, 181–182, 185–187, 197, 224–225
   positive   181–182
Femoral   6, 51, 154, 243
   artery   95–96, 205
   nerve   73, 75
Femorotibial joint   4, 34, 50, 52. *See also* Stifle
Femur   4, 6, 30, 33–34, 42–43, 51–52, 59–61, 63, 153–155, 243
Fenestration   71, 86, 193–194
Fermentation   115, 227–229
Fetlock   50, 52
Fetus   3, 80, 90, 92, 234–235, 237
Fibrin   155
Fibroblasts   187
Fibrous joint   vi, 48, 50–51, 53, 159–161
   gomphosis   48, 109, 160, 162
   suture joint   36, 44, 48, 50, 53–54, 159, 162
   syndesmosis   48, 159, 162–163
Fibrous layer   25, 151

Fibula   33–35, 42–43, 159, 162
Fight or flight   161, 179, 207
Filtration   86, 131, 193, 197–198, 246
Fimbriae   120–121
Flank   6, 114
Flat bone   29, 31, 34, 36, 38, 44, 153–154
Flea   20, 67
Flehmen response   150
Flexion   47, 50, 53–54, 61, 159, 161
Flexor carpi radialis   61
Flexor carpi ulnaris   61
Floating teeth   222
Follicle:
   hair   14–17, 20, 138, 140–142
   ovarian   119, 184, 189, 231–233, 236
   thyroid   78, 184, 186
Follicle stimulating hormone (FSH)   183–185, 189, 232–234, 236
Fontanelle   159, 162
Foramen   29, 40–41
   jugular   38
   magnum   38–39, 72
   mental   36
   nutrient   31
   obturator   34, 61
   ovale   92, 235
   supracondylar   32
   supratrochlear   32
   trochlear   32
Forelimb   4–5, 9, 13, 31, 48, 142
Fossa   29, 31, 33–34, 51, 77, 83, 155
Fovea   29, 32
Frog   18, 142
Frontal bone   36, 48, 58
Functional residual capacity   213
Fundic   26
Fur   13, 16, 137
Furcula   43

g
Ganglion   68, 73, 172, 177
Gas   x, 14, 105–106, 130, 132, 211–212, 214–218, 227
Gastr/o   10, 12
Gastric artery   95
Gastrin   80, 185, 189, 224, 228
Gastrocnemius   34, 63, 65, 168, 243
G cell   80–81, 224, 228
Gelatinous   24–27, 146, 148–149, 151
Gelding   120
Gemelli   61
Genital   16, 86, 94
Genital fold   86

Gestation period   235, 252
Gib   120
Gilt   120
Gingiv/o   10
Gingiva   108–109, 111
Gland:
  accessory reproductive   124
  adrenal   x, 11, 78–81, 175, 181, 183–185, 187–188, 195,
    207, 232, 240, 252–253
  anal   15, 61, 114, 140, 143–144
  bulbourethral   124
  endocrine   x, 77–79, 81, 181–183, 185, 190
  lacrimal   25
  mammary   10, 15, 122, 125, 141, 169, 183
  meibomian   25, 148, 152
  parathyroid   x, 78–79, 81, 154, 186
  pineal   vii, 78, 81
  salivary   107–108, 221
  sebaceous   14–16, 20, 74, 114, 123, 140–142, 144, 150, 254
  sweat (sudoriferous)   14–15, 138, 140–143
  tail   140, 143
  thyroid   x, 8, 78, 184, 186
  vesicular   124
Glaucoma   147
Glenoid fossa   31, 51
Glial cell   67, 71, 74, 174
  astrocyte   71, 74
  oligodendrocyte   67, 174
  schwann cell   67, 174, 179
Globe   25, 139, 146–147, 149
Glomerular filtrate   193, 196, 198
Glomerular filtration rate (GFR)   193, 246
Glomerulus   80, 86, 93, 188, 193–194, 196–199, 209
Gloss/o   10
Glottis   102
Glucocorticoid   79–80, 185, 187–188, 191
Gluconeogenesis   187, 226
Glucose   94, 130, 134, 167, 171, 173, 175, 185, 187–189,
    194, 225–226
Glucosuria   194
Gluteal   60, 62, 95–96, 243
Glyc/gluc/o   10
Glycogen   167, 170, 188, 226
Glycolipid   14
Gnath/o   10
Goblet cell   224
Gomphosis   48, 109, 160, 162
Gonads   vii, 78–79, 119, 185, 189
Gracilis   62, 64, 243
Granulocyte   133, 135
Gray matter   67, 69–70, 72, 252
Greater trochanter   33, 243

Gross anatomy   3, 55
Ground substance   137
Growth hormone (GH)   141, 183–185, 235
Growth plate   49, 54, 153, 156, 160. *See also* Epiphyseal plate
Guard hair   16–17, 20, 141–142
Gubernaculum   123
Gustatory   ix, 22, 145, 150–152
Gyri   69

h
Hair   viii, 3, 8, 11, 13–18, 20, 24–25, 47, 67, 77, 83, 108,
    137–143, 149, 151, 165, 181, 246, 251, 254
Hair cell   24–25, 149, 151
Haircoat   v, 16–18, 81, 138–141, 187, 198
Hairless   18, 138, 140–141
Hardware disease   115
HCO_3 224–225
Head (skeletal):
  femur   33–34, 51, 154
  fibula   34
  humerus   31–32, 51, 154
  long bone   6, 30
  radius   33, 156
Hearing   v, 21, 23–24, 37, 58, 70, 145, 149, 178
Heart   vii, x, 3, 7–9, 55, 70, 80–81, 83, 89–96, 98, 103, 105,
    115, 138, 156, 167, 169, 173, 176–177, 179, 186, 188,
    196–197, 201–209, 214–215, 222, 226–228, 234–235, 237,
    241, 246–247, 251, 253–254
Heart murmur   89, 169, 206, 209
Heart rate (HR)   8, 70, 156, 176–177, 179, 186, 188, 204,
    227–228, 237, 247
Heartworm   204
Heat   150, 231, 236. *See also* Estrus
Heel   18
Heifer   120
Hemat/o   10
Hemes   215
Hemi-   7
Hemoglobin (Hb)   x, 132–133, 139, 215–219, 247
  methemoglobin   216
  oxyhemoglobin   215
Hemolytic   139
Hepat/o   10
Hepatic artery   95
Hepatic vein   97
Hetero-   7
Hiatus:
  aortic   95, 104
  esophageal   104, 110
Hip dysplasia   34, 51, 161
Hippocampus   176, 179
Histamine   133, 169, 224

Hob   120
Hock   4, 45
Home/o-   7
Homeostasis   7, 9, 70, 77, 130, 171, 193, 252
Homeotherm   138
Hoof   7, 15, 18–19, 42–43, 61, 142, 227
Hooves   v, viii, 13, 16, 18, 137, 142, 254
Hormone   x, 31, 77–80, 112–113, 122–123, 132, 141,
    154–155, 157, 169, 171, 175, 184–191, 194–197,
    206–207, 225, 231–233, 235–236, 245–246, 248,
    252, 254
  bound   182, 186
  free (unbound)   182
  inhibiting hormone   183
  monoamine hormone   182–183
  peptide hormone   182–183, 190
  releasing hormone   182–183, 190
  steroid hormone   182–183, 187, 190
Horn   v, viii, 13, 16, 18–20, 120–121, 125, 137, 142–144, 234
Humeroradioulnar joint   4–6, 32, 51, 53, 61, 94, 161. *See also*
    Elbow; Radiohumeral joint
Humerus   30–32, 34, 43, 51, 59, 154, 156, 162, 243
  deltoid tuberosity   32, 59, 243
  greater tuberosity   32
  supracondylar foramen   32
  supratrochlear foramen   32
Husbandry   19
Hydration   viii, 15, 105, 137, 139, 184, 221, 225, 254
Hydrochloric acid (HCl)   224
Hydrolysis   225
Hydrophilic   182–183, 252
Hydrophobic   182–183, 252
Hydrostatic pressure   206
Hyoid   102
Hypaxial muscle   60
Hyper-   7
Hyperadrenocorticism   187, 189
Hypercalcemia   186
Hyperglycemia   8, 194
Hyperparathyroidism   187
Hyperplasia (adrenal)   187
Hyperpolarization   173
Hyperthermia   7, 11, 212, 218, 236
Hyperthyroidism   8, 78, 81, 186, 206
Hypertonic   131, 134
Hypo-   7
Hypoadrenocorticism   188
Hypodermis   13–15, 139, 252, 254
Hypoglycemia   10, 134, 171, 188
Hypophysis   77, 81. *See also* Pituitary
Hypothalamus   vii, v, 70, 77–78, 81, 138, 175–176, 182–187,
    190, 207, 232

Hypothermia   7, 212
Hypotonic   131, 134
Hypsodont   222, 229

i

Iatro   10
Iatrogenic   10, 188, 252
Icterus   139, 144
Ile/o   10
Ileocolic junction   113
Ileus   113
Iliac:
  artery   95–96
  common iliac vein   97
  crest   34
  external iliac artery   95
  external iliac vein   96
  internal iliac artery   95–96
  internal iliac vein   96–97
  vein   96–97
Iliacus   60
Ilium   34, 51, 155, 156, 160, 243
  wing of the ilium   34–35
Immune system   14, 20, 80–81, 123, 133, 143, 156, 184,
    187, 251
Immunocompromised   20
Incise   239
Inclusion   129
Infra-   7
infraorbital   7, 140
Infraspinatus   59
Infraspinous   31
Infundibulum   120–121, 125
Ingesta   107, 110, 113, 222, 224–225, 253
inguinal   94, 99, 111, 123, 140
inguinal sebaceous   140
Inhale   213
Inhibitory impulse   174
Integration   146, 148, 176
Integument   v, viii, 10, 13–14, 16, 18–20, 137–140,
    142–144, 254
Inter-   7
Intercalated disc   56, 167, 201–202
Intercondylar:
  eminence   34
  fossa   33
Intercostal muscle   104
Interdigital   7, 15, 43, 45, 140
Intermediate filament   168
Internal abdominal oblique   60, 64
Internal carotid artery   216
Internal ear   23

Internal intercostal muscle   104
Internal thoracic artery   94
Interparietal bone   37
Interphalangeal joint   50, 52
Interstitial:
   cell   79, 184
   fluid   89, 93
   space   93, 194, 253
Interstitial cell stimulating hormone (ICSH)   184. *See also*
      Luteinizing hormone
Intestine   viii, xi, 9–10, 22, 63, 78, 80, 86, 92–95, 107,
      111–115, 117, 185, 189, 217, 224–228, 239, 252–253
Intra-   7, 233
Intraosseous membrane   160, 163
Intrinsic factor   224, 228
Intromission   233, 237
Intubated   212
Intussusception   113
Invertebrate   7, 29
Iridocorneal angle   147
Iris   25–28, 63, 146–147, 169
Iron   132–133, 155, 215–216, 218
Irregular bone   29, 31, 34, 40, 44–45, 153
Ischiatic nerve   73, 75. *See also* Sciatic
Ischium   34, 61, 160, 243
Islets of Langerhans   79, 81, 188–189
Iso-   7
Isosthenuria   7, 193
Isotonic   131, 134

j

Jack   120
Jacobson's organ   22–23
Jejun/o   10
Jenny   120
Jill   120
Jugular vein   38, 96–97
Juxtaglomerular cells   80, 197

k

Keel   43–44
Keratin   13, 17–19, 137
Keratinization   14, 137
Keratinocytes   13–14, 137, 144
Keratoconjunctivitis sicca (KCS)   148, 247
Ketone   226
Kidney   vii, v, 3, 8, 10–11, 78–81, 83–88, 93, 95, 99, 111, 113,
      116, 119, 150, 155, 169, 185–189, 193–199, 206, 217, 225,
      240, 251–253
   caudal pole   83
   cranial pole   79, 83
Krebs cycle   130

l

Labia   121–122
Laceration   5, 11, 20
Lacrimal apparatus   148
Lacrimal bone   36
Lactation   119, 141, 184–185, 233, 235
Lactic acid   131, 167, 170
Lactose   225
Lagomorph   114, 227
Lamina   40–41
Laminitis   19, 42, 227
Langerhans   13–14, 79, 81, 188
Lanolin   140
Laparotomy   9, 124
Large intestine   9, 107, 111, 114, 117, 225. *See also* Colon
Laryngopharynx   110
Larynx   vii, 94, 102–103, 106, 110, 211
Lateral condyle   30, 32–34
Lateral digital extensor   61, 63
Lateral saphenous vein   97
Latissimus dorsi   59–61, 64, 243
Laxative   226
Left atrioventricular (AV) valve   91, 205
Left bundle branch   202
Lens   25–28, 146–147, 151, 241
Lesion   4
Lesser trochanter femur   34
Lethargy   83, 129, 165, 188
Leuk/o-   7
Leukocyte   7–8, 12, 132
   basophil   132–133, 135, 169
   eosinophil   132–133, 135, 169
   lymphocyte   9, 132–133, 135
   monocyte   132–133, 135
   neutrophil   132–133, 135
Levator ani   61, 243
Ligament   32, 34, 37, 43, 49–50, 63, 80, 112, 124, 160–163,
      235, 253–254
   apical   124
   broad   86, 119–121
   caudal cruciate   52
   cranial cruciate   52
   gastrosplenic   112
   periodontal   160
   round   86
   sacrotuberous   51
   suspensory   26, 28, 61, 121, 146
Ligamentum arteriosum   90
Limbic system   176, 179, 181
Linea alba   57, 60, 240, 243
Linear motion   25
Lingu/o   10

Lipase   224, 227–228
Lipid soluble   129, 131
Lith-   7
Liver   viii, xi, 7, 10–11, 80, 93, 95, 97, 107, 112, 139, 188, 195, 198, 206, 225–226, 228, 253
Lobes   149, 251, 253
    brain   69–70
    liver   112
    lung   89–90, 103–106
    pituitary   77–78
    thyroid   78
Long bone   29–34, 44–45, 48, 153–154, 156
Longitudinal fissure   69
Loop of Henle   86, 194–196, 198
Lubricate   25, 104, 140, 148, 161, 224
Lumen   92–93, 114, 225, 253
Luminal:
    alveoli   214
    duodenum   113
    esophagus   111
    stomach   111, 223–224
Lung parenchyma   214, 217
Luteal phase   232
luteinizing hormone (LH)   183–185, 189–190, 231–233, 236
Lymph   89, 93–94, 96, 99, 111, 114, 161, 208–209, 254
Lymph node   89, 111, 114, 161, 208
    axillary lymph node   94
    inguinal lymph node   94, 99
    popliteal lymph node   94, 96, 99
    prescapular lymph node   94, 99
    submandibular lymph node   94, 99
Lymphatic   vii, v, 14, 57, 89, 93–95, 111–112, 114, 121, 123, 161, 208–209, 252
Lymphatic vessel   57, 89, 93–95, 111, 208
Lymphocyte   9, 132
    B-lymphocyte   133
    natural killer (NK) cells   133, 135
    T-lymphocyte   133, 135
Lymphoma   93

m
Macro-   7
Macrophages   133, 135, 139, 208
Macula   24–25, 148, 151, 197
Macula densa   197
Malassezia   27
Malignant   9, 134
Malleolus   34
Malocclusion   222
Malodorous   27
Mammary   10, 15, 122, 125, 141, 169, 183

Mammo/mast   10
Mandible   36–37, 49–50, 58, 73, 94, 107–109, 116, 143, 160, 162, 187, 243
Mandibular symphysis   8, 36–37, 49–50, 53, 160
Manubrium   40
Manus   33, 52, 253
Mare   119–120
Mass   3–4, 11, 15, 81, 114, 168, 203
Masseter   58, 94, 107, 243
Mast cell   169, 247
Maxilla   36, 58, 108–109, 143, 187
Maxillary artery   94
Meatus   29, 37–38, 102, 106
Mechanical receptor   142, 145
Medial condyle   32–34, 243
Medial gluteal   60
Medial saphenous vein   97
Median:
    artery   94
    nerve   73
Mediastinum   80–81, 103, 105, 133, 253
Medulla:
    adrenal   79–80, 185, 188
    hair   17
    renal   83–88, 193, 199
Megakaryocyte   132–134
Meissner's corpuscle   15, 139
Melan/o-   7
Melanin   13–14, 25, 137–138
Melanocyte stimulating hormone (MSH)   183
Melanocytes   13, 137, 144
Meninges   vi, 68, 72, 74
Meniscus   50, 52, 161, 163
Merkel:
    cell   13, 139, 144
    disc   139
Mesenteric artery   95, 99, 113–114
Mesentery   95, 111, 113–114, 116
Meso-   7
Mesocephalic   9, 38
Mesoductus   124
Meta-   7
Metabolism:
    aerobic   130–131, 167
    anaerobic   130–131, 134, 167, 170
Metacarpal   15, 31–34, 42, 52, 61, 142, 243
Metacarpophalangeal joint   32, 50
Metacarpus   7, 9, 32, 243
Metaphysis   31, 153–154
Metatarsal   15, 33–34, 42, 45, 52, 142, 243
Metri/o/a   10
Micro-   7

Middle ear   23–24, 50, 149, 254

Milk   29, 36, 115, 122, 125, 141, 154, 183–186, 232, 235–236

Milk let down   184–185

Mineralocorticoid   79–80, 185, 187–188

Miosis   177

Mitochondria   55, 130, 134, 170

Mitral valve   91–92, 94, 99, 205–206. *See also* Left Atrioventricular (AV) valve

Modified neurons   21–22, 24

Mononuclear   129–130, 133

Motor unit   169

Mucocutaneous border   101, 107

Mucous membrane   7, 22–23, 25, 101–102, 124, 137, 139, 169, 198, 211, 222, 247, 252

Multinuclear   129–130

Multipotent cell   132

Muscarinic   177, 207

Muscle:

  belly (head)   57, 65

  cardiac   ix–x, 55–57, 64, 91, 165, 167, 170, 201–202, 204, 207, 209

  condition score (MCS)   168

  fasciculation   167

  fast twitch   168

  fiber   55, 57–58, 147, 165–170, 202–203, 252

  insertion   55, 57, 59

  muscle twitch   58, 167–168, 171

  origin   57, 59, 61, 243

  skeletal   vi, ix, 21, 55–58, 61, 63–65, 88–89, 104, 165–170, 176–177, 203, 207, 217

  slow twitch   168

  smooth   vi, 55, 57, 63–65, 86–87, 89, 92, 111–112, 165, 168–170, 176–177, 206, 211, 214, 222, 226

Muscle cell   55–57, 63, 131, 165–170, 201–202, 254

Musculotendinous   213

Myelin sheath   67–68, 74, 174, 178

Myelinated   67, 174

Myo-   7

Myofibril   55, 165

Myogenic muscle   107

Myoglobin   131, 167–168, 217

Myometrium   121, 182

Myosin   57, 165–168, 170

Myosin head   166–167

n

Nares   22–23, 101–102, 105–106, 211–212

Nasal   44, 71, 108, 149–150

  alae   101

  bone   36

  cavity/passage   10–11, 22–23, 36, 38–39, 44, 71, 101–106, 110, 146, 149–150, 211, 222

  conchae   23, 38, 102, 106

  philtrum   101–102, 106

  planum   101, 106, 137, 140, 143

  septum   22, 36, 38, 101

  turbinates   22–23, 102

  vestibule   101

Nasopharynx   110, 211, 253

Navicular bone   43

Neck (anatomical marker):

  bladder   86–87

  bone   32

  tooth   109, 111

Necro-   7

Neo-   7

Neonate   7, 15, 104, 106, 122, 140

Neonate terms   120

Nephro   10

Nephron   vii, v, 10, 80, 84–86, 88, 93, 193–198, 225, 253

Nervous layer   25–26, 151

Nervous sytem:

  autonomic   ix–x, 63, 68, 71–72, 138, 147, 168–169, 172, 174–176, 181, 187, 202, 204, 206–207, 211, 214, 219, 241

  central (CNS)   21, 25, 67–68, 73–74, 77, 139, 145, 149–150, 162, 171, 178, 181–182, 186, 188, 207, 213–214, 246, 252, 254

  craniosacral   177

  nucleus   68, 74

  parasympathetic   176–177, 188, 219, 223

  peripheral   vii, 67, 73–74, 174, 176

  somatic   219

  sympathetic   161, 176–177, 179, 185, 188, 190, 204, 207, 219, 233

  thoracolumbar   177

Neuro   10

Neurocranium   159

Neurogenic muscle   167

Neurohormone   77

Neurohypophysis   78, 183

Neuromuscular junction   166

Neuron   vi, ix, 21–22, 24, 67–68, 74, 138, 166, 168–169, 171–175, 177–178, 252–254

Neurotransmitter   67–68, 74, 79, 81, 166–170, 173–175, 177–179, 183, 188, 190–191, 207, 214, 252, 254

Neuter   10, 119, 124, 253. *See also* Orchiectomy

Nicotinic   177

Nictitating membrane   25, 146

Nipple   16, 122–123, 141

Nociception   150, 253

Nociceptor   162–163

Nodes of Ranvier   67, 172, 174

nonsteroidal anti-inflammatory drugs (NSAID)   189, 191

Non-striated muscle   165, 168, 170. *See also* Smooth muscle

Norepinephrine 168, 170, 177, 185, 188, 190, 207
Nose 4, 11, 16, 22, 29, 36–38, 44, 69, 101, 104, 137, 146, 149, 211, 246, 254
Nostril 22, 101, 105, 149, 211
Nucleus (cellular) 57, 129–130, 132–135, 182–183
Nystagmus 149

O

Obturator muscle 60
Occipital:
  bone 36, 38
  condyle 38, 69
  crest 36
  lobe 69
Ocul/o 10
Olecranon 32, 61, 92, 156
Olfactory 102, 108, 145, 149, 253
  bulb 22, 69, 150, 176
  sense 22, 171, 241
Omasum 115, 227
Omentum 112, 240
Omotransversarius 59, 61
Onych/o 10
Onychectomy (declaw) 18
Ophthalm/o 10
Ophthalmic 148 151
Optic:
  optic chiasm 71, 147, 176
  optic disc 26, 28
  optic nerve 25–26, 71, 147, 176
Orbicularis oculi 58
Orbicularis oris 58
Orchi/o 10
Orchiectomy 8, 10, 119, 253
Organelle 55–57 129, 134, 137, 165–166
Organ of Corti 24–25, 28, 149, 151
Organophosphate 178
Oro 10
Oropharynx 10, 102, 110, 211, 222, 253
Orthopneic 211, 253
Os cordis 91
Os coxae 34
Os penis 124–125
Osmosis 131, 194, 198, 253
Osseo, oste/o 10
Ossicle 28, 37, 50
  incus 24
  malleus 24
  stapes 24, 149, 151
Ossification 49, 53, 157, 160
Ossify 31, 49
Osteoarthritis 161–163, 247
Osteoblast 8, 153–154, 156
Osteochondritis dissecans 51
Osteoclast 153, 156
Osteology ix, 8, 153–156
Osteons 154–155
Otitis 10, 27
Oto 10
Otolith 25, 148, 151
Otoscope 27–28
Oval window 24, 149, 151
Ovarian artery 96, 121, 123
Ovaries 78–80, 96, 120–121, 123, 184–185, 189, 253. *See also* Ovary
Ovariohysterectomy 60, 86, 121, 231, 236, 247, 253
Ovary 86, 119, 125, 231–233. *See also* Ovaries
Oviduct 86, 120–121, 125, 234, 237
Ovulation 184, 231–233, 236, 252
Ovum 120–121, 231–232, 234
Oxidation 130, 167, 215–216
Oxidation-reduction 130
Oxygen (O_2) 7, 38, 68, 89–90, 93–96, 99, 101, 108, 123, 130–132, 134, 139, 167, 169–171, 177, 189, 193, 196, 203, 205–208, 211–212, 214–219, 227, 234, 252
Oxygenation xi, 204, 215, 217–218
Oxyhemoglobin dissociation curve 215
Oxytocin 122, 141, 169, 182–185, 232, 234–236

P

Pacinian corpuscle 139, 144
Packed cell volume (PCV) 248
Pads v, viii, 14–16, 50, 138, 142, 160–161
Pain 8, 14, 18–19, 21, 25, 28, 53, 73, 88, 95, 97, 139, 150, 161–162, 217–218, 221–222, 227
Palate:
  cleft palate 36, 38, 44
  hard palate 38, 44, 108, 254
  soft palate 105, 108, 116
Palatine bone 36, 38, 44, 108
Palatoglossal arch 107
Palmar 6, 15–16, 18, 62, 142, 243, 253–254
Palpebrum 146
Pan- 7
Pancreas vii, v, 78–79, 81, 95, 107, 113, 116, 181, 185, 188–189, 191, 224–225, 227–228
Pancreatitis 12, 79, 227
Panniculus 58
Papillae:
  dermal 14
  duodenal 113
  gustatory 22, 108
Papillary muscle 91
Para- 8

Parafollicular cell (C-Cell)   186
Parathyroid hormone (PTH)   154, 185–187, 190, 194, 248
Parietal:
  bone   36, 48
  cell   224, 228
  lobe   69
  serosa   106
Partial pressure   214
Parturition   xi, 121–122, 141, 182, 232, 235, 237, 253
Passive immunity   141
Pastern:
  long pastern   42–43, 52
  short pastern   42–43, 52
Patella   33–34, 45, 52, 63, 161, 243
Patellar surface   34
Patellar tendon   30, 52, 63, 175, 243
Pectoantebrachialis   59
Pectoral deep   58–59
Pectoral girdle   43
Pectoral superficial   58–59
Pectoralis major   58–59
Pectoralis minor   58
Pelvic girdle   59, 80
Pelvis   v–vi, 6, 10, 34–36, 40, 42, 49, 51, 53, 59–62, 74, 86–88,
     119, 124, 160, 193, 196, 199, 235, 243
Penis   87, 96, 121, 124–125, 233
Pepsinogen   224, 228
Peri-   8, 122
Pericardial effusion   89
Pericardium   8, 90, 94
  fibrous pericardium   89
  serous pericardium   89, 98
Perilymph   28, 151
Perimetrium   121
Perimysium   57
Perineum   61, 74, 114
Periosteum   31, 49, 68, 153
Peripheral circulation   vii, 204
Peristalsis   63, 169, 222, 225
Peritoneal membrane   6, 83
Peritoneum   6, 83, 111, 114, 121, 253
Peritubular capillaries   194, 198
Pes   35, 253
Phalange   9, 31–35, 42–43, 243
Phalanx   18, 33, 35, 42–43, 248, 253
Phalanx:
  P1   33, 35, 42, 52
  P2   33, 35, 42, 52
  P3   18, 33, 35, 42–43, 52, 248
Pharyng/o   10
Pharynx   viii, 8, 10, 24, 38, 94, 102, 107, 110, 211, 253
Pheromones   v, 15, 23, 28, 141, 149–150, 152, 189, 191, 233

Phleb/o   10
Phospholipid   129, 134, 182
Photoperiod   233
Photoreceptor   26–28, 145, 147, 151
  cone cell   26–27
  rod cell   26–27
Pigment   7, 13, 26, 28, 137–140, 146, 215
Pinna   4, 23–24, 49, 53, 58, 73, 108, 139, 146, 149, 155, 253
Pituitary   141, 169, 175, 195, 197
  anterior   v, 77–78, 80, 182–187, 190, 232, 236. *See also*
     Adenohypophysis
  intermediate   78
  posterior   77–78, 81, 183–185, 232. *See also* Neurohypophysis
  stalk   77, 183
Placenta   80, 232, 234–236
  retained   235
Plantar   6, 15–16, 18, 62, 142, 243, 254
Plantigrade   142
Plasma   7, 132–133, 135, 161, 182–183, 193, 197, 208, 215
Platelet   viii, 89, 132, 134, 153. *See also* Thrombocyte
Platysma   58
Pleura   vii, 103–104, 213, 254
Pleural effusion   104
Pleural membrane   6
Pleuritis   104
Plexus   161, 254
  brachial   73, 75, 95
  cervical   73
  lumbar   73
  pampiniform   123
  periarticular   161
  venous   93, 121
Pneum/o   10
Pneumatized   43, 155
Pod/o   10
Poiesis   10
Poikilo   10
Poikilotherm   138, 144
Polarized   130, 166, 201–202
Poly-   8
Polydactyl   8, 10, 12, 18, 254
Polydipsia (PD)   10–11, 187–189, 236, 248
Polyestrous   233
Polyuria (PU)   187–189
Popliteal artery   96
Portal circulation   226
Portal system   77, 183
Portal vein   97, 112–114
Post-   8, 197
Posterior chamber   27, 146–147
Postganglionic   177
Postsynaptic   68, 74, 173–175, 178, 254

Pre- 8, 197
Preauricular   58
Preganglionic   175
Prehensile   221
Preload   204, 210
Premature atrial contraction (PAC)   203
Premature ventricular contraction (PVC)   203
Prepuce   96, 124
Presynaptic   68, 173–174, 178, 254
Primary hair   16, 141. *See also* Guard hair
Proenzyme   224, 228
Proestrus   231, 236
Progestin   80
Prolactin   141, 183–185, 190, 232–233, 235–236
Pronate   62, 254
Pronator quadratus   61
Pronator teres   61
Proprioception   ix, 21, 28, 148, 162, 254
Propulsion   225
Prostaglandin   v, 189, 191, 232, 235
Prostate   84, 124–125, 197
Prostatic artery   96
Protection   viii, 31, 69, 71, 123, 137, 141, 143–144, 153, 161
Proventriculus   115
Proximal convoluted tubule (PCT)   86, 194, 198–199
Pruritus   13, 19–20
Pseudo-   8
Pseudopregnancy   8, 233
Puberty   233
Pubic brim   111
Pubic symphysis   8, 49, 51, 160
Pubis   34, 160
Pudendal artery   96, 114
Pudendal nerve   74, 87
Pulmo/n   10
Pulmonary artery   90–91, 96, 204–205, 209
Pulmonary Circuit   92, 204
Pulmonary valve   91–92, 99, 205
Pulmonary vein   90, 96, 205
Pulse deficit   95, 205
Pupil   26, 146–147, 176–177, 241
Purkinje fiber   202, 209
Pyelo   10
Pygostyle   43
Pyo   11
Pyometra   10, 236

q

Quadratus femoris   61
Quadriceps   63, 243
  rectus femoris   63
  vastus intermedius   63
  vastus lateralis   62–63
  vastus medialis   63
Quarters   19
Queen   120
Quick   18, 20

r

Radial bone   32
Radial nerve   73, 75, 95
Radioactive iodine   186
Radiograph (X-Ray)   3, 42–43, 53, 64, 98, 105, 113, 115, 153, 161–162, 213, 217, 227, 245–246, 248, 254. *See also* X-Ray
Radiohumeral joint   32. *See also* Elbow; Humeroradioulnar joint
Radius   31–33, 43, 48, 61–62, 156, 159–160, 243
Ram   120
Ramus of the mandible   36, 50, 107–108
Re-   8, 23
Receptor adaptation   146
Rectum   61, 74, 87, 95–97, 107, 114, 121, 124
Rectus abdominis   60
Redox balance   130
Referred upper airway noise   105
Reflex   67, 175, 222, 254
  myotatic   175
  patellar   175
Refractory period:
  absolute refractory period   173, 179
  relative refractory period   173–174
Relaxin   80, 235, 237
Ren/o   11
Renal:
  artery   83, 86, 88, 95, 99, 193, 197–199
  corpuscle   86, 88
  cortex   83–88, 193, 199
  hilus   83, 88, 199
  medulla   83–88, 193, 199
  pelvis   10, 86, 88, 193, 196, 199
  threshold   194
  vein   88, 97, 99
Renin   80, 185, 188–189, 196–197, 199
Renin-Angiotensin-Aldosterone (RAA) System   185, 196, 199
Reperfusion injury   130
Repolarization   v, 173, 202–203, 209
Reptile   3, 18, 78, 90, 119, 132, 187
Respiratory acidosis   216–217
Respiratory alkalosis   216, 218
Respiratory tract   38, 169, 177, 188, 211–213, 218
  lower   103, 211
  upper   211, 213
Rest and digest   177, 179, 208, 219

Resting potential   173, 178
Rete   93
Reticular   14–15
Reticulum   55, 115, 165–166, 170, 227, 229, 252, 254
Retina   10, 25–27, 71, 146–147
Retro-   8
Rhamphotheca   143
Rhin/o   11
Rhomboideus   59, 64
Right atrioventricular (AV) valve   205. *See also* Tricuspid
     valve (Right AV valve)
Right bundle branch   202
Rongeur   222
Rostral plate   105–106
Rotary motion   25, 28, 148
Round window   24
Rubber jaw   187
Rugae   108, 111, 116, 223, 254
Rumen   115, 227, 229
Ruminant   15, 19, 34, 52, 60, 63, 91, 112, 114–115, 123–124,
     142, 216, 227–228

S
Sacroiliac joint   51
Sacrum   42, 45, 51, 73–74, 177
Saddle thrombus   95
Saliva   152, 221, 227, 241
Salivary gland   107–108, 221
   mandibular   108
   parotid   108
   sublingual   108
Saphenous artery   96
Saphenous nerve   73
Saphenous vein   96–97, 99, 168
Sarcolemma   55, 165–166, 170, 254
Sarcomere   55–56, 166–167
Sarcoplasm   165, 170, 254
Sarcoplasmic reticulum   55, 165–166, 170, 254
Sarcoptic Mange   20
Sartorius   62, 64, 243
Scalenus   59, 213
Scales   13, 17, 78
Scalpel blade   20, 239
Scapula   31–32, 40, 43, 51, 58–59, 61, 243
Scapulohumeral joint   31, 51. *See also* Shoulder
Scent   16, 140–141, 143
Sciatic   62, 73
Sclera   25, 139, 146
Scrotum   79, 123–124, 140
Scruff   15, 139
Sebaceous gland   14–16, 20, 74, 114, 123, 140–142, 144,
     150, 254

carpal   140
circumanal   140
circumoral   140
cutaneous pouch   140, 143
interdigital sebaceous   15, 140
sebaceous   140
tail   140
Sebum   15, 17, 140, 254
Secondary hair   16–17, 141. *See also* Wool hair
Secondary renal hyperparathyroidism   18. *See also*
     Hyperparathyroidism
Secretin   80, 185, 189, 224
Segmentation   225
Seizure   129, 150, 188
Sella turcica   77, 81
Semen   87, 124, 233, 237
Semi-   8
Semicircular canal   24–25, 28, 148, 151–152
Semilunar valve   91, 205
Semimembranosus   62, 243
Seminiferous tubule   123, 233–234, 237
Semitendinosus   62–63, 65, 73, 243
Sensory nerve   139, 162
Septum   202–203
   atrioventricular   92
   interatrial   92
   nasal   22, 36, 38, 101
   ventricular   92, 202
Serosa   106, 111
Serratus dorsalis   59
Serratus muscle   59
Serratus ventralis   59, 65, 243
Sertoli cell   123
Sesamoid bone   29–32, 34, 43, 45
Sex hormone   79–80, 122, 182, 185, 187–188, 252
Shaft   14, 16, 31, 45, 153, 156
Short bone   29–32, 43–45, 153
Shoulder   vi, 4, 6, 31, 43, 51, 59, 61, 92, 251. *See also*
     Scapulohumeral joint
Shunt   226
Sigmoid flexure   124
Signalment   28, 64
Sinister/o   11
Sinoatrial node (SA node)   201–202
Sinus   17, 77, 97, 247
   frontal   19, 102, 143
   maxillary   102
Sinusoid   93
Sire   120, 233
Skull   vi, 4, 9–10, 19, 22–23, 31, 36–39, 41, 43, 48,
     50–51, 53, 68–69, 77, 102, 142–143, 151,
     159, 162

Small intestine   xi, 9, 78, 80, 107, 185, 189, 252
  duodenum   79, 95, 113–114, 116, 224–226, 228
  ileum   10, 95, 113–114, 116, 225
  jejunum   10, 95, 113, 225
Smell   v, 21–22, 27, 69, 102, 108, 145, 149–150, 152, 221,
    241, 253
Smooth muscle   vi, 55, 57, 63–65, 86–87, 89, 92, 111–112,
    165, 168–170, 176–177, 206, 211, 214, 222, 226
  multiunit   63, 65, 169–170
  single unit   63, 169, 181
Sodium Potassium pump   173
Sole   18
Soma   67–68, 74, 171–172, 174, 177–178
Somatostatin   183–185, 188
Sow   120–121
Sperm   79, 86, 123–124, 184–185, 231, 233–234, 237. *See also*
    Spermatozoa
Spermatic cord   84, 123, 125
Spermatogenesis   123, 233, 237
Spermatozoa   122–125, 184, 233–234, 237.*See also* Sperm
Sphenoid   38
Sphincter   121, 176–177, 206, 222
  anal   61, 74, 114, 226
  lower esophageal   111
  pyloric   112–113, 224
  upper esophageal   110, 116
Spine   4, 29, 31, 40, 53, 59, 64, 124, 142, 160, 181, 243, 252
Spine of the scapula   31, 59, 243
Spinous process   40–42
Splenic contraction   217
Splint bone   42, 45, 52
Sprite   120
SQ   15, 248. *See also* Sub Q; Subcutaneous
Stallion   120
Stay apparatus   61, 63
Steer   120
Stenotic   105
Stercobilin   226
Stercobilinogen   226
Sternocephalicus   58
Sternum   vi, 31, 38–40, 43–44, 58, 89–90, 240, 243
Stertor   105
Stifle   4, 6, 11, 44, 45, 50, 52, 62–63, 94, 96, 175, 243. *See also*
    Femorotibial joint
Stimulated (induced) ovulator   232
Stoma   11
Stomach   viii, xi, 8–12, 78, 80–81, 95, 107, 110–116, 170,
    185, 189, 222–225, 227–228, 239–240, 254
  cardia   112, 115
  fundus   26, 112, 116
  greater curvature   112, 116, 240
  lesser curvature   112

pyloric antrum   112, 224
  pylorus   112
  ruminant   115, 228
Stomach serosa   111
Stratum basale   14
Stratum corneum   14
Stratum granulosum   14
Stratum lucidum   14, 20
Stratum spinosum   14
Stretch receptor   21, 28, 150, 207, 214
Striated   ix, 57, 83, 111, 114, 165–170, 201, 222, 226
Striated involuntary muscle   170. *See also* Cardiac muscle
Striated voluntary muscle   57, 170
Stridor   105
Stroke volume   204, 218
Styloid process   32
Sub Q   15. *See also* SQ; Subcutaneous
Sub-   8, 15
Subarachnoid space   68–69
Subclavian artery   94
Subclavian vein   96, 99
Subcutaneous   8, 13–15, 58, 139, 248, 252, 254. *See also* SQ
Subdural space   68
Sublingual   8, 10, 108
Sublumbar muscles   60
Suborbital   15
Sulci   69
Superficial brachial artery   94
Superficial digital flexor   61, 243
Superficial gluteal   60, 62
Supernumerary nipple   122–123
Supinate   61–62, 254
Supinator muscle   61
Supporting cell   24–25
Supra-   8
Suprahamate process   31
Supraspinatus   59, 64, 243
Supraspinous   31
Surface area   22, 69, 83–84, 111, 123, 129, 212, 223, 245
Surfactant   214, 219
Suture   60, 248
Suture joint   36, 44, 48, 50, 53–54, 159, 162
  coronal suture   48, 162
  sagittal suture   48
Sweat   14–15, 20, 123, 138, 140–144
Sy/syl/sym-   8
Symphysis   8, 36–37, 49–51, 53–54, 160, 163, 243
Synapse   vi, 67–68, 166, 173–175, 254
Synaptic bulb   67
Synaptic terminal   174
Synchondrosis   49, 54, 160, 163
Syncope   208

Syndesmosis   48, 159, 162–163
Synovial
  cavity   49, 160–161
    condyloid (ellipsoidal)   50, 54
    fluid   49, 161, 163
    hinge   50, 54
    joint   vi, ix, 48–53, 159–161, 163
    pivot   50, 54
    plane   50, 54
    saddle   50, 54
    spheroidal   50, 54
Systemic circuit   92
Systemic lupus erythematosus (SLE)   140, 143
Systole   204–205

t

Tachy-   8
Tactile   ix, 15, 17, 20–21, 139–140, 142, 145, 150,
    175–176, 254
Tactile hair   15, 17, 20, 139–140, 142, 254
Talus   34
Tapetum lucidum   25, 146–147
Tapeworm   20
Target   71, 173, 175–177, 182, 236, 251
Tars/o   11
Tarsal   15, 34, 42, 142
Tarsometatarsus   43, 45
Tarsus   4, 6, 11, 15–16, 31, 33–35, 42, 45, 52, 62–63, 73, 142
Taste   v, 21–22, 108, 145, 149–150, 175, 189, 241
Taste bud   22, 150
Teat   122, 125, 141, 183
Tectorial membrane   24–25, 149, 151
Teeth   xi, 23, 39, 48, 94, 160, 229
  canine teeth   23, 109
  carnassial   109
  deciduous   109, 116, 222
  incisors   36, 108–109, 114, 116, 222
  molar   109, 116
  premolar   108–109, 116
  retained deciduous   109
Telogen   141
Temperature   x, 7, 11, 21, 28, 70, 123, 138–139, 141–142,
    144–145, 150, 175, 183, 208, 212, 215–218, 233, 248
  ambient temperature   138
  core temperature   138, 208, 212, 217
Temporal bone   36–37, 50, 58
Temporalis   58
Temporomandibular joint   50–51
Tendon   30, 32, 34, 43, 49–50, 52, 57, 61, 63, 142, 160–163,
    175, 213, 243, 254
Tensor fasciae latae   62, 243
Teres major   59, 61

Teres minor   61
Terminal bouton   67–68, 166, 173–174. *See also*
    Synaptic bulb
Testicles (testes)   78–79, 81, 84, 119, 123–125, 184–185,
    189, 233–234
Tetraiodothyronine (T4)   182, 184–186, 190
Thalamus   70, 176, 179
Therm/o   11
Thermoreceptor   145, 150
Thermoregulation   viii, 14, 16, 18, 137–140, 142, 175, 222
Thick filament   165. *See also* Myosin
Thin filament   165, 168. *See also* Actin
Third Eyelid   25, 146
Thorac/o   11
Thoracic girdle   59, 65
Thorax   vi, 6, 11, 40, 53, 58–59, 64, 90, 94, 97, 103–105, 213,
    217, 254
Thrombocyte   132. *See also* Platelet
Thrombopoiesis   132
Thymopoietin   80
Thymosin   80
Thymus   vii, 78, 80, 89, 133
Thyroglobulin   184
Thyroid slip   78
Thyroid stimulating hormone (TSH)   182–186
Thyroxine   182, 184, 190
Tibia   4, 33–35, 42–43, 52, 63, 160, 162, 243
Tibial tuberosity   34, 52, 63
Tibiotarsus   43, 155
Tidal volume   212, 215, 217–218, 253–254
Toe   10, 18, 33, 43
Tom   120
Tongue   8, 10, 22, 58, 102, 107–109, 116, 150, 152, 221–222,
    229, 241, 251, 253
  apex   108
  genioglossus   58
  hyoglossus   58
  root   108
  styloglossus   58
Tonsil   94
Tooth   48, 109–111, 160, 162, 222–223, 251
  cementum   109
  crown   109, 111, 222
  dentin   109
  enamel   109, 111
  pulp   109, 111
  root   109, 111, 160
Tooth surface:
  apical   109
  buccal   109
  coronal   109
  distal   109

labial   109
  lingual   109
  mesial   109
  occlusal   109
  palatal   109
Topcoat   16
Trache/o   11
Trachea   vii, 7, 9, 11, 78–79, 81, 102–103, 105–106, 110, 211–212, 214, 222, 251–253
Tracheostomy tube   212
Trans-   8
Transduction   146
Transit time   226
Transitional cell   87–88
Transitional cell carcinoma   87–88
Transitional epithelial cell   86
Transport, active   131, 194, 225
Transport, passive   131, 194, 225
Transverse abdominis   60
Transverse process   40–42, 60
Transverse tubules   55, 165
Trapezius   58–59, 61, 64, 243
Tremor   74, 171, 177. *See also* Fasciculation
Triadan chart   110, 222–223
Triceps brachii   61
Trich   11
Tricuspid valve   91–92, 98, 205 *See also* Right atrioventricular (AV) valve
Trigone   87–88, 240
Triiodothyronine (T3)   40, 182, 184–186, 190
Trochlear notch   32, 51
Tropomyosin   156, 170
Troponin   166, 170
Trunk   6, 59, 72, 90–94, 96, 112, 124, 147, 167, 176, 205, 221, 252, 254
Trypsin   224
Tubercle   29
Tuberosity   29, 32, 34, 51–52, 59, 63, 243
Tubular filtrate   194, 196, 198
Tubular secretion   194
Tunic   92–93, 113, 123
Turbulent blood flow   206, 209
Turgor   139, 144, 236, 254
Tympanic bulla   37, 149
Tympanic membrane   23–24, 27–28, 50, 149, 254

u

Ulna   31–33, 43, 48, 51, 62, 159–160
Ulnar bone   32
Ulnar nerve   73
Ultra-   8
Umbilical artery   86, 95

Undercoat   16, 141
Ungual crest   33, 35
Ungulate   18, 142, 254
Unguligrade   142
Unilateral   81, 105, 123
Unmyelinated   67
Urachus   86
Ure/uro   11
Uremia   x, 197
  post-renal   197
  pre-renal   197
  renal   197
Ureter   vii, 83, 86–88, 111, 197, 240
Ureter ectopic   86
Urethra   vii, 11, 83–84, 87–88, 96, 114, 121, 124, 197, 233
Urethra external   87
Urethral process   124
Urethralis muscle   87, 124
Urinary system   3–4, 83–84, 88, 197
Urobilinogen   198
Uterine horn   120–121, 125, 234
Uvea   25

v

Vagina   87, 114, 121, 125, 231, 235–236
Vaginal artery   96
Vaginal tunics   123
Valve   8, 89, 91–94, 96, 99, 205–206, 222, 254
Vas deferens   123–124
Vasa vasorum   93
Vascular layer (eye)   25, 146, 151
Vasoconstriction   93, 138, 143–144
Vasodilation   138, 143–144, 207
Vasopressin   183–185, 189, 195, 197, 207
Vein   vii, 10–11, 18, 38, 57, 71, 73, 79, 83, 88–90, 92–93, 95–97, 99, 104, 112–114, 123, 168, 177, 205–208, 240, 249, 251, 253–254
Velvet   19, 142
Ven   11
Vena cava   90, 96–97, 123, 201, 205, 208–209, 226
Ventilation   x, 211–213, 253
  minute volume   212, 218
  ventilation perfusion (V/Q) mismatch   212
Ventral horn   173
Ventral nerve root   173
Ventricle   69–70, 72, 78, 89–93, 96, 98–99, 202–206, 209–210, 216
Ventricular tachycardia   203, 208, 249
Ventriculus   115
Ventrum   4, 6
Venule   11, 93, 205–206, 214, 251

Vertebrae   vi, 31, 40–43, 49, 51, 58–60, 69, 83, 160, 243
  caudal   40, 42–43
  cervical   40–41, 59, 243
  lumbar   40, 42, 60, 69, 83
  sacral   40, 42. *See also* Sacrum
  thoracic   40–42, 58, 243
Vertebral artery   94
Vertebrate   29, 90, 171
Vesicle   68, 74, 254
Vesicular sound   105
Vessel   3–4, 10, 14–15, 25, 31, 57, 63, 68, 70–71, 77, 83, 86,
    89–99, 111–112, 114, 123, 125, 138, 154–155, 161, 163, 168,
    175–177, 183, 196–199, 205–209, 211–212, 226, 240, 251–254
Vestibular   87, 145, 148–149
Vestibular apparatus   148–149
Vestibule:
  inner ear   24–25, 28, 148, 151
  nasal   101
  oral   107, 110
  vaginal   121
Vibrissae   17, 142, 254. *See also* Whiskers
Villi   224–225
Virus   176, 246, 253
Viscera   95, 112, 240, 254
Visceral smooth muscle   63
Viscerocranium   159, 162
Vision   v, 10, 21, 25–26, 70, 147, 149
Vitamin D   139, 154, 157, 194
Vitreous:
  compartment   27
  humor   27, 146–147

Vocal fold   102, 108
Vomeronasal organ   22–23, 108, 150, 152
VPC   203, 208
Vulva   9, 121–122
  recessed   122
Vulvoplasty   9, 122. *See also* Episioplasty

W
Waterproof   13–14, 140
Waxy   15, 25, 27, 140, 148, 254
Wether   120
Wheezes   105
Whelping   129
Whisker   13, 17–18, 142, 254. *See also* Vibrissae
White matter   67, 69–70, 72, 74, 77, 254
Whorls   16
Wool hair   16, 141–142. *See also* Secondary hair

X
X-ray   53, 64, 153, 236 *See also* Radiograph
Xiphihumeralis   59
Xiphoid   40

Z
Z-line   167
Zonule   26, 146–147, 151
Zoonotic disease   254
Zygomatic arch   36, 58, 243
Zygomatic bone   36
Zygote   234, 236